MANUAL OF
PULMONARY FUNCTION TESTING

MANUAL OF PULMONARY FUNCTION TESTING

GREGG L. RUPPEL, M.Ed., R.R.T.

Director, Pulmonary Function Laboratory,
St. Louis University Hospital,
St. Louis University Medical Center,
St. Louis, Missouri;
Instructor, Forest Park Community College,
St. Louis, Missouri

FIFTH EDITION

With 94 illustrations

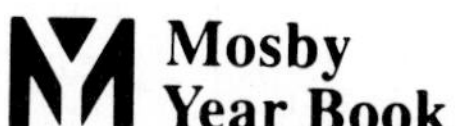

St. Louis Baltimore Boston Chicago London Philadelphia Sydney Toronto

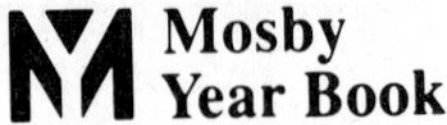

Dedicated to Publishing Excellence

Publisher: David T. Culverwell
Developmental Editor: Christi Mangold
Editorial Assistant: Cecilia F. Reilly
Editorial Project Manager: Jolynn Gower
Production Assistant: Pete Hausler
Book Design: Gail Morey Hudson

FIFTH EDITION

Printed in the United States of America

Mosby–Year Book, Inc.
11830 Westline Industrial Drive, St. Louis, Missouri 63146

Library of Congress Cataloging-in-Publication Data

Ruppel, Gregg, 1948-
Manual of pulmonary function testing / Gregg L. Ruppel. — 5th ed.
p. cm.
Includes bibliographical references.
Includes index.
ISBN 0-8016-5319-3
1. Pulmonary function tests—Handbooks, manuals, etc. I. Title.
[DNLM: 1. Respiratory Function Tests. WB 284 R946m]
RC734.P84R86 1991
616.2′4075—dc20
DNLM/DLC
for Library of Congress 90-13261
CIP

UG/D/D 9 8 7 6 5 4 3 2 1

Preface

The primary function of the lung can be stated as twofold: first, the oxygenation of mixed venous blood; second, the removal of carbon dioxide from that same blood. These two functions depend on the integrity of the airways, the pulmonary vascular system, the alveolar septa, the respiratory muscles, and the respiratory control mechanisms. Ideally, tests designed to assess the status of each part of the pulmonary system separately would be most appropriate. Most lung function tests, however, measure the condition of the component systems in an overlapping way.

The evaluation of pulmonary function in the laboratory or at the bedside may be indicated for the following reasons:

1. To determine the *presence* of lung disease or abnormality of lung function
2. To determine the *extent* of abnormalities
3. To determine the *extent of impairment* caused by abnormal lung function
4. To determine the *progression* of the disease
5. To determine the *nature of the physiologic disturbance*
6. To determine a *course of therapy* for treatment of a particular lesion

This text presents, as concisely as possible, explanations of many commonly used pulmonary function studies, the testing techniques used, and the significance of individual tests in regard to pulmonary disease. Also included are sections on pulmonary exercise evaluation, metabolic testing, pediatric pulmonary function testing, test regimens for specific purposes (disability, preoperative evaluation, and so on), pulmonary function testing equipment, computers, and quality assurance.

The fifth edition enlarges on the material presented in the first four editions, and reflects the suggestions of users of those texts. The chapters on pulmonary function equipment and computers have been expanded to reflect some of the new technologies in common use. Chapter 11, dealing with quality assurance issues, has been expanded to include recommendations of the American Thoracic Society and the Centers for Disease Control regarding testing protocols and safety.

As in the previous edition, Chapters 1 through 11 are followed by self-assessment questions. Most of the self-assessment questions are new to this edition, and answers may be found in the Appendix. Entries in the selected bibliographies at the end of each chapter are arranged according to specific topics within the chapter. As with previous editions, prediction regressions and nomograms for normal values are contained in the Appendix, along with information on the use of predicted values. Sample calculations for some of the more complicated measurements (lung volumes, plethysmography, diffusion, and exercise) are also included in the Appendix.

This manual is intended to serve as a text for students of pulmonary function testing and as a handy reference for technicians and physicians alike. Because of the diversity of testing methods and equipment currently in use, some aspects of certain tests are treated in a general way. For this reason, readers are encouraged to make use of the bibliographies provided. The presentation of the significance of various tests presumes a rudimentary knowledge of the pulmonary anatomy and physiology. Again, readers are urged to refer to the General References included in the selected bibliography to refresh or support their background in lung function. The terminology used is that of the American College of Chest Physicians-American Thoracic Society Joint Committee on Pulmonary Nomenclature. In some instances test names reflect very common usage that does not follow the ACCP-ATS recommendations.

Gregg Ruppel

Acknowledgments

My thanks to Drs. William Kistner, John Winter, and James Wiant for their encouragement in the development of the original text. My special thanks to Drs. Roger Secker-Walker, Susan Marshall, Gerald Dolan, and Cesar Keller for comments and constructive criticisms in the preparation of the revised editions. Special thanks also go to Ronald Gilmore and Jack Tandy for their contributions to the illustrations in this and previous editions. A note of thanks also to Thomas Anderson, MEd, RRT, David Shelledy, MA, RRT, Patricia Dent, BS, MS, RPT, and Barbara Disborough, MA, RRT for their reviews of and suggestions for the 4th edition. Louis Metzger, RPFT, Donald Barker, BS, PA, RPFT, David Hoover, RRT, RPFT, Barbara Disborough, MA, RRT, Randall Krohn, James Kemp, MD, Alan Hibbett, RPFT, and Michael Snow, RPFT all provided guidance and suggestions for the 5th edition. My appreciation for materials and illustrations provided goes to Warren E. Collins Inc., Gould Inc., Radiometer America, Jones Medical Instrument Co., Vitalograph Medical Instrumentation, Instrumentation Laboratories, Medical Graphics Inc., Hewlett Packard, Hans Rudolph Inc., Biochem International, Ohmeda, and Abbott Critical Care Systems.

To

Carol

for her patience and encouragement

Contents

1

Lung Volume Tests

VITAL CAPACITY (VC)

Description

The vital capacity (VC) is the volume of gas measured on a slow, complete expiration after a maximal inspiration, without forced or rapid effort (Fig. 1-1). The VC is normally recorded in either liters or milliliters, and reported at body temperature, pressure, saturated with water vapor (BTPS). The vital capacity is also sometimes referred to as the slow vital capacity (SVC), in distinction to the forced vital capacity (FVC) as discussed in Chapter 3.

Technique

The VC is measured by having the subject inspire maximally and then exhale completely into a spirometer capable of recording change in lung volume, with no time limit imposed on the maneuver. The VC can also be measured from maximal expiration to maximal inspiration. The value resulting from the latter method is sometimes termed the inspiratory vital capacity (IVC) or (SVC), while the value resulting from the former method is simply called the VC or SVC.

Significance

Normal values for VC, as well as for many other lung function parameters, are computed using the following linear equation:

$$VC = xH - yA - z$$

where

H = Height in centimeters (cm)
A = Age in years
x,y,z = Constants

Nomograms and regression equations for men, women, and children appear in the Appendix. The VC may vary as much as 20% from predicted normal values in healthy individuals and may vary from time to time in the same individual, depending on the position of the body or time of day. The VC in adults varies directly with height and inversely with age and is

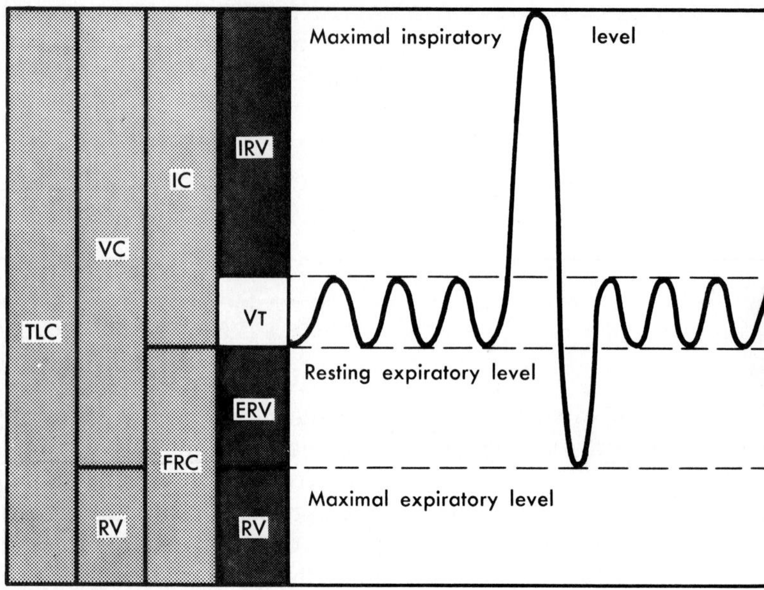

Fig. 1-1 Lung volumes and capacities—diagrammatic representation of various lung compartments, based on a typical spirogram. *TLC*, Total lung capacity; *VC*, vital capacity; *RV*, residual volume; *FRC*, functional residual capacity; *IC*, inspiratory capacity; *VT*, tidal volume, *IRV*, inspiratory reserve volume; *ERV*, expiratory reserve volume. Shaded areas indicate relationships between the subdivisions and relative sizes, as compared to the TLC. The resting expiratory level should be noted, since it remains more stable than other identifiable points during repeated spirograms. Hence, it is used as a starting point for FRC determinations. (Modified from Comroe JH, Jr et al: The lung: clinical physiology and pulmonary function tests, ed 2, Chicago, 1962, Year Book Medical Publishers, Inc.)

generally smaller in females than in males. Recent evidence indicates that lung volumes may differ significantly according to race or ethnic origin, so that interpretation of the measured volumes in regard to predicted normal values should consider these factors, in addition to age, height, weight, and sex (see Selecting and Using Predicted Values in the Appendix).

Decreases in VC can be caused by a loss of distensible lung tissue, as in bronchogenic carcinoma, bronchiolar obstruction, pulmonary edema, pneumonia, atelectasis, pulmonary restriction, pulmonary congestion, or surgical excisions. In general, restriction may be the result of tissue destruction, space-occupying lesions, or changes in the composition of the parenchyma itself. Tissue loss may be illustrated by resection, as in a lobectomy, where the decrease in VC is roughly proportional to the tissue removed. A good example of a space-occupying lesion is a tumor, which directly displaces lung tissue. Fibrotic diseases, such as silicosis, may cause changes in the elastic properties of the parenchyma. The vital capacity is often reduced in obstructive lung disease, while other lung compartments show increased volumes (see Residual Volume). Some causes of decreases in VC are not related to lung lesions, such as depression of the respiratory centers or neuromuscular diseases; reduction of available thoracic space caused by pleural effusion, pneumothorax, hiatus hernia, or cardiac enlargement; limitation of movement of the diaphragm that may result from pregnancy, ascites, or a tumor; and limitation of thoracic movement that may occur because of scleroderma, kyphoscoliosis, or pain.

When the measured VC value is less than 80% of the predicted VC or less than the 95% confidence limit (see the Appendix), the interpretation of the measured VC value should be corrlelated with the history and physical findings. The terms "mild," "moderate," and "severe" may be used to qualify the extent of reduction of the VC, and should be based on a statistical comparison (i.e., confidence intervals) of the measured VC versus the predicted VC. Spuriously low estimates of the VC may result from poor subject effort or inadequate instruction in the performance of the test maneuver. Reproducible values for at least three maneuvers should provide acceptable results (see Chapter 11).

The VC can be subdivided into the inspiratory capacity and the expiratory reserve volume.

INSPIRATORY CAPACITY (IC) AND EXPIRATORY RESERVE VOLUME (ERV)

Description

The inspiratory capacity and expiratory reserve volume are subdivisions of the VC. The IC is the largest volume of gas that can be inspired from the resting expiratory level (Fig. 1-1). The IC is sometimes further divided into the tidal volume (V_T) and the inspiratory reserve volume (IRV). The ERV is the largest volume of gas that can be expired from the resting end-expiratory level (see Fig. 1-1). Both the IC and ERV are recorded in liters or milliliters and corrected to BTPS.

Technique

The IC may be measured by having the subject breathe normally for several breaths and then inhale maximally. The volume inspired from the resting expiratory level is measured from an appropriate spirogram, usually as part of an SVC maneuver. The IC may also be estimated by subtracting the ERV from the VC.

The ERV may be measured by having the subject breathe normally for several breaths and then exhale maximally, while recording the changes on a spirogram and measuring the volume exhaled from the average end-expiratory level. Likewise, the ERV may be estimated by subtracting the IC from the VC. The accuracy of the measurement of both the IC and ERV depends on the determination of the passive end-expiratory level. This is best accomplished by recording at least three tidal breaths that vary by less than 100 ml before the slow vital capacity maneuver.

Significance

The IC and ERV normally comprise approximately 75% and 25% of the VC, respectively. Changes in the absolute volumes of the IC or ERV usually parallel increases or decreases in the VC. Increased tidal volume, in response to exertion or acid-base disorders, may encroach on both the IRV and ERV since both the end-inspiratory and end-expiratory levels are altered. This pattern may also be seen when subjects are asked to breathe into a spirometer through a mouthpiece with nose clips in place. Changes in the IC or ERV are of minimal diagnostic significance when considered alone. Reduction of either the IC or ERV is consistent with restrictive defects. Erroneous estimates of ERV may confound the measurement of residual volume (RV) (described in the next section), because the ERV is usually subtracted from the functional residual capacity (FRC) to calculate the RV. An underestimated ERV causes the computed RV to appear larger than the actual RV.

FUNCTIONAL RESIDUAL CAPACITY (FRC) AND RESIDUAL VOLUME (RV)

Description

The functional residual capacity (FRC) is the volume of gas remaining in the lungs at the end-expiratory level. The residual volume (RV) is the volume of gas remaining in the lungs at the end of a maximal expiration (see Fig. 1-1). Both are recorded in liters or milliliters, corrected to BTPS.

Technique

The two gas dilution methods of measuring the FRC employ foreign gases (i.e., gases not normally present in the lungs).

Open-circuit method. The FRC and its subdivision the RV must be measured indirectly because the gas filling these compartments cannot be exhaled from the lungs. The concentration of nitrogen (N_2) in the lungs is presumed to be in equilibrium with the atmosphere, or approximately 80%. By having the subject breathe 100% oxygen (O_2) for several minutes, the N_2 in the lungs can be gradually washed out. Since all of the N_2 cannot be washed out, the test is usually continued until the concentration of alveolar N_2 is less than 1%; then an alveolar sample is taken. The exhaled gas is collected in a spirometer or bag that has been flushed previously with pure O_2. First, the concentration of N_2 is measured; then, the original volume of gas in the lungs at the end-expiratory level can be computed using the following formula (Fig. 1-2):

$$\text{FRC} = \frac{F_{E}N_{2_{final}} \times \text{Expired volume} - N_{2_{tiss}}}{F_{A}N_{2_{alveolar\ 1}} - F_{A}N_{2_{alveolar\ 2}}}$$

where

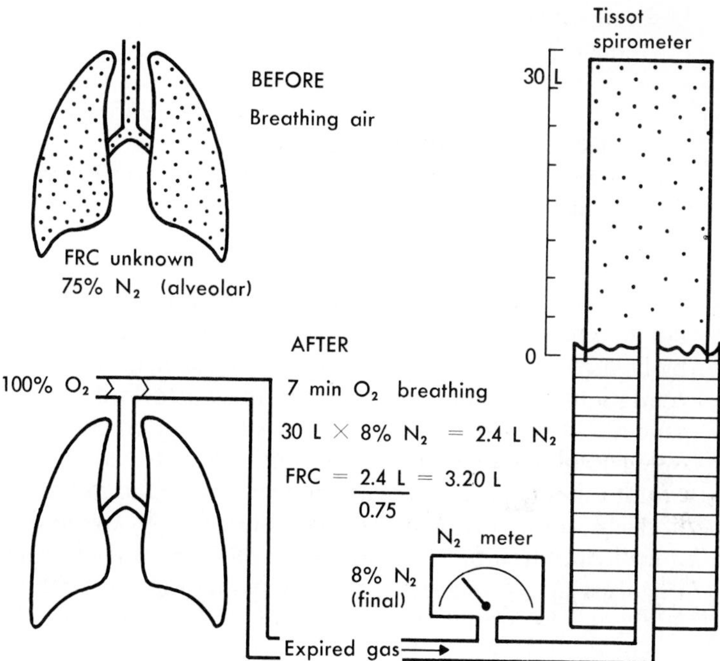

Fig. 1-2 Open-circuit determination of RV. In a patient breathing air, the alveolar N_2 concentration is assumed to be equal to atmospheric N_2 pressure minus water vapor and CO_2, or approximately 75%. Alternatively, the fractional concentration of alveolar N_2 can be measured at the beginning and at the end of the O_2 breathing. After the subject breathes 100% O_2 for 7 minutes and exhales all gas into a large-volume Tissot spirometer, the entire gas sample is analyzed for N_2 concentration and the FRC is computed as indicated. The switch from breathing room air to pure O_2 must come at precisely the end-expiratory level to ensure that the volume actually measured is the FRC. The RV is determined by subtracting the ERV from the FRC. (Modified from Comroe JH, Jr et al: The lung: clinical physiology and pulmonary function tests, ed 2, Chicago, 1962, Year Book Medical Publishers, Inc.)

$F_EN_{2_{final}}$ = Fraction of N_2 in volume expired
$F_AN_{2_{alveolar\ 1}}$ = Fraction of N_2 in alveolar gas initially
$F_AN_{2_{alveolar\ 2}}$ = Fraction of N_2 in alveolar gas at end of test (determined from an alveolar sample)
$N_{2_{tiss}}$ = Volume of N_2 washed out of blood/tissues

Corrections for the amount of N_2 washed out of the blood and tissue and for small amounts of N_2 in "pure" O_2 must be made when computing the FRC. For each minute of O_2 breathing, approximately 30 to 40 ml of N_2 are removed from blood and tissue, so that $0.04 \times (T) = N_{2_{tiss}}$, where T is time of the test, is subtracted from the volume of N_2 in the spirometer.

Since all of the N_2 in the lungs may not be washed out, even after 7 minutes of O_2 breathing, the $FAN_{2_{alveolar\ 2}}$ may be measured by taking an alveolar N_2 sample near the end of the test, and subtracting this value from the alveolar N_2 present at the beginning. The FRC must be corrected to BTPS (see the Appendix).

To obtain the RV, the previously determined ERV is subtracted from the FRC as just measured:

$$RV = FRC - ERV$$

A newer method for performing the open-circuit procedure uses a rapid N_2 analyzer in combination with a spirometer to provide a "breath-by-breath" analysis of expired N_2. Analog signals proportional to N_2 concentration and volume (or flow) are integrated to derive the exhaled volume of N_2 in each breath. The values from all breaths are added to compute a total volume of N_2 washed out. The test is continued for 7 minutes or until the N_2 in alveolar gas has been reduced to less than 1%. The FRC is calculated by dividing the total volume of N_2 washed out by the fractional concentration of alveolar N_2 at the beginning of the test and making the necessary corrections (i.e., blood/tissue washout and temperature). In addition, a breath-by-breath plot of the $\%N_2$ (or log $\%N_2$) versus volume or number of breaths can be obtained to derive indices of the distribution of ventilation (see Fig. 4-2.)

In systems employing a pneumotachometer, a device sensitive to the composition of gas (see Chapter 9), corrections must be made for changes in the viscosity of the gas as O_2 replaces N_2 in the expirate. This is usually easily accomplished by software or electronic correction of the analyzer output.

Closed-circuit method. The FRC can also be calculated indirectly by diluting the gas in the lungs with a gas of known concentration. A suitable spirometer is filled with a known volume of gas to which helium (He) has been added. The amount (usually about 600 ml) and concentration of He (usually about 10%) are measured and recorded before the test is begun. Then the subject rebreathes the gas in the spirometer, with a CO_2 absorber in place, until the concentration of He falls to a stable level. This usually requires less than 7 minutes. Oxygen is added to the spirometer system to maintain the fractional concentration at a level near or above that of room air and to keep the system volume relatively constant.

An older method added a large bolus of O_2 at the beginning of the procedure and allowed the patient to gradually consume the O_2. Because of the possibility of equilibrium not being attained before the added O_2 was depleted, this method is no longer commonly used.

If the 10% He mixture is prepared in an appropriate system volume (usually 6 to 8 L), equilibration between the normal lungs and the rebreathing system takes place quickly, typically in about 3 minutes. The final concentration of He is then recorded. The system volume (i.e., the volume that was in the spirometer before the test began) can then be calculated:

$$\text{System volume} = \frac{\text{He}_{\text{added}}\ (\text{milliliters})}{F_{\text{He}_{\text{initial}}}}$$

where

$$F_{\text{He}_{\text{initial}}} \text{ is the \%He converted to a fraction (\%He/100)}$$

Once the system volume is known, the FRC and RV can be computed

$$\text{FRC} = \frac{(\%\text{He}_{\text{initial}} - \%\text{He}_{\text{final}})}{\%\text{He}_{\text{final}}} \times \text{System volume}$$

Either percent or fractional concentration of He may be used because the term is a ratio.

Some automated systems employ the same method to calculate the system volume; a small amount of He is added to the closed system, followed by a known volume of air. The change in He concentration after the addition of the air is used to determine the system volume, as described previously. As in the open-circuit technique:

$$\text{RV} = \text{FRC} - \text{ERV}$$

Rebreathing is normally continued until the He concentration changes by no more than 0.02% per 30 seconds (see Chapter 11 for criteria for acceptability of lung volumes).

Several corrections are frequently made to the FRC value obtained using the above equation. Because a small volume of He dissolves in the blood during the test, the final He reading is lower than it would have been had the decrease in He been due solely to dilution by the subject's FRC. The loss of He to the blood results in a slight increase in the apparent FRC. A volume of 100 ml is usually subtracted from the measured FRC to correct for this effect. The dead space volume of the breathing valve should likewise be subtracted from the measured FRC.

Most manufacturers recommend a "switch-in" error correction to be applied when the subject is turned into the system at a point either above or below the actual end-expiratory level or FRC. Depending on the subject's breathing pattern, a volume difference of several hundred milliliters may result. However, the effect of the switch-in error may be insignificant, because equilibrium does not occur instantaneously at switch-in, and because the total volume of the spirometer and lungs is constantly changing with tidal breathing, removal of CO_2, and addition of O_2. If the switch-in error is large, or if the patient's end-expiratory level appears to be changing or irregular during the maneuver, the test should be restarted after allowing the patient to breathe air for several minutes to clear any residual He from the lungs. The FRC must be converted to BTPS (Fig. 1-3). Sample calculations of both the open-circuit and closed-circuit techniques can be found in the Appendix.

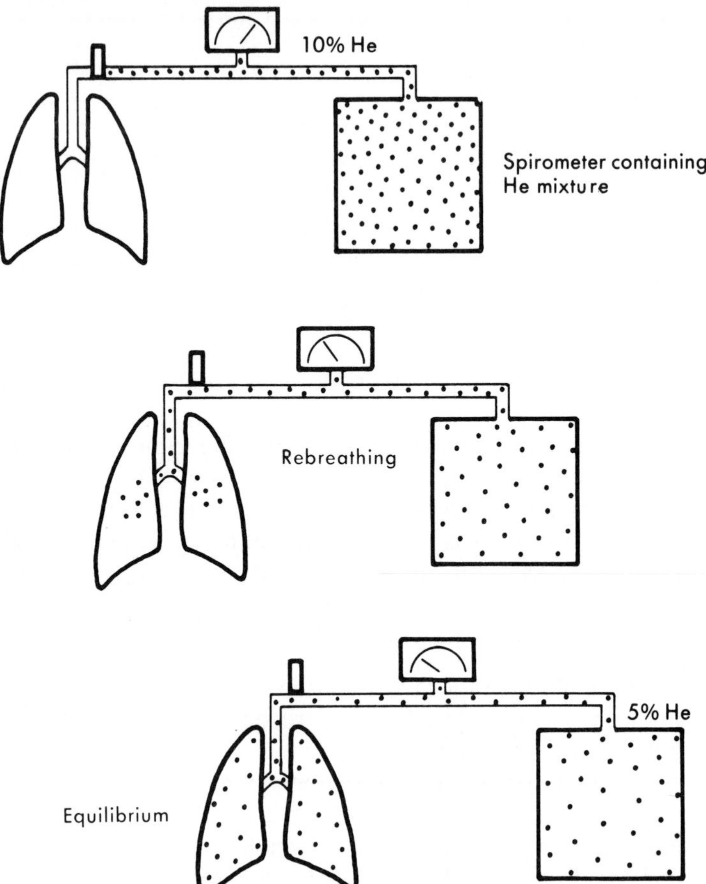

Fig. 1-3 Closed-circuit determination of RV. The lungs of a person breathing air contain no He. The person then rebreathes a mixture of He and air (O_2), of which the volume and He% are known. He is diluted until an equilibrium is reached. The volume of He initially present and its concentration are known, and the volume of the rebreathing system can be calculated. At the end of the test, the same volume of He has been diluted in a larger volume (rebreathing system plus lungs), and the total volume is computed from the initial He volume ($V\text{He}_{initial}$) and the final He concentration ($F\text{He}_{final}$) values, as follows:

$$\text{Total volume of system (after rebreathing)} = \frac{V\text{He}_{initial}}{F\text{He}_{final}}$$

The FRC is derived by subtracting the rebreathing system volume (see text). The switch from air to the He mixture must be made at the end-expiratory level for accurate measurement of FRC. RV is derived by subtracting the ERV from the FRC. (Modified from Comroe HJ, Jr et al: The lung: clinical physiology and pulmonary function tests, ed 2, Chicago, 1962, Year Book Medical Publishers, Inc.)

Significance

In both the open- and closed-circuit techniques, the RV is measured indirectly as a subdivision of the FRC. This is the preferred method because the resting end-respiratory level is more reproducible than the points of complete inspiration or complete expiration. The end-expiratory level and the ERV must be accurately measured; if the tidal breathing pattern is irregular, the ERV value may be overestimated or underestimated thus affecting the calculation of the RV.

The validity of both techniques depends on the assumption that all parts of the lung are reasonably well ventilated. In subjects who have obstructive disease, a 7-minute test period may not be long enough to wash N_2 out or mix He to a stable level in the poorly ventilated parts of the lungs. Hence, the measured FRC, RV, and total lung capacity (TLC) values will be less than the true values. Prolongation of the test improves results somewhat but will not account for completely trapped gas, as in bullous emphysema.

In either of the foreign gas techniques, leaks in the valving or circuitry or at the connection to the subject will affect gas concentrations and cause erroneous estimates of FRC. Most commonly, leaks result in overestimates of lung volumes. Likewise, malfunction of the gas analyzer in either method will produce spurious values. Integrity of the breathing circuit or analyzer should be questioned whenever FRC values appear inconsistent with the subject's clinical history, or with other lung function parameters, such as spirometry results or carbon monoxide diffusing capacity (DL_{CO}), discussed in Chapter 5.

An increase in the FRC is considered pathologic. An FRC value of greater than approximately 120% of the predicted represents hyperinflation, which may result from emphysematous changes, asthmatic or bronchiolar obstruction, compensation for surgical removal of lung tissue, or, in some instances, from thoracic deformity. An increase in FRC usually results in muscular and mechanical inefficiency, causing an increase in the effort required to breathe.

An increase in RV indicates that, despite the subject's maximal expiratory effort, the lungs still contain an abnormally large amount of gas. This type of change may appear in young asthmatics and is usually reversible. Increases of RV are also characteristic of emphysema and bronchial obstruction, both of which may cause chronic air trapping. RV and FRC usually increase together. As RV becomes larger, more ventilation may be required to adequately exchange O_2 and CO_2 in the lung. This usually requires an increase in tidal volume, rate, or both. At the same time the work of breathing is increased. Patients with increased RV often display gas exchange abnormalities, such as hypoxemia or CO_2 retention.

FRC and RV, and the total lung capacity derived from them, are typically decreased in restrictive diseases that interfere with the bellows action of the chest or the lungs. Such decreased values are seen in those diseases associated with extensive fibrosis, such as sarcoidosis, asbestosis, and complicated silicosis. Restrictive disorders affecting the chest wall include kyphoscoliosis, pectus excavatum, neuromuscular weakness, and obesity. FRC and RV values may also be lower than normal in diseases that occlude many alveoli, such as pneumonia.

Table 1-1 lists typical lung volume values for a normal adult male, a patient with hyperinflation (as in emphysema), and a patient with restriction (as in sarcoidosis). It should be noted that generalized restrictive processes cause the lung volumes to be reduced approximately equally. Thus the proportional relationship between different lung volume compartments, such as the RV/TLC ratio, may be relatively normal.

In obstructive patterns, one of two changes in the proportions of the various compartments is usually observed. The RV may be increased; this increase may be at the expense of a reduction in VC (see Fig. 1-7), with the TLC remaining close to the expected value. In other cases, the RV may increase, while the VC remains fairly well preserved, so that the TLC value is actually greater than the predicted value. The term "air trapping" is sometimes used to describe the increase in FRC and RV, while the term "hyperinflation" is often used to describe the absolute increase in TLC.

THORACIC GAS VOLUME (VTG)

Description

The thoracic gas volume (VTG) is the volume of gas contained in the thorax, whether in communication with open airways or trapped in any compartment of the thorax. VTG is usually measured at the end-expiratory level, and is then equal to the FRC. It also may be measured at other lung volumes and then corrected to relate to the FRC. The VTG is recorded in liters or milliliters.

Technique

The VTG is measured using the body plethysmograph (Fig. 1-4). The technique is based on Boyle's law, which states that the volume of gas varies in inverse proportion to the pressure to which it is subjected, if the temperature is held constant. At the start of the test, the patient has an unknown

Table 1-1 Comparative lung volumes for a normal adult male, a subject with hyperinflation, and a subject with restriction

Value	Normal	Hyperinflation	Restriction
VC (ml)	4800	3000	3000
FRC (ml)	2400	3600	1500
RV (ml)	1200	3000	750
TLC (ml)	6000	6000	3750
RV/TLC (%)	20	50	20

volume of gas in the thorax (i.e., the FRC). By occluding the airway and allowing the patient to decompress the gas in the chest by making an inspiratory effort, a new volume and a new pressure are generated. The change in pulmonary gas pressure is easily measured at the airway, since mouth pressure theoretically equals alveolar pressure when there is no air flow. The change in pulmonary gas volume is measured by monitoring the change in pressure in a constant-volume plethysmograph, or by measuring the flow of gas into and out of a flow box (see Plethysmographs, Chapter 9). In a constant-volume plethysmograph, the transducer measuring box pressure is calibrated directly in terms of volume change by introducing a small, known volume of gas into the sealed chamber and expressing the pressure change as an index of volume.

In a constant-volume plethysmograph, the subject breathes against a closed airway, which has been occluded by means of an electrical shutter. The air within the chest is alternately compressed and decompressed by the action of the ventilatory muscles. The transducer measuring mouth pressure (which equals alveolar pressure) is plotted on the vertical axis of

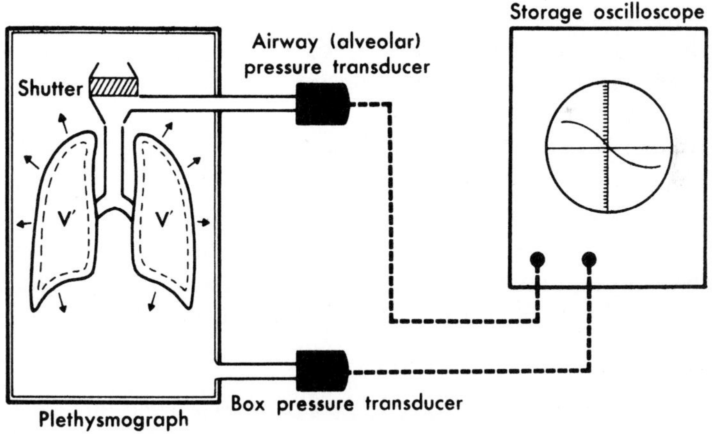

Fig. 1-4 Thoracic gas volume (VTG). The body plethysmograph is used to measure VTG. Boyle's law states that the volume varies inversely with the pressure if the temperature is held constant. A "pressure" type of plethysmograph, with pressure transducers for measurements of box pressure and airway (alveolar) pressure, is shown. An electronic shutter momentarily occludes the airway, so that airway pressure is approximately equal to alveolar pressure. Simultaneously, the alveolar gas is decompressed because of enlargement of the thorax, without gas flow. This change in alveolar volume is reflected by an increase in box pressure, and an estimation of the volume change can be derived by calibration. When the original pressure (P), the new pressure (P′), and the new volume (V′ or V + ΔV) are known, the original volume V or VTG) can be computed using Boyle's law. (See text and Appendix.)

an oscilloscope or computer screen, while the transducer measuring box pressure (calibrated as volume change) is plotted on the horizontal axis (see Fig. 1-4). Changes in each parameter are graphed continuously and appear as a sloping line, which is equal to $\Delta P/\Delta V$, where ΔP equals change in alveolar pressure and ΔV equals change in alveolar volume. The change in alveolar volume is measured indirectly by noting the reciprocal change in plethysmograph volume.

The original VTG can then be obtained from the slope of the tracing by applying a derivation of Boyle's law:

$$V_{TG} = \frac{P_B}{\lambda V_{TG}} \times \frac{P_{box}cal}{P_{mouth}cal} \times K$$

where

V_{TG} = Thoracic gas volume
P_B = Barometric pressure minus water vapor pressure
λV_{TG} = Slope of the oscilloscope trace equal to $\Delta P/\Delta V$
$P_{box}cal$ = Box pressure transducer calibration factor
$P_{mouth}cal$ = Mouth pressure transducer calibration factor
K = Correction factor for volume displaced by the subject

For the complete derivation of the equation and sample calculations, see the Appendix.

The measurements are usually made with the subject panting shallowly at a rate of 1 to 2 breaths/second with an open glottis. This type of breathing allows small pressure changes to be recorded at or near FRC, and eliminates some artifact related to temperature fluctuations. Some plethysmograph systems allow VTG measurements by occluding the airway during normal breathing without panting. If the mouth shutter is closed at precisely end-expiration, VTG equals FRC. Several determinations can be made quickly to obtain an average for the slope of $\Delta P/\Delta V$.

Significance

The VTG is a quick and precise means of measuring FRC and is used in combination with simple spirometry to derive other lung volume compartments. The plethysmograph's obvious advantage is that it measures the volume of gas in the thoracic cavity, whether the gas is in ventilatory communication with the atmosphere or not. The VTG measurement of FRC is often larger than the FRC values derived using the He dilution or nitrogen washout techniques, especially in emphysema and other diseases characterized by air trapping and in the presence of uneven distribution of ventilation. When gas dilution tests are extended beyond 7 minutes, the results for FRC determinations approach the VTG figure.

Recent evidence suggests that, in severe obstructive patterns, the FRC may actually be overestimated when the VTG technique is used, primarily because of inaccuracies in measuring alveolar pressure at the mouth during airway occlusion. Normal lungs, however, produce similar results when either method is used.

When two or more methods of determining lung volumes are employed, it is often instructive to compare the FRC determined by each method, particularly in subjects with suspected obstructive disease. The ratio of FRC_{box}/FRC_{gas} may be used as an index of gas trapping. The ratio value is usually near unity (i.e., one) in persons having normal lungs or in subjects who have a mild restriction. Values greater than one indicate gas volumes detectable by the plethysmograph but "hidden" to the gas techniques. Care must be taken to ensure that lung volume measurements determined by the two methods are reliable before the values are expressed as a ratio.

By appropriate integration of the pneumotachometer flow signal, spirometric indices (i.e., FVC, FEV, and SVC) may be obtained using the same equipment normally used in plethysmography, allowing measurements of both lung volumes and flows in a single sitting.

The VTG maneuver requires that the technician carefully instruct and monitor the subject to obtain acceptable data (see Chapter 11). VTG cannot be measured in subjects who have claustrophobia or physical limitations that preclude entry into the box, or those who are unable to perform the panting maneuver acceptably.

RADIOLOGIC ESTIMATION OF TOTAL LUNG CAPACITY (TLC)

Description

TLC can be determined according to several methods using standard posterior-anterior (P-A) and lateral radiographs of the chest. A common procedure involves dividing the films into ellipsoidal segments and estimating the volumes of each segment. A planimeter can also be used to estimate the thoracic volume.

Technique (ellipsoid segment method)

P-A and lateral chest radiographs are shot at a standard distance of 72 inches. The borders of the lungs, heart, and diaphragms are outlined using a china marker or similar pencil. Fig. 1-5 illustrates the necessary outlines for the measurements. If the lung apex is not visible on the lateral film, it can be determined after some preliminary measurements are made. The P-A film is first subdivided (Fig. 1-5), as follows:

1. A horizontal line is drawn 2.75 cm from the apices (line #1).
2. A second line is drawn 2.75 cm below the first (line #2).
3. A horizontal line is drawn through the upper diaphragm dome (line #4).
4. A horizontal line is drawn midway between lines #2 and #4 (line #3). These lines determine segments I through IV.

The lateral film is then subdivided (Fig. 1-5), as follows:

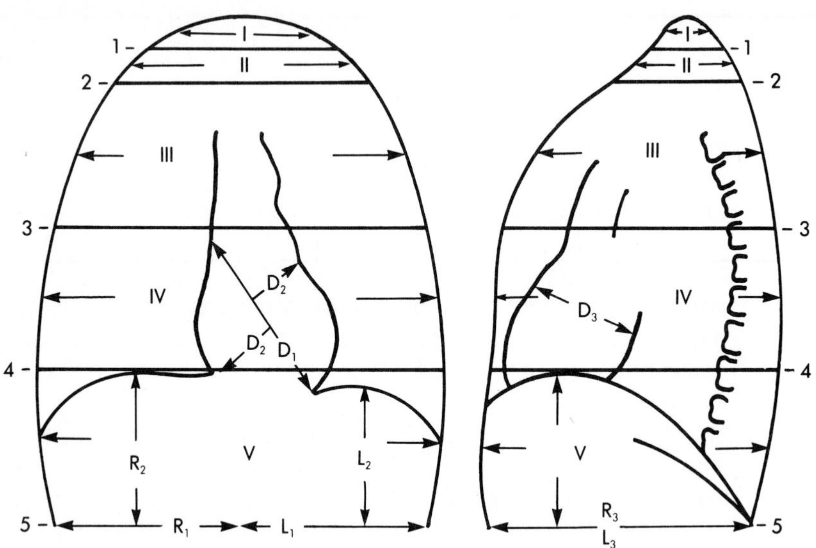

Fig. 1-5 Radiologic estimation of total lung capacity (TLC). Standard posterior-anterior (P-A) and lateral x-ray films are outlined as indicated with wax pencil or marker. Lines 1, 2, 3, 4, and 5 divide each film into five segments (I to V). R_1, R_2, and R_3 define the volume under the right diaphragms. L_1, L_2, and L_3 are taken from the left diaphragm; $R_1 = L_1$, $R_3 = L_3$, and L_2 is the height of the left hemidiaphragm while R_2 is the height of the right hemidiaphragm. D_1, D_2, and D_3 allow the calculation of the volume occupied by the heart. All measurements are made in centimeters, and each respective segment is measured at the point indicated by the arrows.

1. A horizontal line is drawn through the upper diaphragm dome (line #4).
2. The apex of the lung on the lateral view can then be determined by measuring the distance from the apex to line #4 on the P-A film and transposing it to the lateral film.
3. Line #1 is drawn 2.75 cm below the apex.
4. Line #2 is drawn 2.75 cm below line #1.
5. Line #3 is drawn midway between lines #2 and #4, as on the P-A film.
6. A fifth horizontal line is drawn through the posterior sulcus forward to the anterior limit of the diaphragm. The distance from line #4 to line #5 is then transposed to the P-A film to determine segment V; perpendicular lines are added from the margins of the diaphragms to line #5 on the P-A film.

The heart is outlined as indicated on Fig. 1-5; line D_1 is drawn through the long axis from the right atrium to the apex. Perpendiculars D_2 to D_1 are drawn to the farthest borders of the heart outline. Line D_3 is drawn to note the longest distance across the heart shadow on the lateral film.

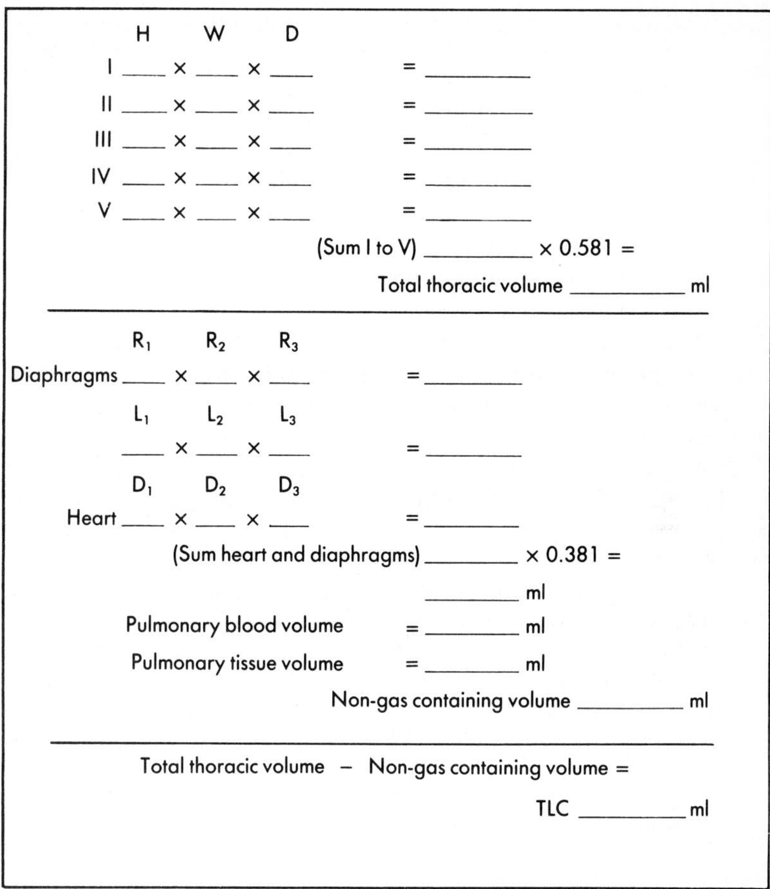

H W D
I ___ × ___ × ___ = ______
II ___ × ___ × ___ = ______
III ___ × ___ × ___ = ______
IV ___ × ___ × ___ = ______
V ___ × ___ × ___ = ______
(Sum I to V) ______ × 0.581 =
Total thoracic volume ______ ml

R_1 R_2 R_3
Diaphragms ___ × ___ × ___ = ______
L_1 L_2 L_3
___ × ___ × ___ = ______
D_1 D_2 D_3
Heart ___ × ___ × ___ = ______
(Sum heart and diaphragms) ______ × 0.381 =
______ ml
Pulmonary blood volume = ______ ml
Pulmonary tissue volume = ______ ml
Non-gas containing volume ______ ml

Total thoracic volume − Non-gas containing volume =
TLC ______ ml

Fig. 1-6 Typical data record sheet for radiologic estimation of TLC. The height (*H*), width (*W*), and depth (*D*) of each of the five thoracic segments (*I* and *V*) are multiplied; these five products are added and multiplied by a factor derived from the equation for the volume of an ellipsoid. A similar procedure is used for the two hemidiaphragms and heart; their volumes are added to those for the pulmonary blood and tissue. The difference between the total thoracic volume and the non-gas volume is the TLC.

Measurements such as the following are then made from each segment and recorded on a data sheet (Fig. 1-6):

1. The width and depth of each segment are recorded in centimeters, measuring from the midpoint of the segment; the height is also recorded.
2. The measurements are then multiplied (width × depth × height) and added together.
3. The sum is multiplied by a factor (0.581) derived from the formula for the volume of an ellipsoidal cylinder and a correction factor for x-ray divergence. This product is the total thoracic volume (TTV).

The non-gas volume (NGV) must be subtracted from the TTV. The volumes under the right and left diaphragms are calculated separately, as follows:

1. R_1 equals half the length of line #5; R_2 is the height of the right diaphragm; and R_3 is the length of line #5 on the lateral film.
2. L_1, L_2, and L_3 are measured similarly, for the left side.
3. The product of these measurements is multiplied by 0.381, a factor for their volumes.
4. The heart dimensions D_1, D_2, and D_3 are treated similarly (Fig. 1-6).

Pulmonary tissue and blood volumes are derived from body measurements (see the Appendix). These volumes and the heart and diaphragm volumes are all subtracted from the TTV to derive the TLC, in milliliters. It is important to note that both the P-A and lateral films should be taken with the subject at TLC; the subject should specifically be instructed to inspire as deeply as possible so that TLC is accurately estimated.

Significance

TLC values determined radiologically correlate well with plethysmographic determinations in healthy persons and in subjects who have obstruction. Radiologic techniques produce more accurate TLC values than gas dilution techniques in subjects who have moderate to severe obstruction. Radiologic determination of TLC offers a means of double-checking volumes determined by other methods, and may be available where the equipment for gas dilution or plethysmographic measurements is not. Also, radiologic determination of TLC may provide lung volume information in subjects for whom other methods are impractical, such as those who have had a tracheotomy. Chest x-ray determination of TLC may be used to "size" the lungs for both the donor and recipient in cases of lung transplantation, provided the films are taken using similar techniques.

As noted previously, subjects must hold their breath at TLC when each film is exposed, or the TLC may be underestimated. The presence of space-occupying lesions, such as masses or atelectasis, may confound the routine method, but more than five segments may be created to subdivide around a well-defined lesion. Diffuse space-occupying lesions, such as pneumonia or pulmonary edema, and diseases that increase pulmonary tissue/blood volume may reduce the accuracy of the radiologic lung volume determination.

TOTAL LUNG CAPACITY (TLC) AND RESIDUAL VOLUME/TOTAL LUNG CAPACITY RATIO (RV/TLC × 100)

Description

The TLC is the volume of gas contained in the lungs at the end of a maximal inspiration. It is measured in liters or milliliters, and corrected to BTPS. The RV/TLC ratio is the fraction of the TLC that can be defined as RV, expressed as a percentage.

Technique

The TLC is normally calculated by a combination of other specific lung volume measurements. The two most common are addition of the FRC and IC, and addition of the VC and the RV. The TLC can be calculated using the radiologic method described earlier. In addition, TLC can be calculated using several single-breath techniques (i.e., single-breath He dilution or single-breath N_2 washout). These techniques are commonly used in conjunction with other measurements when a lung volume determination is required for the calculation of a particular parameter (i.e., alveolar volume for the calculation of DL_{CO} discussed in Chapter 5). Although single-breath lung volume determinations correlate well with multiple-breath techniques in healthy individuals, single-breath lung volume values tend to be lower than true values in the presence of moderate to severe obstruction.

The RV/TLC ratio is calculated by dividing the residual volume by the total lung capacity and multiplying by 100. Either ambient temperature, pressure, saturated with water vapor (ATPS) or BTPS values may be used

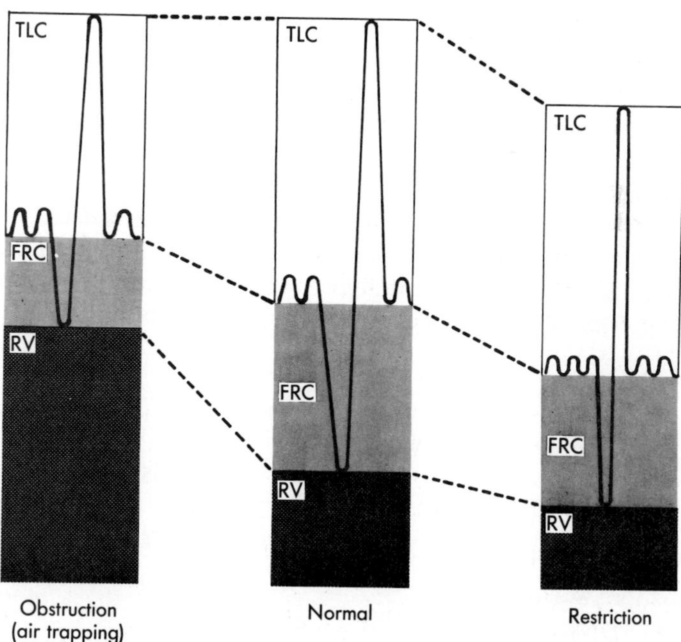

Fig. 1-7 Lung volume alterations in obstructive and restrictive patterns. A comparison of the changes in lung volume compartments in obstruction and restriction shows the following: in obstruction, with air trapping, the FRC and RV are both increased at the expense of the VC, and hence TLC remains relatively unchanged; in restrictive patterns, the FRC, RV, and VC are all decreased proportionately, resulting in a decrease in the TLC.

in the ratio, but both volumes must be expressed in the same units before performing the division.

Significance

The TLC may be decreased by processes that occupy space in the lungs, such as edema, atelectasis, neoplasms, or fibrotic lesions. Other diseases that commonly result in decreased TLC include pulmonary congestion, pleural effusions, pneumothorax, and thoracic deformities. Pure restrictive defects show proportional decreases in most lung compartments (Fig. 1-7), as described previously in this chapter for FRC and RV, although it is possible for one or more lung volume subdivisions to be reduced more than others. When the TLC value is less than 80% of the predicted or less than the 95% confidence limit, a restrictive process should be suspected. TLC may be either normal or increased in subjects who have asthma, chronic bronchitis, bronchiectasis, cystic fibrosis, or emphysema (see Table 1-1 and Fig. 1-7). A normal or increased TLC value does not mean that ventilation or the surface area for diffusion is normal. A normal TLC value in conjunction with an increased RV value is consistent with air trapping (i.e., the RV increased at the expense of the VC). When the TLC value is greater than 120% of the predicted TLC or above the 95% confidence limit as a result of increased RV, hyperinflation is present, and the work of breathing is usually increased. For predicted normal values, see the Appendix.

In healthy young adults, the RV/TLC ratio may vary from 20% to 35%. Since this is a ratio, values greater than 35% may result from absolute increases of the RV, as in emphysema, or from a decrease in the TLC, because of a loss of VC. Values greater than 35% do not indicate dysfunction but are of greatest diagnostic value when correlated with the absolute values of RV and TLC. A large RV/TLC in the presence of an increased TLC is often indicative of hyperinflation, while an increased RV/TLC with a normal TLC indicates that air trapping is present.

SELF-ASSESSMENT QUESTIONS

1. Calculate the FRC from the open-circuit method using the following data. (Refer to the Appendix.)

$\%N_{2_{Final}}$	5.9% (0.059 as a fraction)
Volume expired	37.0 L
$\%N_{2_{Alveolar\ 1}}$	80% (0.80 as a fraction)
$\%N_{2_{Alveolar\ 2}}$	1% (0.01 as a fraction)
Time	6.5 minutes
Blood/tissue washout factor	0.04 L/min
Breathing circuit dead space	1.0 L
Spirometer temperature	24°C
FRC = ______________________	(BTPS)

2. A patient has these lung volumes:

	Measured	Predicted
VC	3.3	3.6
FRC	3.2	2.2
RV	2.8	1.7
TLC	6.1	5.3

   These values are consistent with:
   a. Normal lung volumes
   b. Obstructive pattern
   c. Restrictive pattern
   d. Combined obstructive and restrictive pattern

3. Calculate the FRC from the closed-circuit method using the following data. (Refer to the Appendix.)

He_{added}	0.6 L
$\%He_{initial}$	9.1% (0.091 as a fraction)
$\%He_{final}$	5.5% (0.055 as a fraction)
He absorption correction	0.1 L
Temperature	25°C

   FRC = ______________________ (BTPS)

4. A patient who has restrictive disease (sarcoidosis) has her FRC measured using the closed-circuit method and by plethysmography; the FRC as measured by the gas dilution method would be expected to be:
   a. Much smaller than the V_{TG}
   b. Approximately equal to the V_{TG}
   c. Much larger than the V_{TG}
   d. Unrelated to the V_{TG} since the methods measure different lung compartments

5. Restrictive lung disease:
   a. Is characterized by an increase in RV
   b. Typically causes a decrease in VC
   c. Causes a decrease in FRC
   d. Results in an RV/TLC % greater than 50%
   e. b and c

6. In a pressure-type plethysmograph, changes in alveolar volume are:
   a. Obtained by measuring changes in box pressure
   b. Obtained by measuring flow at the mouth during panting
   c. Obtained by measuring mouth pressure with the shutter closed
   d. Considered to be zero

7. Total lung capacity (TLC) can be calculated using which of the following equations?

I. RV + VC
II. FRC + IC
III. VC − ERV + RV
IV. FRC − IC + VC
a. I, II, III
b. I, II only
c. III, IV only
d. II, IV only

8. Which of the following methods of lung volume determination correlate best with the plethysmographic value in a patient who has moderate to severe airways obstruction:
a. Radiologic (chest x-ray film)
b. Open-circuit (N_2 washout)
c. Closed-circuit (He dilution)
d. Single-breath He dilution

9. Increased RV and RV/TLC ratio would be expected in:
a. A subject who has pneumonia
b. A subject who has emphysema
c. A subject who has pulmonary fibrosis
d. All of the above
e. b and c only

10. Determination of the VTG in body plethysmography is based on the principle that:
a. Flow is proportional to the square of the pressure
b. Pressure and volume vary inversely
c. Gas volumes expand as temperature increases
d. Volume varies directly with flow

11. Which of the following are true when measuring FRC using the gas dilution techniques:
I. The open-circuit method uses O_2
II. The closed-circuit method is influenced by the evenness of ventilation
III. The closed-circuit method requires rebreathing
IV. The open-circuit method requires an N_2 analyzer
a. I, II, III, IV
b. II, III, IV
c. I, III only
d. II, IV only

12. When calculating TLC from chest x-rays, which of the following must be subtracted from the total thoracic volume:
I. Pulmonary blood volume

II. Volume of the heart
III. Volume under the bony structures
IV. Pulmonary tissue volume
a. I, II, III
b. I, II, IV
c. III, IV only
d. I, IV only

SELECTED BIBLIOGRAPHY

General references

Altman PL and Dittmer DS, editors: Respiration and circulation, Bethesda, Md, 1971, Federation of American Societies for Experimental Biology.

Briscoe WA: Lung volumes. In Fenn WO and Rahn H, editors: Handbook of physiology—respiration II, Washington, DC, 1965, American Physiological Society.

Crapo RO et al: Lung volumes in healthy nonsmoking adults, Bull Eur Physiopathol Respir 18:419, 1982.

Forster RE: The lung: clinical physiology and pulmonary function tests, ed 3, Chicago, 1986, Year Book Medical Publishers, Inc.

Goldman HI and Becklake MR: Respiratory function tests: normal values at median altitudes and the prediction of normal results, Am Rev TB and Pulm Dis 79:457, 1959.

Grimby G and Soderholm B: Spirometric studies in normal subjects. III. Static lung volumes and maximal voluntary ventilation in adults with a note on physical fitness, Acta Med Scand 173:199, 1964.

Hepper NGG, Black LF, and Fowler WS: Relationships of lung volume to height and arm span in normal subjects and in patients with spinal deformity, Am Rev Respir Dis 91:356, 1965.

Pare PD, Wiggs BJR, and Coppin CA: Errors in the measurement of total lung capacity in chronic obstructive lung disease, Thorax 38:468, 1983.

West JB: Pulmonary pathophysiology: the essentials, ed 3, Baltimore, 1987, Williams & Wilkins.

West JB: Respiratory physiology: the essentials, ed 3, Baltimore, 1985, Williams & Wilkins.

Thoracic gas volume

Begin P and Peslin, R: Influence of panting frequency on thoracic gas volume measurements in chronic obstructive pulmonary disease, Am Rev Respir Dis 130:121, 1984.

Bohadana AB et al: Influence of panting frequency on plethysmographic measurements of thoracic gas volume, J Appl Physiol 52:739, 1982.

Brown R et al: Influence of abdominal gas on the Boyle's law determination of thoracic gas volume, J Appl Physiol 44:469, 1978.

Dubois AB et al: A rapid plethysmographic method for measuring thoracic gas volume: a comparison with a nitrogen washout method for measuring functional residual capacity, J Clin Invest 35:322, 1956.

Habib MP and Engel LA: Influence of the panting technique on the plethysmographic measurement of thoracic gas volume, Am Rev Respir Dis 117:265, 1978.

Leith DE and Mead J: Principles of body plethysmography, DLD-NHLBI, Nov, 1974.

Lourenco RV and Chung SYK: Calibration of a body plethysmograph for measurement of lung volume, Am Rev Respir Dis 95:687, 1967.

Rodenstein DO, Stanescu DC, and Francis C: Demonstration of failure of body plethysmography in airway obstruction, J Appl Physiol 52:949, 1982.

Shore SA et al: Effect of panting frequency on the plethysmographic determination of thoracic gas volume in chronic obstructive pulmonary disease, Am Rev Respir Dis 128:54, 1983.

Foreign gas lung volumes

Hathirat S, Renzetti AD, and Mitchell M: Measurement of the total lung capacity by helium dilution in a constant volume system, Am Rev Respir Dis 102:760, 1970.

Hickham JB, Blair E, and Frayser R: An open circuit helium method for measuring functional residual capacity and defective intrapulmonary gas mixing, J Clin Invest 33:1277, 1954.

McMichael, J: A rapid method of determining lung capacity. Clin Sci 4:167, 1939.

Meneely GR et al.: A simplified closed circuit helium dilution method for the determination of the residual volume of the lungs. Am J Med 28:824, 1960.

Rodenstein DO and Stanescu DC: Reassessment of lung volume measurements by helium dilution and by body plethysmography in chronic airflow obstruction, Am Rev Respir Dis 126:1040, 1982.

Schaaning CG and Gulsvik A: Accuracy and precision of helium dilution technique and body plethysmography in measuring lung volume, Scand J Clin Invest 32:271, 1973.

Radiologic estimation of total lung capacity

Barnhard JH et al: Roentgenographic determination of total lung capacity Am J Med, 28:51, 1960.

Barrett WA et al: Computerized roentgenographic determination of total lung capacity Am Rev Respir Dis, 113:239, 1976.

Bencowitz HZ: Program for calculation of radiographic total lung capacity, Am Rev Respir Dis 128:576, 1983.

Campbell SC: Estimation of total lung capacity by planimetry of chest radiographs in children 5 to 10 years of age, Am Rev Respir Dis 127:106, 1983.

O'Brien RJ and Drizd TA: Roentgenographic determination of total lung capacity: normal values from a national population survey, Am Rev Respir Dis 128:949, 1983.

Wehr KL and Masferrer R: Clinical usefulness of planimetric estimation of total lung capacity, Respir Care 20:966, 1975.

2

Ventilation and Ventilatory Control Tests

TIDAL VOLUME (V_T)

Description

The tidal volume (V_T) is the volume of gas inspired or expired during each respiratory cycle, usually measured in milliliters and corrected to BTPS (Fig. 2-1). Conventionally, the volume expired is expressed as the V_T.

Technique

The V_T can be measured directly by simple spirometry (see Fig. 1-1). The subject breathes into a volume-displacement or flow-sensing spirometer. The volume change is measured from the excursions directly or integrated from the flow signal, and is recorded as a spirogram either on paper or on a computer graphic screen. Since no two breaths are identical, the V_T inhaled or exhaled should be measured for at least 1 minute, then divided by the rate to determine the average volume:

$$V_T = \dot{V}/f$$

where

$\dot{V}$ = Volume expired ($\dot{V}_E$) or volume inspired ($\dot{V}_I$) during a given interval; usually the $\dot{V}_E$

f = Number of breaths for the same interval (i.e., the respiratory rate)

The $\dot{V}_I$ and V_T are normally slightly greater than the $\dot{V}_E$, because the body at rest produces a slightly lower volume of CO_2 than the volume of O_2 it consumes. This exchange difference is termed the respiratory exchange ratio (RER), and is calculated as the $\dot{V}CO_2/\dot{V}O_2$, where $\dot{V}CO_2$ is the volume of CO_2 produced and $\dot{V}O_2$ is the volume of O_2 consumed per minute. The RER is usually assumed to be about 0.8 at rest. For most clinical purposes the expired volume is measured to calculate tidal volume.

Tidal volume (V_T) may also be estimated by means of respiratory inductive plethysmography (RIP) discussed in Chapter 9. RIP uses coils of wire as transducers that respond to changes in the cross-sectional area of the rib cage and abdominal compartments. With appropriate calibration, inductive plethysmography can be used to measure tidal volume without connections to the airway.

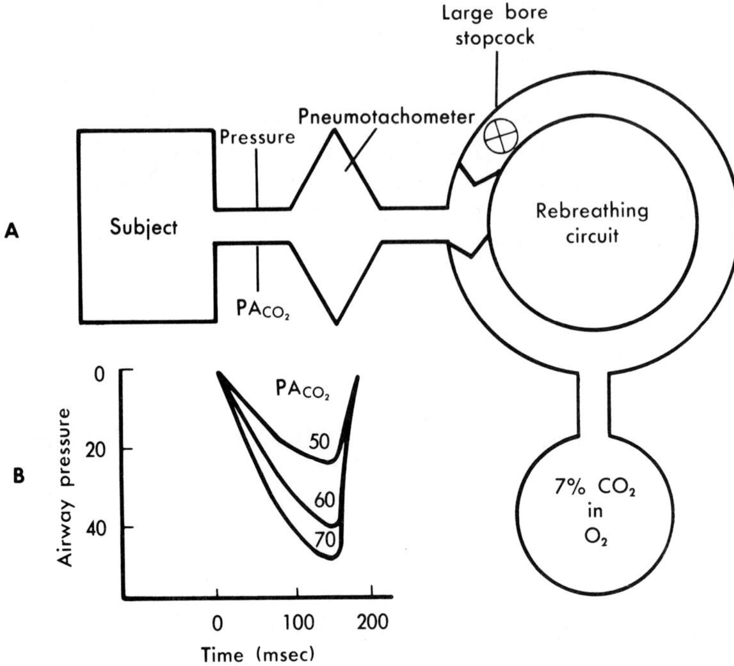

Fig. 2-1 **A,** Apparatus for measurement of occlusion pressure (P_{100}). A rebreathing circuit as diagrammed can be used for measurement of P_{100} and ventilation during progressive hypercapnia. Hypercapnia is produced at full arterial saturation by rebreathing 7% CO_2 in O_2 from a reservoir approximately equal to the subject's VC plus 1 L. Ventilation is measured by integration of the signal from the pneumotachometer. PA_{CO_2} and pressure are monitored from taps at the mouthpiece. A large-bore stopcock, shutter, or similar device is placed in the inspiratory line to occlude flow for single breaths. One-way valves allow the large-bore stopcock to be closed during expiration so that the subsequent inspiration occurs against the occluded airway at FRC. **B,** Representative tracings of the airway pressure developed during occlusion at various levels of hypercapnia (PA_{CO_2} 50, 60, 70) for the first 100 ms.

Significance

Average tidal volumes for healthy adults range from 400 to 700 ml, but there is considerable variation even from these values. Decreased tidal volumes occur in many types of pulmonary disorders, such as particularly severe restrictive patterns, pulmonary fibrosis, and neuromuscular diseases such as myasthenia gravis. Decreased tidal breathing caused by mechanical changes in the lungs or chest wall (i.e., compliance and/or resistance) is almost always accompanied by an increased respiratory rate, which is required to maintain alveolar ventilation. Decreases in both V_T and respiratory rate are usually associated with respiratory center depression, and typically result in alveolar hypoventilation. Some subjects who have pulmonary disease may exhibit increased VT values, particularly at rest. The VT alone is not an adequate indicator of alveolar ventilation, and should never be considered outside the context of rate and minute volume. Rapid rates and small tidal volumes may suggest increased dead space or hypoventilation, but must be correlated with arterial pH and partial pressure of CO_2 (P_{CO_2}) values (see Chapter 6) to be definitive. Many subjects who have little or no pulmonary disease display increased tidal volumes as a result of breathing into the pulmonary function apparatus with the nose occluded; hence, measurements of ventilation may be spuriously increased when measured during pulmonary function testing.

RESPIRATORY RATE (f)

Description

The respiratory rate, frequency of breathing (f), is the number of breaths per unit of time, usually per minute.

Technique

The respiratory rate may be determined by counting the chest movements or the excursions of a spirometer. Counting the rate for several minutes and taking an average produces a more accurate value than shorter measurements.

Significance

The normal respiratory rate ranges from 10 to 20 breaths per minute. Increased demand for ventilation, such as during exercise, usually results in increases in both the rate and depth of breathing, so that respiratory frequency is often a good indicator of the stimulus to ventilate.

Increases or decreases in the respiratory rate are indications of a change in the ventilatory status. Breathing frequency, when evaluated with the tidal volume, may be used as an index of ventilation. Hypoxia, hypercapnia, metabolic acidosis, conditions that cause decreased lung compliance, and exercise all result in increases in respiratory rate, in the presence of a normal respiratory drive. Decreased breathing frequency is common in central nervous system depression and in CO_2 narcosis. Measurements of both tidal volume and respiratory rate may be artifactually elevated in subjects breathing through mouthpieces and other unfamiliar breathing circuits, and/or using a nose clip.

MINUTE VOLUME ($\dot{V}_E$)

Description

The total volume of gas expired per minute ($\dot{V}_E$) includes both the alveolar and dead space ventilation. It is recorded in liters per minute, BTPS.

Technique

The $\dot{V}_E$ may be determined by allowing the subject to breathe either into or out of a volume-displacement or flow-sensing spirometer, or a similar metering device, for at least 1 minute. Measuring expired gas volume for a period of several minutes and dividing by the time gives an average $\dot{V}_E$. Because it is measured from expired gas, the $\dot{V}_E$ is usually slightly smaller than the $\dot{V}_I$ as a result of the respiratory exchange ratio. In most clinical situations, this difference is negligible. BTPS corrections should be made.

Significance

Normal minute ventilation values range from 5 to 10 L/min, with wide variations in normal subjects. The $\dot{V}_E$ is the primary index of ventilation when used in conjunction with blood gas values. Since the $\dot{V}_E$ is the sum of both the dead space and effective alveolar ventilation, absolute values for $\dot{V}_E$ do not necessarily indicate either hypoventilation or hyperventilation.

A large minute ventilation at rest (i.e., greater than 20 L/min) may result from an enlarged dead space volume, since an increase in total ventilation is required to provide adequate alveolar ventilation. $\dot{V}_E$ increases in response to hypoxia, hypercapnia, metabolic acidosis, anxiety, and exercise. Decreased $\dot{V}_E$ may result from hypocapnia, metabolic alkalosis, respiratory center depression, or neuromuscular disorders that involve the ventilatory muscles.

Hypoventilation is defined as inadequate ventilation to maintain a normal arterial P_{CO_2}, and the respiratory acidosis that results. Hyperventilation is ventilation in excess of that needed to maintain adequate CO_2 removal, with a resulting respiratory alkalosis. The diagnosis of either hyperventilation or hypoventilation requires blood gas analysis (see Chapter 6).

CHEMICAL CONTROL OF VENTILATION

Description

Ventilatory response to CO_2 is the measurement of the increase or decrease in $\dot{V}_E$ caused by breathing various concentrations of CO_2 under normoxic conditions (Pa_{O_2} = 90 to 100 mm Hg). It is recorded as L/min/mm Hg P_{CO_2}.

Ventilatory response to O_2 is the measurement of the increase or decrease in $\dot{V}_E$ caused by breathing various concentrations of O_2 under isocapnic conditions (Pa_{CO_2} = 40 mm Hg).

Occlusion pressure (P_{100}) or $P_{0.1}$ is the pressure generated at the mouth during the first 100 ms of an inspiratory effort while breathing against an occluded airway. It is usually measured in centimeters of water (cm H_2O).

Technique

CO_2 response can be measured in two ways, as follows:

1. Open-circuit technique. When using this method, various concentrations (1% to 7%) of CO_2 in air or O_2 are breathed from a demand valve or reservoir until a steady state is reached. Measurements of

end-tidal PCO_2 (PET_{CO_2}), arterial PCO_2, P_{100}, and $\dot{V}E$ may be made at each concentration.

2. Closed-circuit or rebreathing technique. The subject rebreathes from a one-way circuit containing a reservoir of 7% CO_2 in O_2 (see Fig. 2-1). The circuit includes valves and pressure taps for monitoring P_{100}, and ports for extracting samples for PET_{CO_2} determinations. A pneumotachometer (see Chapter 9) is placed in line to record $\dot{V}E$. Similarly, the gas reservoir bag may be placed in a rigid container or box, and volume change measured by connecting a spirometer to the container (i.e., "bag-in-box" setup). The subject rebreathes until the concentration of PET_{CO_2} exceeds 9%, or until 4 minutes have elapsed. The rebreathed gas is also analyzed to ascertain that the FI_{O_2} remains above 0.21. The subject's oxygen saturation (Sa_{O_2}) may also be monitored by means of a pulse oximeter (see Chapter 9). Changes in $\dot{V}E$ are monitored and plotted against PET_{CO_2} to obtain a response curve.

O_2 response can also be measured using either open- or closed-circuit techniques:

1. Open-circuit technique. The subject breathes gas mixtures containing O_2 concentrations between 12% and 20% to which CO_2 is added to maintain alveolar PCO_2 (PA_{CO_2}) at a constant level. Once a steady state is reached, Pa_{O_2}, $\dot{V}E$, and P_{100} can be measured. This procedure, often called a step test, is repeated at various O_2 concentrations to produce the response curve. Continuous monitoring of PET_{CO_2} is necessary to titrate the addition of CO_2 to the system to maintain isocapnia (as in Fig. 2-3). Pa_{O_2} should be monitored, since it often varies from the PA_{O_2}. Pulse oximetry may be used to monitor changes in saturation. CO_2 response curves are sometimes measured at widely varying PA_{O_2} values, and the subsequent difference in ventilation or P_{100} at any particular PCO_2 is attributed to the response to hypoxemia.
2. Closed-circuit technique (progressive hypoxemia). The subject rebreathes from a system similar to that used for the closed-circuit CO_2 response, but which also contains a CO_2 scrubber. CO_2 can be added to the inspired gas to maintain isocapnia, or a variable blower may be used to direct a portion of the rebreathed gas through the scrubber to maintain isocapnia (as in Fig. 2-3). Response to decreasing inspired PO_2 is monitored by recording $\dot{V}E$ or P_{100}, and the Pa_{O_2} or saturation is measured either directly by indwelling catheter or indirectly by pulse oximetry.

P_{100} (or $P_{0.1}$) is measured using a system similar to that in Fig. 2-1. A pressure tap at the mouth records pressure changes versus time on a storage oscilloscope or high-speed recorder, or by computer. A large-bore stopcock or electronic shutter mechanism is included in the inspiratory line so that inspiratory flow can be randomly occluded. The unidirectional breathing

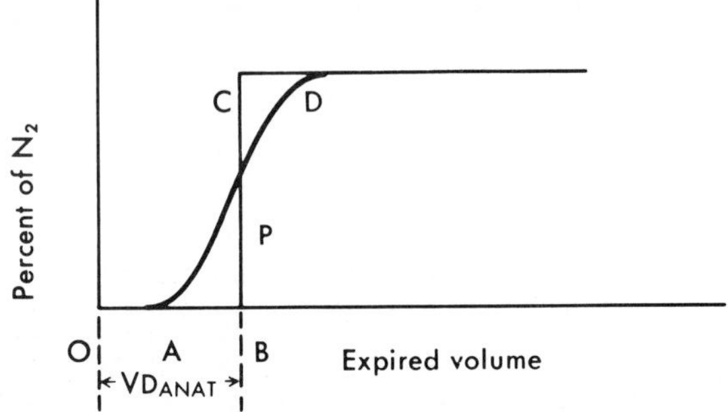

Fig. 2-2 Anatomic dead space determination. The rise in concentration of N_2 during a single expiration, after a breath of 100% O_2, is illustrated. Only the initial portion of the breath is included. As the subject expires, the N_2 concentration rises slowly at first as pure dead space gas is exhaled; then as bronchial air is expired, the N_2 concentration rises abruptly. Since different parts of the lungs empty at different rates, the change from pure dead space air to alveolar gas appears as an S-shaped curve. By constructing a square wave front (*BC*) so that the areas *ABP* and *DCP* are equal, the anatomic dead space can be estimated as being equal to the volume expired up to point B.

circuit allows the stopcock or shutter to be closed during expiration, so that the subsequent inspiration can occur against complete occlusion, starting at FRC. The entire apparatus is usually hidden from the subject so that he or she is unaware of the impending airway occlusion. A pressure-time curve is recorded either from the oscilloscope or by means of a high speed (i.e., 50 to 100 mm/sec) recorder. The P_{100} is usually measured at varying $P_{ET_{CO_2}}$ values or levels of desaturation to assess the effect of changes in the stimuli to ventilation. P_{100} and $\dot{V}_E$ are usually graphed against $P_{ET_{CO_2}}$ (i.e., CO_2 response) or versus Sa_{O_2} (i.e., O_2 response).

Significance

The response to an increase in $P_{A_{CO_2}}$ in the healthy individual is a linear increase in $\dot{V}_E$ of approximately 3 L/min/mm Hg P_{CO_2}. The normal range of response varies from 1 to 6 L/min/mm Hg P_{CO_2} and some variation is present in repeated testing of the same individual. The response to CO_2 in subjects who have obstructive disease may be reduced; this is partially attributable to increased airway resistance, which has been shown to reduce ventilatory response in healthy individuals. It is not yet clear why some subjects who have obstructive disease increase ventilation to maintain a normal Pa_{CO_2} while others tolerate an increased Pa_{CO_2}. A plot of minute ventilation versus $P_{ET_{CO_2}}$ may be used to determine a slope or response curve.

The normal response to a decrease in Pa_{O_2} appears to be exponential

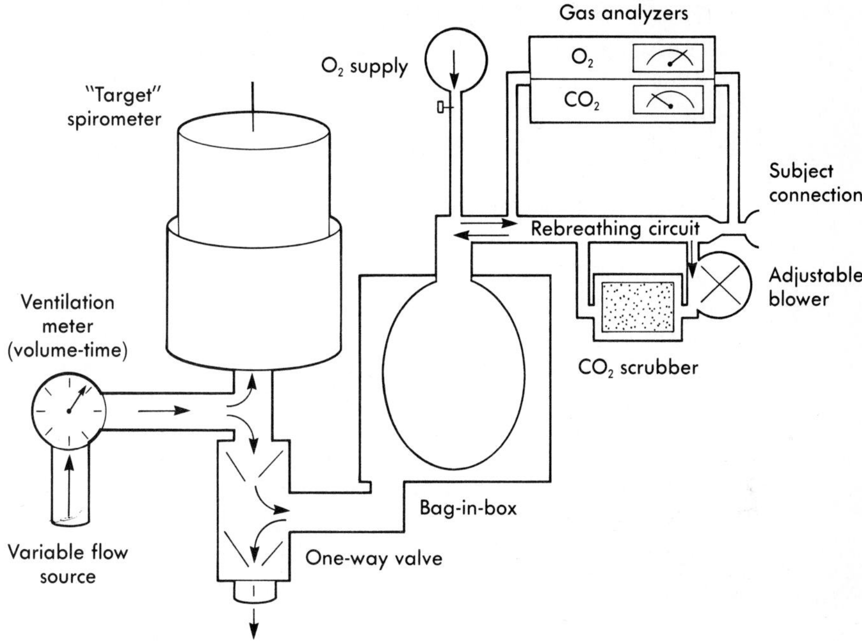

Fig. 2-3 Apparatus for measuring maximum sustained ventilatory capacity (MSVC). The subject breathes through a rebreathing system that consists of a bag-in-box apparatus, to which an O_2 supply, gas analyzers for O_2 and CO_2, and a CO_2 scrubbing device are attached. The analyzers allow continuous monitoring of the O_2 and CO_2 concentrations; the O_2 supply is adjusted to maintain a normal FI_{O_2}, while an adjustable blower on the CO_2 scrubber regulates the CO_2 concentration in the system to avoid hypercapnia or hypocapnia. Connected to the box via a one-way valve is a volume-displacement spirometer. A variable flow source is adjusted to deliver a fixed volume of gas to the "target" spirometer per minute. As the subject inspires, gas is removed from the bag and the spirometer falls; on exhalation, gas is forced from the box out the one-way valve, and the spirometer rises. As long as the subject's minute ventilation matches the flow of gas entering the target spirometer, the spirometer's volume remains fairly constant. Flow is gradually adjusted to obtain the maximal flow that the subject can maintain over an extended interval.

once the Pa_{O_2} has fallen to the range of 40 to 60 mm Hg. Again, there are wide variations in responses among individuals. The hypoxic response is increased in the presence of hypercapnia and decreased in hypocapnia. Subjects who have severe chronic obstructive lung disease and chronic CO_2 retention receive their primary respiratory stimulus from the hypoxemic response. This group of subjects may suffer severe or even fatal respiratory depression if that response is obliterated by uncontrolled oxygen therapy.

Some subjects with minimal intrinsic lung disease show markedly decreased response to hypoxemia or hypercapnia. These include subjects who have myxedema, obesity-hypoventilation syndrome, obstructive sleep apnea, and idiopathic hypoventilation. CO_2 and O_2 response measurements, along with tests of pulmonary mechanics, may be particularly valuable in the evaluation and treatment of these types of subjects.

The P_{100} ($P_{0.1}$) has been suggested as a measurement of ventilatory drive independent of the mechanical properties of the lungs. Since no air flow occurs during occlusion of the airway, significant interference from mechanical abnormalities, such as increased resistance or decreased compliance, is omitted. Reflexes from the airways and chest wall are also of little influence during the first 100 ms of the occluded breath. Therefore, the pressure generated can be viewed as proportional to the neural output of the medullary centers that drive the rate and depth of breathing. This proportionality may be influenced by other factors, however, such as body position and the contractile properties of the respiratory muscles.

Subjects whose Pa_{CO_2} values are normal have P_{100} values in the range of 1.5 to 5 cm H_2O. P_{100} has been shown to increase in hypercapnia and hypoxia, and appears to correlate well with the observed ventilatory responses. Increasing P_{CO_2}, and thereby inducing hypercapnia, in healthy subjects typically results in an increase in the occlusion pressure of 0.5 to 0.6 cm H_2O/mm Hg P_{CO_2}, with as much as 20% variability. Some subjects who have chronic airway obstruction demonstrate little or no increase in P_{100} in response to an increase in their P_{CO_2}, even with increased airway resistance, whereas healthy persons increase their P_{100} when breathing through artificial resistance on challenge with high P_{CO_2} or low P_{O_2}. This failure to respond to increased resistance in the airways may predispose individuals with chronic obstructive pulmonary disease (COPD) to respiratory failure when lung infections occur. Similarly, patients maintained on mechanical ventilation may experience difficulty in weaning if their ventilatory drive is compromised, as demonstrated by failure to increase the P_{100} when challenged with increased P_{CO_2}. Determination of the P_{100} may prove helpful in determining the effects of treatment in subjects who have abnormal ventilatory responses.

RESPIRATORY DEAD SPACE (V_D)

Description

Respiratory dead space (V_D) is that volume of the lungs that is ventilated but not perfused by pulmonary capillary blood flow. The dead space can be divided into the conducting airways, or anatomic, dead space; and the nonperfused alveoli, or alveolar, dead space. The combination of alveolar and anatomic dead space volumes is the respiratory, or physiologic, dead space, or V_D. V_D is recorded in liters or milliliters, BTPS.

Technique

Anatomic dead space may be estimated from an individual's body size, but the total wasted ventilation, or respiratory dead space, is of greater importance clinically. The V_D can be calculated in two ways. The first uses Bohr's equation defining V_D:

$$V_D = \frac{(F_{A_{CO_2}} - F_{E_{CO_2}})}{F_{A_{CO_2}}} V_T$$

where

V_T = Tidal volume
$F_{A_{CO_2}}$ = Fraction of CO_2 in alveolar gas
$F_{E_{CO_2}}$ = Fraction of CO_2 in expired gas

Since the concentration of CO_2 in the alveoli is difficult to measure, the partial pressures of the component gases may be substituted and the equation written as follows:

$$V_D = \frac{(Pa_{CO_2} - P_{E_{CO_2}})}{Pa_{CO_2}} V_T$$

where

V_T = Tidal volume
Pa_{CO_2} = Arterial P_{CO_2}
$P_{E_{CO_2}}$ = P_{CO_2} of expired gas sample

Note that the arterial P_{CO_2} is substituted for the alveolar P_{CO_2}; this presumes that equilibration is perfect between the alveoli and pulmonary capillaries, which may not be true in certain diseases. The test is based on the fact that there is practically no CO_2 in the atmosphere; therefore the partial pressure of CO_2 in the expired gas is inversely proportional to the physiologic dead space, or V_D. By collecting gas over several respiratory cycles and obtaining simultaneous Pa_{CO_2}, all the variables are supplied, and a reasonably accurate physiologic dead space calculation can be made by applying the previous equation. The estimate becomes more accurate as more expired gas is collected. The accuracy depends on the measurement of $\dot{V}_E$, as well as the partial pressures of CO_2 both in the expired gas and in the arterial sample. The mixed expired gas sample is usually collected in a bag or balloon after filling and emptying it several times with expired gas to "wash out" room air from the valves, tubing, and bag itself. The volume of gas in the bag can be measured either during collection, by inclusion of an appropriate volume transducer, or by emptying the contents into a Tissot spirometer. If minute ventilation and rate are recorded during collection, the absolute volumes of the V_D and V_T can be determined. Without measuring the actual $\dot{V}_E$, only the dilution ratio can be determined; this is referred to as the V_D/V_T ratio.

A second method calculates the anatomic dead space from the single-breath analysis method, or Fowler's method (see also Chapter 4). This technique requires continuous analysis of the concentration of N_2 in the expired gas plus simultaneous measurement of the V_E. After inhaling 100% O_2, the subject breathes out through the recording apparatus. During the first part of the breath, pure O_2 is exhaled, and the N_2 concentration remains at zero (see Fig. 2-2) until a volume equal to the anatomic dead space has been exhaled. Then, the N_2 concentration rises rapidly to the level of alveolar N_2, diluted with O_2. Because the conducting airways have different lengths and volumes, the curve depicting the change in N_2 concentration does not present a "square front." By numerical methods, a square front can be constructed, and the anatomic dead space is the VE up to the square front. Bohr's equation can be modified as follows to apply to the data obtained from a single-breath analysis:

$$V_D = \frac{(F_{A_{N_2}} - F_{E_{N_2}})}{F_{A_{N_2}}} V_E$$

where

V_E = Volume expired

$F_{A_{N_2}}$ = Fraction of N_2 in alveolar gas (read from N_2 meter at end of breath)

$F_{E_{N_2}}$ = Fraction of N_2 in expired sample (computed by measuring area under $\%N_2$ curve and dividing by VE)

The difficulty in obtaining the $F_{E_{N_2}}$ restricts this type of calculation to more sophisticated laboratory setups.

Significance

The measurement of VD, although difficult, yields important information regarding the ventilation/perfusion characteristics of the lungs. *Anatomic dead space* is larger in men than in women because of differences in body size; it increases along with the VT during exercise and in certain forms of pulmonary disease, such as bronchiectasis. It may be decreased in asthma or in diseases characterized by bronchial obstruction or mucus plugging. Because of the difficulty in measuring the anatomic dead space, estimates based on age, sex, FRC, or body size may be used; for clinical purposes, the anatomic dead space in milliliters is sometimes equated with the subject's ideal body weight in pounds.

Of greater clinical significance is the measurement of VD, which is accomplished reasonably well by applying the Bohr equation. The volume of ventilation wasted on the conducting airways and poorly perfused alveoli is usually expressed as a fraction of the tidal volume, VD/VT, and is considered normal if the derived value is between 0.2 and 0.4. Expressing dead space in this way eliminates the necessity of measuring the $\dot{V}_E$ in the application of the Bohr equation. Physiologic dead space measurements are a good index of ventilation/blood flow ratios, because all CO_2 in expired gas comes from perfused alveoli (see Chapter 6). The VD/VT ratio decreases in healthy subjects during exercise because of increases in the cardiac output and the increased perfusion of alveoli at the lung apices. This occurs despite absolute increases in the VD itself. Increases in dead space and in the VD/VT ratio may be observed in pulmonary embolism and in pulmonary hypertension. In pulmonary embolism, large numbers of arterioles may be blocked, resulting in little or no CO_2 removal in the associated alveoli. In pulmonary hypertension, increased pulmonary arterial pressure causes most alveoli to be perfused, so there is little or no "recruitment" of under-perfused gas exchange units. This is most notable during exercise, when the VD/VT normally falls.

ALVEOLAR VENTILATION ($\dot{V}_A$)

Description

The $\dot{V}_A$ is that volume of gas that participates in gas exchange in the lungs. $\dot{V}_A$ can be considered equal to the $\dot{V}_E$ minus the dead space ventilation per minute ($\dot{V}_D$). For a single breath, VA equals the VT minus the VD. The $\dot{V}_A$ is usually expressed as volume per unit time, normally liters per minute, BTPS.

Technique

The $\dot{V}_A$ can be calculated in two ways:

1.
$$\dot{V}_A = f(V_T - V_D)$$

where

VT = Tidal volume
VD = Respiratory dead space
f = Respiratory rate

Often, for the sake of convenience, the VD is estimated as being equal to the anatomic dead space. This method is valid only when there is little or no alveolar dead space, such as in individuals who do not have pulmonary disease.

2. Since atmospheric gas contains almost no CO_2, $\dot{V}_A$ can be calculated on the basis of CO_2 elimination from the lungs. A volume of expired gas is collected in a bag, balloon, or spirometer, then analyzed to determine the volume of CO_2 contained (see Chapter 7). The following equation can then be used:

$$\dot{V}_A = \frac{\dot{V}_{CO_2}}{F_{A_{CO_2}}}$$

where

$\dot{V}_{CO_2}$ = Volume of CO_2 produced in milliliters per minute, (STPD)
$F_{A_{CO_2}}$ = Fraction of CO_2 in alveolar gas

If an end-tidal CO_2 monitor is used, a close approximation of the concentration of $P_{A_{CO_2}}$ is easily obtained and the equation simplified as follows:

$$\dot{V}_A = \frac{\dot{V}_{CO_2}}{\%\ \text{alveolar}\ CO_2} \times 100$$

End-tidal CO_2 may not equal alveolar CO_2 in subjects who have grossly abnormal patterns of ventilation/perfusion (see Chapter 6).

The same equation can be used with a substitution of the arterial P_{CO_2} for the alveolar P_{CO_2} (i.e., $P_{A_{CO_2}}$), again presuming that arterial blood and alveolar gas are in equilibrium. The equation then becomes:

$$\dot{V}_A = \frac{\dot{V}_{CO_2}}{Pa_{CO_2}} \times 0.863$$

where

$\dot{V}_{CO_2}$ = Volume of CO_2 produced in milliliters per minute (STPD)
Pa_{CO_2} = Partial pressure of arterial CO_2
0.863 = Factor for converting from concentration to partial pressure and correcting $\dot{V}_{CO_2}$ to BTPS

Significance

Both methods are suitable for calculating the $\dot{V}_A$. The CO_2 elimination method is more accurate than the equation, $V_A = f(V_T - V_D)$, when anatomic dead space is used in place of V_D. The differences become more apparent in situations where there are pronounced ventilation/blood flow imbalances. $\dot{V}_A$ at rest is about 4 to 5 L/min, with wide variations in healthy individuals. The adequacy of the $\dot{V}_A$ can only be determined by performing arterial blood gas studies. Low $\dot{V}_A$ associated with acute respiratory acidosis (i.e., Pa_{CO_2} greater than 45 and pH less than 7.35) defines hypoventilation. Excessive $\dot{V}_A$ (i.e., Pa_{CO_2} less than 35 and pH greater than 7.45) defines hyperventilation. Chronic hypoventilation and hyperventilation are associated with abnormal P_{CO_2} values, but near normal pH values. Decreased $\dot{V}_A$ can result from absolute increases in dead space as well as decreases in total ventilation ($\dot{V}_E$).

MAXIMUM SUSTAINED VENTILATORY CAPACITY (MSVC)

Description

The maximum sustained ventilatory capacity (MSVC) is the maximum level of ventilation that can be maintained for a specified interval, usually 15 minutes, under isocapnic conditions. Because a rebreathing circuit is used, the ventilation measurement is typically *not* corrected to BTPS (see following Technique section). The MSVC is recorded in liters/minute.

Technique

The MSVC is measured by allowing the subject to ventilate in a rebreathing system, such as that in Fig. 2-3. A bag-in-box apparatus is connected to a spirometer or other volume transducer via a large one-way valve. A large valve is required to minimize resistance at higher flow rates. A variable flow generator supplies gas to the spirometer at selectable flow rates. As the subject inspires from the bag-in-box system, gas is removed from the spirometer into the box, then into the atmosphere when the subject exhales. Connected to the rebreathing circuitry are O_2 and CO_2 analyzers, as well as taps for addition of O_2 and a scrubber for CO_2 removal. Using readings from the gas analyzers, O_2 can be added to maintain an acceptable F_{IO_2}, normally greater than 15%. When a variable speed blower is attached to the CO_2 scrubber, the fraction of CO_2 in the circuit can be maintained close to baseline levels. The subject rebreathes and attempts to keep the spirometer at a "target" level. As long as the subject ventilates at a flow equal to the flow rate from the generator, the spirometer volume remains relatively constant. If the subject cannot match the flow, the spirometer rises and the flow must be further adjusted. The subject is usually allowed to choose the most efficient tidal volume/breathing rate combination. Several short trials may be necessary to establish the level of ventilation that can be maintained for the desired interval, usually 15 minutes. Some learning may occur so that repeat runs may be needed to establish the subject's highest or "best" MSVC.

Significance

Normal maximum voluntary ventilation (MVV) values (see Chapter 3) range from 100 to 200 L/min, while normal resting ventilation is usually 5 to 10 L/min. The MSVC falls between these extremes, usually at 65% to 70% of the MVV. A subject who has an MVV of 100 L/min would typically have an MSVC of about 70 L/min. The MSVC represents a level of ventilation that can be sustained for an extended period, and is determined by the status of the respiratory control mechanisms, the respiratory muscles, and the total work of breathing (i.e., compliance and resistance).

MSVC measurements are particularly useful for evaluating the endurance of the respiratory muscles, and have been used to assess various therapies aimed at training or reconditioning this group of muscles. The MSVC is reduced in subjects who have obstructive disease, because of the increased work of breathing associated with ventilation at higher flow rates. Despite this absolute reduction, the MSVC may be above 70% of the same subject's MVV. Because of the low absolute levels of sustainable ventilation in subjects who have obstruction, it is clear why exercise limitations may occur with normal activities such as walking. The MSVC may also be reduced in subjects who have defects influencing the neuromuscular aspects of ventilation, such as myasthenia gravis. The MSVC, as an index of respiratory muscle endurance, is often used in conjunction with maximal inspiratory and expiratory pressures (see Chapter 3), which relate to respiratory muscle strength.

SELF-ASSESSMENT QUESTIONS

1. Assessing a subject's ventilatory response to hypoxemia by the rebreathing method requires:
   a. Special low concentration O_2 gas mixtures

b. A variable rate CO_2 scrubbing device
c. A fast (50 to 100 mm/sec) recording device
d. All of the above

2. A subject performs a closed-circuit CO_2 response test. The results show a change in ventilation at the rate of 0.5 L/min for each mm Hg change in $P_{ET_{CO_2}}$. This is:
   a. Markedly reduced
   b. Only slightly reduced
   c. Within normal limits
   d. Consistent with pulmonary fibrosis

3. Exhaled gas is collected in a large-volume spirometer for 7 minutes; during this period the subject breathes 61 times. If the total volume collected is 36.6 liters (BTPS), what is the:
   a. V_T ____________________
   b. Rate (f) ____________________
   c. $\dot{V}_E$ ____________________

4. A subject's $\dot{V}_E$ is measured as 4.5 L/min (BTPS). Blood gases in the same subject reveal a pH of 7.21 and a P_{CO_2} of 57; this level of ventilation is:
   a. Within normal limits
   b. Consistent with hypoventilation
   c. Consistent with hyperventilation
   d. Inconsistent with the reported blood gases

5. Which of the following parameters are commonly reported in assessing the response to increasing carbon dioxide tensions (CO_2 response test):
   I. Occlusion pressure (P_{100})
   II. Physiologic dead space (V_D)
   III. Oxygen saturation (Sa_{O_2})
   IV. Minute ventilation ($\dot{V}_E$)
   a. I, II, III, IV
   b. I, II, III
   c. I, IV only
   d. III, IV only

6. The response to an increased $P_{A_{CO_2}}$ in normal individuals is to:
   a. Decrease $\dot{V}_E$ slightly
   b. Increase $\dot{V}_E$ by 20 L/min for each mm Hg increase in P_{CO_2}
   c. Increase $\dot{V}_E$ by 1 to 6 L/min for each mm Hg increase in P_{CO_2}
   d. Maintain a constant $\dot{V}_E$ until the $P_{A_{CO_2}}$ rises to between 55 and 60 mm Hg

7. The V_D (respiratory dead space) may be increased
   a. By pulmonary embolism
   b. During exercise
   c. In pulmonary hypertension
   d. All of the above

8. The P_{100} measures:
   a. The endurance of the diaphragm
   b. The response of the respiratory muscles to CO_2
   c. The $\dot{V}_E$ when the Pa_{O_2} is 100 mm Hg
   d. The output of the respiratory centers

9. A subject has arterial blood drawn and expired gas collected; $\dot{V}_E$ is 9.5 L/min (BTPS), Pa_{CO_2} is 40 mm Hg, and partial pressure of CO_2 in the expired sample ($P\bar{E}_{CO_2}$) is 27 mm Hg; the respiratory rate is measured as 15 breaths/min. What is the:
   a. V_T ____________________
   b. V_D ____________________
   c. V_D/V_T ____________________

10. A subject has a $\dot{V}_E$ of 9.0 L/min BTPS and a respiratory rate of 18; if the subject's V_D/V_T is 0.40, what is his
    $\dot{V}_A$ = ____________________ L

11. A subject has a maximum sustained ventilatory capacity (MSVC) that is 83% of her MVV, but the MVV is only 27% of the predicted value; these findings are:
    a. Consistent with normal lung function in an older adult
    b. Consistent with an obstructive disease pattern
    c. Consistent with a mild restrictive pattern
    d. Physiologically impossible

12. Hyperventilation is:
    a. A respiratory rate greater than 25 breaths/minute
    b. Inadequate ventilation to maintain a normal P_{CO_2}
    c. A minute ventilation greater than 25 L/min, BTPS
    d. A level of ventilation that produces respiratory alkalosis

SELECTED BIBLIOGRAPHY

General references

Forster RE: The lung: clinical physiology and pulmonary function tests, Chicago, 1988, Year Book Medical Publishers, Inc.

West JB: Pulmonary pathophysiology: the essentials, ed 3, Baltimore, 1987, Williams & Wilkins.

West JB: Respiratory physiology: the essentials, ed 3, Baltimore, 1985, Williams & Wilkins.

Ventilation

Gray JS, Gracius FS, and Carter ET: Alveolar ventilation and dead space problem, J Appl Physiol 2:307, 1956.

Riley RL and Cournand A: 'Ideal' alveolar air and the analysis of ventilation-perfusion relationships in the lungs, J Appl Physiol 1:825, 1949.

Severinghaus JW and Stipfel M: Alveolar dead space as an index of distribution of blood flow in pulmonary capillaries, J Appl Physiol 10:335, 1957.

Chemical control of ventilation

Cherniak NS et al: Occlusion pressure as technique in evaluating respiratory control, Chest (suppl) 70:137, 1976.

Read DJC: A clinical method for assessing the ventilatory response to carbon dioxide, Aust Ann Med 16:20, 1967.

Rebuck AS and Campbell EJM: A clinical method for assessing the ventilatory response to hypoxia. Rev Respir Dis 109:345, 1974.

Shaw RA, Schonfeld SA, and Whitcomb, ME: Progressive and transient hypoxic ventilatory drive tests in healthy subjects, Am Rev Respir Dis 126:37, 1982.

Respiratory muscles

Black LF and Hyatt RE: Maximal respiratory pressures: normal values and relationship to age and sex, Am Rev Respir Dis 99:696, 1976.

Brody AW et al: Correlations, normal standards, and interdependence in tests of ventilatory strength and mechanics, Am Rev Respir Dis 89:214, 1964.

Leith D and Bradley M: Ventilatory muscle strength and endurance training, J Appl Physiol 41:508, 1976.

3

Pulmonary Mechanics

FORCED VITAL CAPACITY (FVC)

Description

The forced vital capacity (FVC) is the maximum volume of gas that can be expired, when the subject tries as forcefully and rapidly as possible, after a maximal inspiration to total lung capacity. A maneuver performed similarly beginning at maximal expiration and inspiring as forcefully as possible is called forced inspiratory vital capacity (FIVC). The FVC and FIVC maneuvers are often performed in sequence to provide a continuous flow-volume loop (see page 50). Both the FVC and FIVC are recorded in liters, BTPS.

Technique

The FVC is measured by having the subject, after inspiring maximally to TLC, expire as forcefully and rapidly as possible into a volume-displacement or flow-sensing spirometer. The volume expired may be read from a direct volume-time tracing such as that produced on a kymograph (Fig. 3-1) or derived from the integration of a flow signal. A spirometer that produces a hard copy tracing of either volume-time or flow-volume is essential for clinical laboratory purposes to allow visual inspection of the maneuver. Devices providing numerical data alone may be helpful for simple screening, but the results should be correlated with data obtained from a spirometer that meets the criteria proposed by the American Thoracic Society (see Chapter 11). Because the FVC maneuver is an effort-dependent test, not all subjects may be able to perform it acceptably. Criteria for judging the validity of spirometric data are detailed in Chapter 11. The reported volumes should be corrected to BTPS.

Significance

The FVC is normally equal to the slow vital capacity (SVC) (see Chapter 1). The FVC and SVC may differ substantially if the subject's effort varies, or in the presence of severe airways obstruction. The FVC may be lower than the SVC in some subjects who have obstructive diseases if the forced expiration causes bronchiolar collapse from which air trapping results. In subjects without obstruction, the FVC and SVC should be within 5% of each other. The FVC may be reduced in emphysema because of loss of

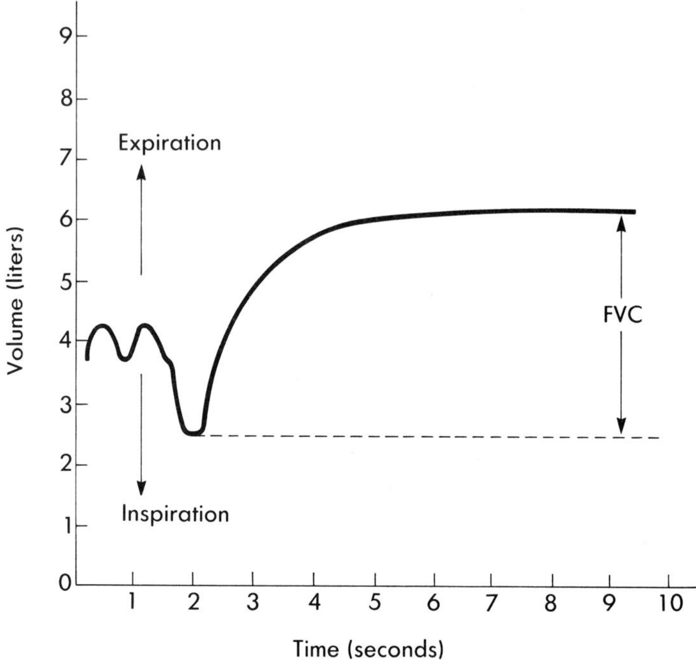

Fig. 3-1 Forced vital capacity (FVC)—Typical spirogram plotting volume against time as the subject exhales forcefully. In this tracing, expiration causes an upward deflection; in some systems, the tracing is inverted. The subject inspires to the maximal inspiratory level (dashed line) at which point the lungs are close to TLC; the subject expires as rapidly as possible to the maximal expiratory level, at which the lungs contain only the RV (see text).

support for the small airways (i.e., airways less than 2 mm in diameter). The forced vital capacity may also be reduced because of mucus plugging and bronchiolar constriction, as found in chronic bronchitis, chronic or acute asthma, bronchiectasis, and cystic fibrosis. Reduced FVC may also be seen in some subjects who have large airway obstructive processes, such as tumors or diseases affecting the patency of the trachea and mainstem bronchi. Not all subjects who have airways obstruction exhibit a reduction in forced vital capacity in relation to their predicted values. However, forced expiratory time (FET), the time required to expire the FVC, is often prolonged well beyond the 4 to 6 seconds seen in healthy individuals, and may exceed 20 seconds in subjects who have severe obstruction.

Accurate measurement of the FVC in subjects who have severe obstruction may be limited by the interval over which the spirometer accumulates volume. Many spirometers allow only 10 seconds of volume recording, hence, the FVC and flow values derived from it may be inaccurate if the subject continues to exhale. An accurate diagnosis of obstruction, however, can usually be made from 10 seconds of recording (see Chapter 11).

Decreased FVC is a common feature of restrictive diseases. A lower than predicted FVC in subjects who have restrictive diseases may result from an increase in fibrotic tissue, as in pulmonary fibrosis; vascular congestion, as in pneumonia or pulmonary edema; space-occupying lesions, such as tumors or pleural effusions; neuromuscular disorders, such as myasthenia gravis; or chest deformities, such as scoliosis. Any disease that affects the bellows action of the chest or the distensibility of the lung tissue itself tends to result in a reduced FVC. Obesity and pregnancy are common causes of reduced FVC, since they interfere with movement of the diaphragm and excursion of the chest wall.

Interpretation of the FVC in patients who have obstructive diseases requires correlation with flows, while in patients who have restrictive patterns, the FVC should be considered in relation to the other lung volume parameters (i.e., RV, TLC) Values less than 80% of predicted values or less than the 95% confidence limit are considered abnormal in both obstruction and restriction. Values less than 50% of expected values denote a marked reduction of FVC, and are often accompanied by a patient's complaint of exertional dyspnea.

The validity of the FVC maneuver depends largely on the subject's effort and cooperation, as well as on the instruction and coaching supplied by the technologist. Because of its central role in routine spirometry, the acceptability of the FVC should be evaluated according to specific criteria (see Chapter 11).

FORCED EXPIRATORY VOLUME (FEV_T)

Description

The FEV_T is the volume of gas expired during a given time interval (T) from the beginning of an FVC maneuver. The time interval is stated as a subscript to FEV. Those intervals in common use are $FEV_{0.5}$, $FEV_{1.0}$, $FEV_{2.0}$, and $FEV_{3.0}$. The FEV_T is normally stated in liters, and T is expressed in seconds (Fig. 3-2). Of the various FEV measurements, the $FEV_{1.0}$ is the most widely used.

Technique

The FEV_T may be measured by introducing a means of timing an FVC maneuver during the described intervals. Normally, this is done by recording the FVC spirogram on graph paper moving at a fixed speed, so that the volume at any interval can be read from the graph. Because accurate measurement of the FEV intervals depends on determination of the *start-of-test*, the spirometer should provide a hard copy tracing or printout; this allows for direct measurement on both the volume and time axes and *back-extrapolation* when necessary (see Chapter 11). Computerized spirometers detect the start-of-test as an incremental change in flow or volume above a certain threshold, then store volume and flow data points in memory. The computer may then generate a representation of the volume-time graph; if only the expiratory data is presented, assessing the start-of-test is

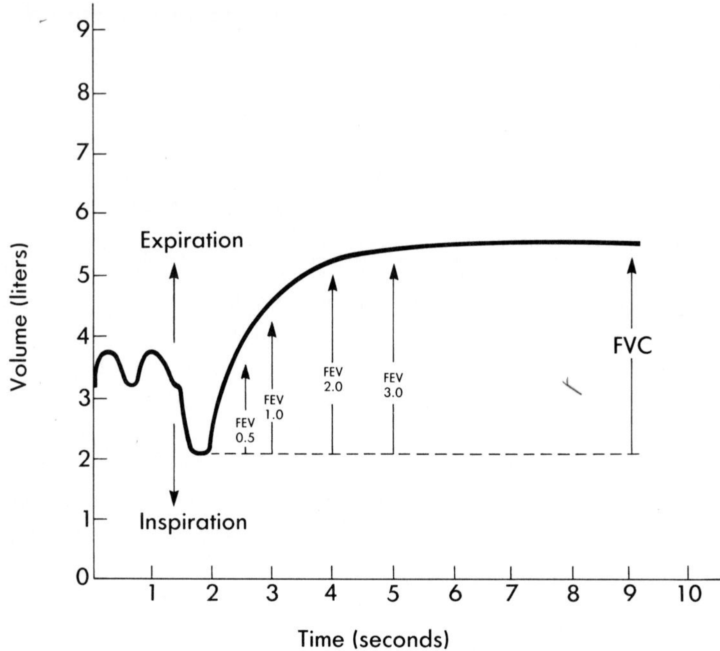

Fig. 3-2 Forced expiratory volume maneuver (FEV)—a spirogram of FEV_T maneuver, with the subject exhaling as forcefully and rapidly as possible, as for the FVC. Arrows indicate the FEV at intervals of 0.5, 1.0, 2.0, and 3.0 seconds. Precise timing and acceptable "start-of-test" are required to determine the FEV_T accurately (see text and Chapter 11).

difficult, and inaccurate FEV values may result. Some flow-sensing devices report the FEV_T only in digital form after integration of the expiratory flow, but such measurements should be used with caution if a hard copy spirogram is not available for correlation. All FEV_T values should be corrected to BTPS.

Significance

Since the FEV_T maneuvers measure the volume of gas expired during various units of time, they are, in reality, measures of the average flow during their respective intervals. Decreased FEV_T values are common in both obstructive and restrictive patterns. The FEV_T may also be reduced due to poor effort or cooperation by the subject.

Airway obstruction due to mucus secretion, bronchospasm, inflammation, or loss of elastic support for the airways themselves (i.e., emphysema) all result in decreased FEV_T values. The $FEV_{1.0}$ and the $FEV_{1.0}$/FVC ratio (see next section) are the most widely used and best standardized indices of obstructive disease. However, the FEV_T may remain relatively well preserved in the early stages of obstruction in the small airways (i.e., airways less than 2 mm in diameter). Other more sensitive tests of small airways function may produce abnormal values, while the $FEV_{1.0}$ and other FEV parameters are within normal limits.

Restrictive processes such as fibrosis, edema, space-occupying lesions, neuromuscular disorders, obesity, and chest wall deformities may all cause reduced FEV_T and FVC values. However, unlike the pattern seen in obstructive disorders in which the FVC may be preserved and the FEV_T reduced, in simple restriction the FVC and FEV_T are proportionately decreased. In many subjects who have moderate or severe restriction, the $FEV_{1.0}$ may equal the FVC; that is, the entire FVC is exhaled in the first second. Distinction between obstructive and restrictive causes of reduced FEV_T is made by relating the FEV_T to the FVC as the FEV_T/FVC ratio, and to other flow measurements.

As previously noted, of all the FEV parameters, the $FEV_{1.0}$ is the most widely used spirometric parameter, particularly for assessment of airway obstruction. The $FEV_{1.0}$ is used in conjunction with the FVC for simple screening, for assessment of response to bronchodilators, for inhalation challenge studies, and for detection of exercise-induced bronchospasm (see Chapters 7 and 8).

The validity of the test depends largely on the cooperation and effort of the subject. This is true of all of the common FEV_T parameters (i.e., $FEV_{0.5}$, $FEV_{1.0}$, $FEV_{2.0}$, and $FEV_{3.0}$) since each of these includes the effort-dependent early portion of the forced exhalation. Reproducibility of the FEV_T should be within 5% for the two best of at least three maneuvers. Accurate measurement of the FEV requires an adequate spirometer, preferably one that allows inspection of the volume-time curve and back-extrapolation (see Chapter 11).

FORCED EXPIRATORY VOLUME/FORCED VITAL CAPACITY RATIO (FEV_T/FVC OR $FEV_{T\%}$)

Description

The $FEV_{T\%}$ is the ratio of the FEV_T to the FVC expressed as a percentage, where T is the interval from the start of the FVC maneuver to a specific time.

Technique

The subject performs the FVC maneuver, and the FVC and FEV_T are computed. The ratio is then derived using the following equation:

$$FEV_{T\%} = \frac{FEV_T}{FVC} \times 100$$

The reported values for FEV_T and FVC may be the maximal values obtained from a series of FVC maneuvers. The FEV_T/FVC ratio based on these values may be different from the ratio obtained on any single maneuver. If other measurements of flow (i.e., either instantaneous or averaged) are to be reported, they should be obtained from the single maneuver with the largest sum of FVC and $FEV_{1.0}$. (see Chapter 11).

Significance

A healthy young adult can expire 50% to 60% of the FVC in 0.5 seconds, 75% to 85% in 1 second, 94% in 2 seconds, and 97% in 3 seconds. The actual expected ratio in an individual may be derived by taking the ratio of predicted FEV_T to predicted FVC, although most studies of healthy subjects have derived regression equations for the ratio itself. The $FEV_{1.0}$/FVC ratio tends to decrease with increasing age, since $FEV_{1.0}$ decreases at a slightly faster rate than FVC. In general, subjects who do not have airways obstruction can expire their entire FVC within 4 seconds. Conversely, subjects who have obstructive disease will have a reduced $FEV_{T\%}$ ratio in most cases; an $FEV_{1.0}$/FVC ratio lower than 65% is the hallmark of obstructive disease. Because the $FEV_{1.0}$/FVC is a ratio, mild to moderate obstructive disease can be identified without reference to absolute predicted values; if the ratio is less than 65%, except in the oldest subjects, then some degree of obstruction is present. The $FEV_{T\%}$ may be as low as 30% is severe obstructive disease.

Subjects who have restrictive disease often have normal or increased $FEV_{T\%}$ values, because air flow may be minimally affected; in restriction, the $FEV_{1.0}$ and FVC are usually reduced in equal proportion. If the restriction is severe, the $FEV_{0.5}$ or $FEV_{1.0}$ may approach the FVC value, and the FEV_T% appears to be higher than normal. The $FEV_{1\%}$ may be 100% when the FVC is severely reduced.

Validity of the FEV_T% depends on the individual's effort and cooperation on the specific FEV_T and on the FVC. Since the values used to derive the ratio may be taken from separate maneuvers, both the FEV_T and FVC should be reproducible within 5% (see Chapter 11). Poor patient effort during the FVC measurement may result in an overestimate of the FEV_T%. Some clinicians prefer to use the largest SVC to calculate the FEV_T% (See Chapter 12, Case Studies). This may be necessary if the SVC is significantly larger than the FVC due to airway compression during maximal effort.

FORCED EXPIRATORY $FLOW_{200\text{-}1200}$ ($FEF_{200\text{-}1200}$)

Description

The forced expiratory flow ($FEF_{200\text{-}1200}$) is the average flow rate for the liter of gas expired after the first 200 ml during an FVC maneuver. The same test was previously called the maximal expiratory flow rate ($MEFR_{200\text{-}1200}$). The $FEF_{200\text{-}1200}$ is usually recorded in liters per second but may be stated in liters per minute (Fig. 3-3).

Technique

The $FEF_{200\text{-}1200}$ is measured from an acceptable FVC maneuver. To obtain the value manually from a spirographic tracing, the time interval from the

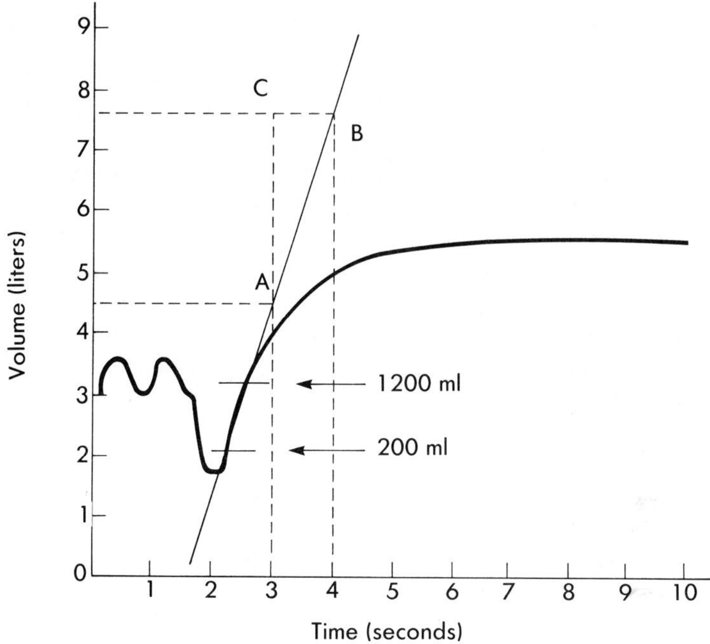

Fig. 3-3 $FEF_{200\text{-}1200}$. An FVC spirogram on which points at 200 ml and 1200 ml above the beginning of the forced expiration have been marked; a line connecting these two points is extended to cross two time lines 1 second apart, points A and B. The flow rate in liters per second can be read as the vertical distance between the points of intersection (A and C) and here is about 3.0 L/sec.

200 ml point to the 1200 ml point is divided into 1 L to obtain the average flow rate for that interval. If the 200 ml and 1200 ml points are marked on the shoulder of the curve, a straight line connecting them may be extended so that it intersects two time lines 1 second apart on the graph paper. The flow rate may then be read as the distance between these two points of intersection (Fig. 3-3). Flow rates must be corrected to BTPS, but volume points may be marked on the uncorrected curve before BTPS corrections are applied. FVC curves that display back-extrapolated volumes (see Chapter 11) greater than 200 ml may yield spurious values for the $FEF_{200\text{-}1200}$. Computerized spirometers store volume and flow data points for the FVC maneuver and calculate the average flow during the 200 ml to 1200 ml volume interval.

Significance

The $FEF_{200\text{-}1200}$ measures the average flow of the early part of a forced expiration. The initial 200 ml of volume may be expired at a slower rate because of inertia of the lung-thorax system, and is usually disregarded for this reason. The average rate of air flow in the initial part of a forced expiration for a healthy adult male typically ranges from 6 to 7 L/sec (≅400

L/min). $FEF_{200\text{-}1200}$ decreases significantly with age and is normally lower in women than in men (see the Appendix).

The $FEF_{200\text{-}1200}$ is a good index of air flow characteristics of the larger airways, but since it is calculated from the first segment of the forced expiration, obstruction of the small airways (i.e., airways less than 2 mm in diameter) may be present when the $FEF_{200\text{-}1200}$ is normal. Obstructive diseases cause a decrease in $FEF_{200\text{-}1200}$, while restrictive disease may result in a normal, or sometimes increased, $FEF_{200\text{-}1200}$. Flow rates as low as 1 L/sec (60 L/min) are not uncommon in obstructive patterns. Low $FEF_{200\text{-}1200}$ values are often seen in conjunction with low peak expiratory flow rate (PEFR) values, since both tests measure flows early in the forced expiration. Similarly, large airway obstruction patterns seen on the expiratory limb of flow-volume curves (see page 53), also accompany decreased $FEF_{200\text{-}1200}$ values. The nature of the obstruction when flow rates are decreased is sometimes clarified by measuring the forced inspiratory flow (FIF) for the same interval from a forced inspiratory volume (FIV) maneuver. Fixed extrathoracic obstructions typically cause decreased flow on both inspiration and expiration.

The validity of the test depends on subject cooperation and effort; low values are often due to poor start-of-test because of poor effort or inadequate explanation of the maneuver.

FORCED EXPIRATORY FLOW$_{25\%\text{-}75\%}$ ($FEF_{25\%\text{-}75\%}$)

Description

The forced expiratory flow$_{25\%\text{-}75\%}$ ($FEF_{25\%\text{-}75\%}$) is the average rate of flow during the middle half of an FVC maneuver. It is usually recorded in liters per second. This test was formerly called the maximum mid-expiratory flow rate (MMFR).

Technique

The $FEF_{25\%\text{-}75\%}$ is measured from a FVC maneuver. The time required for the subject to expire the middle 50% of the FVC is divided into 50% of the FVC. To calculate the $FEF_{25\%\text{-}75\%}$ manually, a volume-time spirogram may be used, with the points at which 25% and 75% of the VC have been expired marked on the curve (Fig. 3-4). A straight line connecting these points is extended to intersect two time lines 1 second apart, and the flow rate can be read directly as the vertical distance between the points of intersection.

Computerized measurement of the $FEF_{25\%\text{-}75\%}$ requires storage of flow and volume data points and calculation of the average flow during the middle portion of the exhalation. The $FEF_{25\%\text{-}75\%}$ is dependent on the FVC; large $FEF_{25\%\text{-}75\%}$ values may be derived from maneuvers producing small FVC values because the "middle half" of the volume is actually gas expired at the beginning of expiration. This effect may be particularly evident if the subject terminates the FVC maneuver before reaching RV. When the

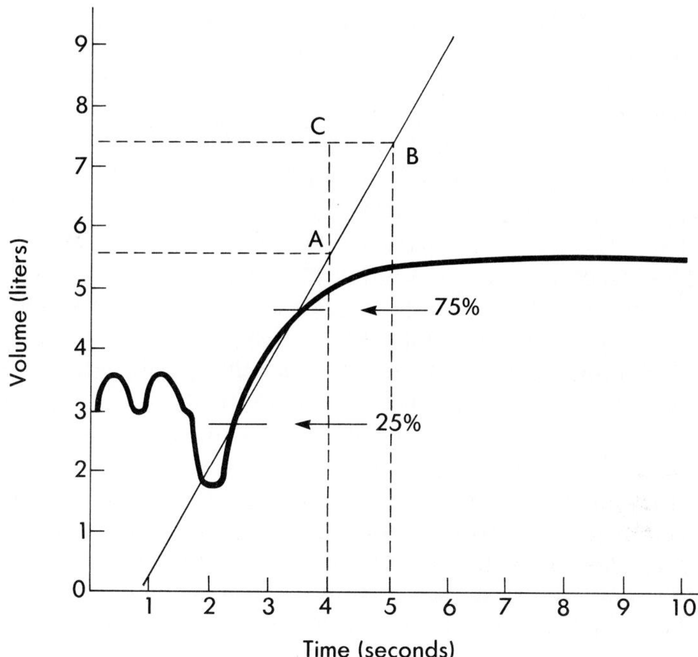

Fig. 3-4 $FEF_{25\%-75\%}$—An FVC spirogram showing the points at which 25% and 75% of the FVC have been expired; these points may be determined by multiplying the FVC by 0.25 and 0.75, respectively. A line connecting these points is extended to intersect two time lines 1 sec apart, points A and B. The flow rate in liters per second can be read as the vertical distance between the points of intersection (A and C), in this case approximately 2 L/sec. Alternatively, the slope of the line connecting the 25% and 75% points can be determined by dividing one-half the FVC by the actual time interval between the points.

$FEF_{25\%-75\%}$ is used for assessing the response to bronchodilator or inhalation challenge, the effect of changes in the absolute lung volumes must be considered. Measuring the $FEF_{25\%-75\%}$ at the same lung volumes in the comparison tests is referred to as the "isovolume" technique, and is typically applied when the FVC changes more than 10%, indicating a change in TLC or RV. The isovolume technique may also be used with other flow measurements that are FVC dependent. The $FEF_{25\%-75\%}$ is recorded from the maneuver producing the largest sum of FVC and $FEV_{1.0}$ values, according to the American Thoracic Society's criteria for the "best test" (see Chapter 11). Flows must be corrected to BTPS.

Significance

The $FEF_{25\%-75\%}$, like the $FEF_{200-1200}$, measures the average flow rate during a given interval (volume), but is based on a segment of the FVC that includes flow from medium-sized and small airways. The values for a healthy young man average between 4 and 5 L/sec, and typically decrease with age. The $FEF_{25\%-75\%}$ varies significantly in healthy subjects, with one standard deviation of approximately 1 L/sec; values as low as 65% of predicted normal values may be statistically within normal limits. This variability limits the usefulness of the $FEF_{25\%-75\%}$ somewhat.

The $FEF_{25\%-75\%}$ indicates the status of the medium-sized and small airways. Decreased flow rates are common in the early stages of obstructive disease, and are seen in asthma and bronchitis. Flow rates as low as 0.3 L/sec are not uncommon in patients with severe obstruction, such as those who have advanced emphysema. Low $FEF_{25\%-75\%}$ values, when found in combination with normal values for other parameters (i.e., FVC, $FEV_{1.0}$), often suggest early small airways abnormality.

Reduced $FEF_{25\%-75\%}$ is sometimes seen in cases of moderate or severe restrictive patterns, when the restrictive lesion causes a decrease in the cross-sectional area of the small airways. Fig. 3-5 shows typical abnormal spirograms comparing obstructive and restrictive patterns. Case study examples of spirometric measurements in both obstructive and restrictive disease patterns are included in Chapter 12. The general descriptions of FVC, FEV_T, and FEF_X measurements in this section may be used to help interpret the numerical data of the case studies.

The accuracy of $FEF_{25\%-75\%}$ values depend on subject effort, but less so than the $FEF_{200-1200}$ or PEFR (see following section). Subjects who perform the FVC maneuver inadequately often produce widely varying flow rates. There is little evidence that the $FEF_{25\%-75\%}$ is more reliable than other flow measurements commonly used in assessing obstructive ventilatory impairments, although it is more commonly used.

PEAK EXPIRATORY FLOW RATE (PEFR)

Description

The peak expiratory flow rate (PEFR) is the maximum flow rate attained during an FVC maneuver. It is usually recorded in liters per second, but may be reported in liters per minute, BTPS.

Technique

The PEFR can be measured by drawing a tangent to the steepest part of a volume-time spirogram, in a manner similar to that used for the $FEF_{200-1200}$. Even with a fast recording device, measurement of this slope is difficult, particularly in subjects whose peak flows are normal. PEFR may be measured more accurately by means of a device that senses flow directly (see Chapter 9) or by deriving flow from the rate of volume change in a volume-displacement spirometer. When either method is used, PEFR is usually represented on a flow-volume display (see Fig. 3-6). The peak inspiratory flow rate (PIFR) is measured similarly. Many portable devices are available to measure maximal flow during a forced expiration; most of

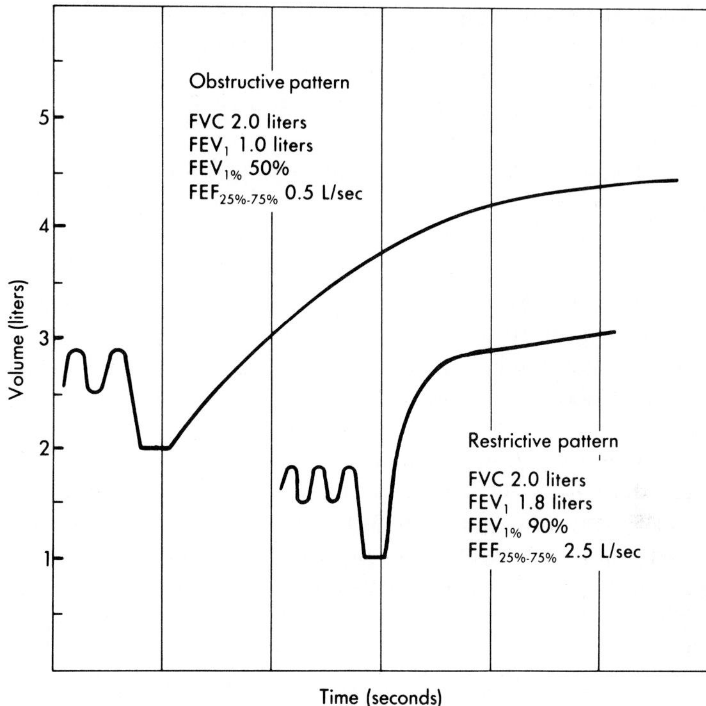

Fig. 3-5 Spirograms showing obstructive versus restrictive patterns. The *obstructive pattern* shows a decreased FVC and reduced flow rates; the volume expired in the first second ($FEV_{1.0}$) is only 50% of the FVC (i.e., $FEV_{1.0}$/FVC or $FEV_{1\%}$). The $FEF_{25\%-75\%}$ is also markedly reduced. The *restrictive pattern* also shows a reduced FVC, approximately equal to that observed in the obstructive defect, but the $FEV_{1.0}$/FVC ratio is increased; almost all of the VC is expired in the first second. The $FEF_{25\%-75\%}$ is not decreased, as in the obstructive pattern. FVC alone cannot be used to distinguish obstructive from restrictive disease patterns; flow rates are typically decreased in obstructive patterns and are decreased significantly in restrictive disease only when the lung volumes are markedly reduced. The $FEV_{1.0}$/FVC ratio, used in conjunction with the actual measured values for $FEV_{1.0}$ and FVC, is helpful in differentiating obstruction from restriction (see text).

these sense flow as bulk movement of gas against a turbine or through an orifice, and record only the PEFR. The PEFR and PIFR, whether reported in liters per second or liters per minute, should be corrected to BTPS.

Significance

The PEFR attainable by healthy young adults may exceed 10 L/sec (600 L/min) BTPS. Even when measured using an accurate pneumotachometer, the value of PEFR measurements may be limited because they are effort dependent. Decreased peak flows should be evaluated for reproducibility before making a diagnostic interpretation. This same effort-dependence, however, also makes the PEFR a good index of subject effort; maximal transpulmonary pressures correlate well with maximal PEFR. Subjects who exert variable efforts during the FVC maneuver are seldom able to reproduce their PEFR.

Subjects who have early small airways obstructive disease may develop an initially high flow rate before airway closing occurs, and may show relatively normal PEFR values. Severe obstruction in the small airways is accompanied by a decrease in peak expiratory flow, although the reduction is often less than in the flows in the small airways themselves. Uniformly decreased PEFR is often associated with upper-airway or large-airway obstruction, but is nonspecific. PEFR and PIFR values assessed from flow-volume loops help to define both the severity and site of large-airway obstruction.

Small, inexpensive devices that measure PEFR as described previously are becoming widely used. The PEFR measured using such portable devices is most useful for following gross changes in airway function in outpatients, or for making bedside assessment of response to bronchodilators. Because simple flow measuring devices may not be accurate (see American Thoracic Society standards, Chapter 11) and because of the effort dependence of the PEFR, such measurements should be compared to spirometry done under laboratory conditions. The primary application of the PEFR used in this way is to follow asthmatics or others susceptible to changes in airway function on a continuous basis or during acute exacerbations.

FLOW-VOLUME CURVES

Description

The flow-volume curve is a graphic analysis of the flow generated during the FVC maneuver plotted against volume change; it is usually followed by an FIV maneuver, plotted similarly (Fig. 3-6). Flow is usually recorded in liters per second and the volume in liters, BTPS. The maximal expiratory flow-volume (MEFV) curve is the expiratory portion of the curve from TLC to RV. The inspiratory component, called the maximal inspiratory flow-volume (MIFV) curve, is plotted from RV to TLC. When both the MEFV and MIFV curves are plotted together, the resulting figure is referred to as a "flow-volume loop."

Technique

The subject performs a standard FVC maneuver, inspiring fully to TLC, then exhaling as rapidly as possible to RV; to complete the loop, an FIV maneuver follows the FVC maneuver, with the subject inspiring as rapidly as possible from RV to TLC. Volume is plotted on the X axis, while flow is plotted on the Y axis. This type of spirogram must be produced either by a recorder capable of plotting flow and volume from their respective

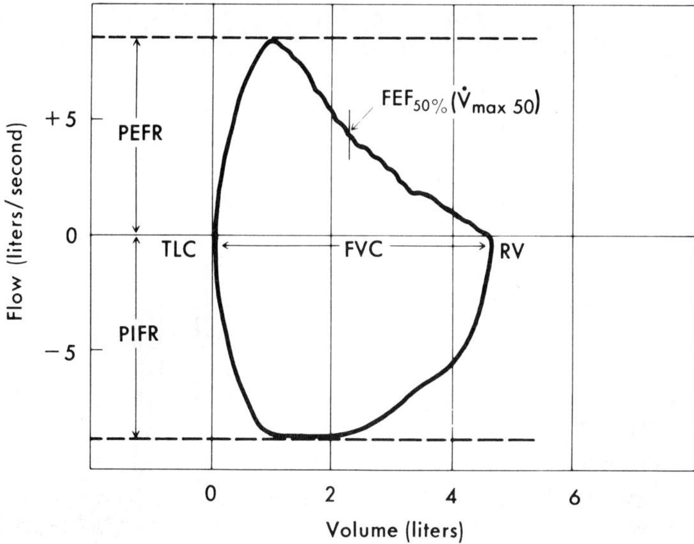

Fig. 3-6 Flow-volume loop—a flow-volume spirogram in which an FVC and an FIVC maneuver are recorded in succession. Flow, in L/sec, is plotted on the vertical axis; and volume, in liters, is plotted on the horizontal axis. The FVC can be read from the tracing as the maximal horizontal deflection along the zero flow line. Peak flows for inspiration (PIFR) and for expiration (PEFR) can be read directly from the tracing as the maximal deflections on the flow axis (positive and negative). The instantaneous flow ($\dot{V}_{max}$) at any point in the FVC can also be measured directly. Plotting devices that are capable of interjecting time marks, or tics, in the tracing allow the FEV_T to be read directly as well (not shown here). Phenomena such as small or large airway obstruction show up as characteristic changes in the flow rate (see Fig. 3-7).

analog inputs (see Fig. 9-27), by a storage oscilloscope, or by computer-generated graphics. From the loop, the peak inspiratory and expiratory flows can be read, as well as the FVC. Commonly used recording sensitivities are 2 L/sec per unit distance on the flow (Y) axis versus 1 L per unit distance on the volume (X) axis, though other scaling factors are sometimes used. The instantaneous flow at any lung volume over the VC can be read directly from the MEFV tracing. Flows at 75%, 50%, and 25% of the VC are commonly reported as the $\dot{V}_{max\ 75}$, $\dot{V}_{max\ 50}$, and $\dot{V}_{max\ 25}$, respectively, with the subscript referring to the percentage of the lung volume (VC) remaining. Flows at the same intervals are also reported as the $FEF_{25\%}$, $FEF_{50\%}$, and $FEF_{75\%}$ respectively, with the subscript in this scheme referring to the portion of the lung volume (VC) that has been exhaled. If automatic timing is available on the graphing device or the computer, the FEV_T and $FEV_{T\%}$ can be determined for specific intervals. Plotting of stored data points allows manipulation of the flow-volume tracings, facilitating comparisons of a series of curves. Computer-generated plots permit bronchodilator or inhalation challenge studies, as well as repetitive maneuvers, to be superimposed or plotted in contrasting colors.

Significance

All of the parameters measured from a standard volume-time tracing of the FVC maneuver can be obtained from a flow-volume curve, provided a timing mechanism is incorporated as described in the previous paragraph. In addition, instantaneous flows at any point in either the forced expiration or forced inspiration can be easily measured. Significant decreases in either flow, indicating obstruction, or in volume, indicating restriction, are easily discernable from a single graphic display. The shape of the expiratory limb of the MEFV tracing from about 75% of the FVC down to RV is largely independent of subject effort; flow during this segment is determined by the elastic recoil properties of the lungs and the flow-resistive properties of the small airways (i.e., airways less than 2 mm in diameter). In healthy subjects, flow, or $\dot{V}_{max}$, during the effort-independent segment decreases linearly with decreasing volume, so that the expiratory curve has a "straight-line" appearance (Fig. 3-6). In subjects who have obstruction in the small airways, flow is decreased, particularly at lower lung volumes; the effort-independent segment of the flow-volume curve takes on a curvilinear or "scooped out" appearance (Fig. 3-7). Values for $\dot{V}_{max\ 50}$ and $\dot{V}_{max\ 25}$ are characteristically decreased. Decreases in $\dot{V}_{max\ 50}$ correlate well with the reduction in $FEF_{25\%-75\%}$ in subjects who have small airways obstructive disease. Because elastic recoil and resistance in the small airways determine the shape of the expiratory limb of the MEFV tracing, quite different lung pathologies can result in similarly decreased flows. Emphysema destroys terminal lung units with a loss of elastic recoil and support for the small airways; bronchitis, asthma, and similar inflammatory processes increase the resistance in the small airways by edema, mucus production, and smooth muscle constriction.

Obstruction of the upper airway, trachea, and mainstem bronchi result in characteristic limitations to either expiratory flow, inspiratory flow, or both, making the flow-volume curve useful in diagnosing these types of abnormalities (Fig. 3-7). Comparison of expiratory and inspiratory flows at 50% of the FVC is helpful in distinguishing the site of the obstruction. Fixed large-airway obstructions typically result in reduced, but approximately equal, flow at 50% of the VC for both inspiration and expiration (Fig. 3-7). Obstructive processes that vary with the phase of breathing also produce characteristic patterns. Variable extrathoracic obstruction usually produces normal expiratory flows with diminished inspiratory flows; the converse is true in the presence of variable intrathoracic obstruction. Airway obstruction associated with abnormality of the muscular control of the posterior pharynx and larynx sometimes produces a "saw-toothed" pattern

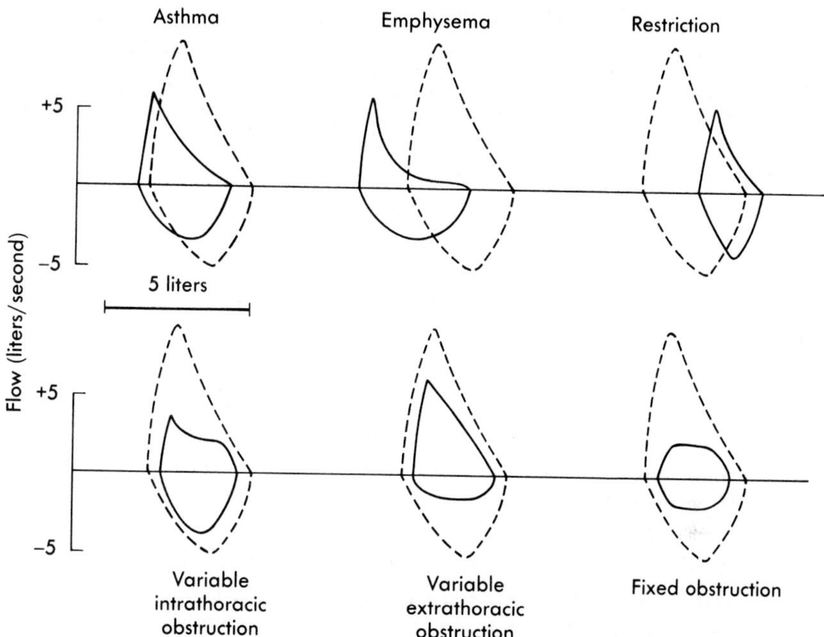

Fig. 3-7 Normal and abnormal flow-volume loops. Six curves are shown plotting flow in liters per second against the FVC. In each example, the expected curve is shown by the dashed lines, while the curve typifying the particular lesion is superimposed. In patients who have asthma and emphysema, the latter portion of the expiratory curve is characteristically "scooped out" and the TLC and RV points are displaced toward higher lung volumes, indicating hyperinflation and/or air trapping. In restrictive patterns, the shape of the loop is preserved but the FVC is decreased, with the TLC and RV displaced toward lower lung volumes than might be expected. The bottom three examples depict types of large airway obstruction. Variable intrathoracic obstruction shows reduced flows on expiration despite near normal flows on inspiration, due to compression of the airways within the chest during a forced expiration. Variable extrathoracic obstruction causes an opposite pattern, with inspiratory flow being reduced while expiratory flow is relatively well preserved. Fixed large airway obstruction is characterized by approximately equal inspiratory and expiratory flows. Comparison of the $FEF_{50\%}$ with the $FIF_{50\%}$ may be helpful in differentiating large airway obstructive processes. Since the magnitude of inspiratory flow is effort dependent, low inspiratory flows should be carefully evaluated.

visible on the inspiratory and expiratory limbs of the MEFV curve. The peak inspiratory flow rate, and the pattern of flow during inspiration are largely effort dependent. Poor subject effort may result in inspiratory flow patterns similar to those seen during variable extrathoracic obstruction. However, if the inspiratory flow pattern is reproducible over repeated efforts, a true obstructive process should be suspected.

In restrictive disease processes, peak expiratory flows may be normal or increased, with linear decreases in flow versus lung volume and the lung volume decreased. Moderate or severe restriction causes equally reduced flows at all lung volumes, and such a curve may appear to be a miniature of the normal MEFV curve.

Before and after bronchodilator MEFV curves can be superimposed, usually by matching at TLC, to facilitate measurement of relative increases in flow at each lung volume. Inhalation challenge studies (see Chapter 8) can be manipulated in a similar manner to assess the reduction in flows at specific lung volumes. Similarly, tidal breathing curves or maximum voluntary ventilation (MVV) curves can be superimposed on the flow-volume curve (i.e., inspiratory and expiratory curves) to evaluate the subject's ventilatory reserve by comparing the areas bounded by each of the curves. Subjects who have severe obstructive lung disease often generate maximal flow-volume curves of only slightly greater dimensions than their tidal breathing curves, consistent with limited ventilatory reserve and usually associated with dyspnea on exertion.

The ability to measure both flow and volume from a single graphic representation of the FVC maneuver is responsible for the widespread popularity of the flow-volume curve. Reproducible MEFV curves, particularly of the PEFR, are good indicators of adequate subject effort. It may be difficult, however, to gauge the validity of the start-of-test from the flow-volume plot; a simultaneous volume-time tracing may be necessary to perform manual back-extrapolation (see Chapter 11).

LOW-DENSITY GAS SPIROMETRY

Description

Low-density gas spirometry may be used to measure maximal expiratory flow volume (MEFV) curves. MEFV maneuvers may be performed using a gas mixture of 80% He and 20% O_2, then comparing changes in flow during this maneuver and the MEFV maneuver performed while the subject breathes air. Two primary sets of values are derived using this technique: the change in maximal flow at specific points in the VC, usually 50% and 25% ($\Delta\dot{V}_{max\ x}$) and the volume of isoflow (Viso$\dot{V}$). The Viso$\dot{V}$ is the portion of the VC remaining in the lungs when gas flow becomes independent of gas density. The Viso$\dot{V}$ is normally expressed as a percentage of the FVC. The $\Delta\dot{V}_{max\ x}$ is recorded as the percent change in flow at the specific point in the VC.

Technique

MEFV curves are obtained as described previously, with the subject first breathing air. Then the MEFV maneuver is repeated after the subject has breathed the He-O_2 mixture. The subject may either breathe the mixture for 10 minutes (i.e., tidal breathing), or take three slow VC breaths of the mixture before performing the maneuver. Both of these techniques yield similar results. The He-O_2 and air curves are then superimposed and

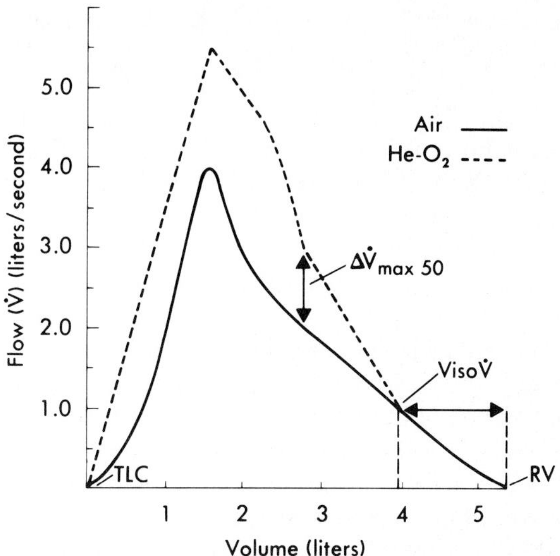

Fig. 3-8 Helium-air MEFV curves. The subject performs two MEFV maneuvers; the first is a simple MEFV maneuver while breathing air; the second MEFV maneuver is performed after the subject has breathed a mixture of 80% He and 20% O_2 for several minutes or for several VC breaths. The two curves are then superimposed by matching at RV. The $\dot{V}_{max\ 50}$, or $\dot{V}_{max}$ at any other lung volume, can then be read directly from each of the tracings. Decreases in the $\dot{V}_{max\ 50}$ are consistent with diseases causing increased resistance in the small airways (i.e., airways less than 2 mm in diameter), but there is apparently little change with loss of elastic recoil. The point at which both curves converge is the Viso$\dot{V}$. At this lung volume, maximum expiratory flow becomes independent of the gas density of the expirate. Diseases that compromise the small airways, either by increased resistance or loss of elastic recoil, tend to increase the Viso$\dot{V}$, so that the curves converge earlier during the expiratory maneuver.

matched at RV if the FVC values are different. The point at which the expiratory curves meet determines the Viso$\dot{V}$, the lung volume at which gas flow becomes independent of gas density (Fig. 3-8).

From the same superimposed tracing, the increase in maximal flow at 50% of the VC ($\dot{V}_{max\ 50}$) can be determined. Since flow in larger airways depends on gas density, measuring the amount of increase in $\dot{V}_{max\ 50}$ while breathing the He-O_2 mixture is a relatively specific test for changes in airway caliber. The increase in $\dot{V}_{max\ 50}$ while breathing the He-O_2 mixture is expressed as a percentage of the $\dot{V}_{max\ 50}$ while breathing air, and is called the $\Delta\dot{V}_{max\ 50}$: It can be computed using the following equation:

$$\Delta\dot{V}_{max\ 50} = \frac{\dot{V}_{max\ 50}\text{He} - \dot{V}_{max\ 50}\text{air}}{\dot{V}_{max\ 50}\text{air}} \times 100$$

where

$\dot{V}_{max\ 50}He$ = Flow at 50% of the VC when breathing He-O_2 mixture
$\dot{V}_{max\ 50}air$ = Flow at 50% of the VC when breathing air

Significance

Normal values for Viso$\dot{V}$ as a percentage of the FVC appear to be in the range of 10% to 20% for persons 20 to 50 years of age. In the absence of obstruction in the small airways (i.e., airways less than 2 mm in diameter) laminar air flow, which is independent of the density of the gas being breathed, occurs near the end of a forced expiration.

An increase in the Viso$\dot{V}$ (i.e., flow limitation in the small airways occurring earlier in the forced expiration) is consistent with obstruction of the small airways. During forced expiration in healthy subjects, the site of flow limitation is in the large airways until low lung volumes are reached. Breathing a gas of low density improves flow in these larger airways, but as flow limitation shifts to the small airways at the end of a forced expiration, air flow becomes laminar, and is independent of gas density. This is the point at which the He-O_2 and air curves converge. Therefore, in diseases of the small airways in which there is increased resistance (i.e., asthma) or in which there is a loss of elastic recoil (i.e., emphysema), flow limitation occurs at a higher lung volume, and Viso$\dot{V}$ is increased.

The $\Delta\dot{V}_{max\ 50}$ may be reduced in diseases that cause increased resistance; as airway diameter is compromised, flow becomes laminar at higher lung volumes and is less dependent on gas density. Loss of elastic recoil does not appear to influence $\dot{V}_{max\ 50}$. Therefore, measurement of $\Delta\dot{V}_{max\ 50}$ may be a relatively specific test for changes in the caliber of small airways. A subject who has early small airways disease would typically have an increased Viso$\dot{V}$; if the $\Delta\dot{V}_{max\ 50}$ is decreased, then a process causing primarily changes in resistance would be suspected. If, however, the $\Delta\dot{V}_{max\ 50}$ is relatively normal despite the abnormal Viso$\dot{V}$, then loss of elastic recoil might be the cause of the small airways abnormality. The Viso$\dot{V}$ is one of the most sensitive tests of small airways obstruction. It may be abnormal even before the FEV_1 or $FEF_{25\%-75\%}$ drop below the lower normal limits.

Low-density gas spirometry is relatively simple to perform. By facilitating evaluation of both the $\Delta\dot{V}_{max\ 50}$ and the Viso$\dot{V}$, it can often help elucidate the pathology causing early small airways disease.

MAXIMUM VOLUNTARY VENTILATION (MVV)

Description

The maximum voluntary ventilation (MVV) is the largest volume that can be breathed during a 10- to 15- second interval with voluntary effort. It is recorded in liters per minute, BTPS.

Technique

The MVV is measured by having the subject breathe deeply and rapidly for 10 to 15 seconds. The subject should set the rate, and should move a

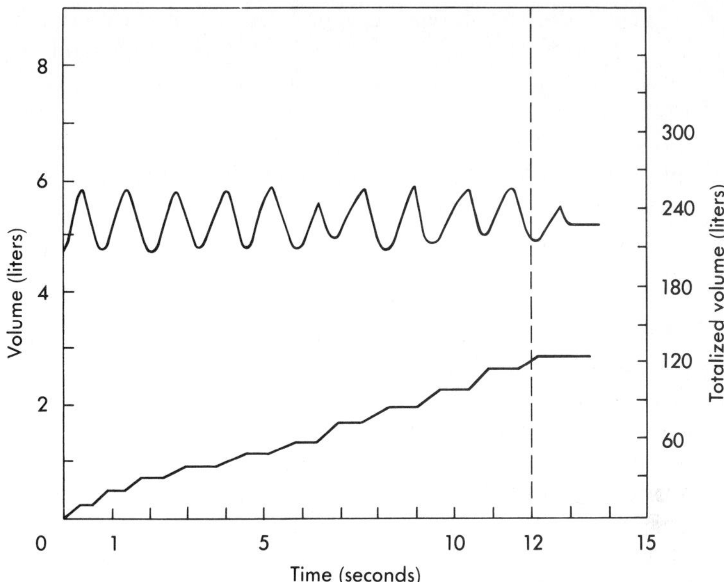

Fig. 3-9 Maximum voluntary ventilation. A composite MVV spirogram on which breath-by-breath volume change and accumulated volume are plotted against time. The top tracing shows the actual volume moved on each breath during a 12-second interval; to calculate MVV, the volumes of individual breaths are added and multiplied by a factor of 5 (i.e., 60 seconds/12 seconds = 5). Since the MVV is stated as a flow rate in liters per minute, the values for 12 seconds must be extrapolated to 1 minute. The lower tracing is computer generated and depicts the totalized volume, in liters per minute, exhaled during the 12-second maneuver (in this example, approximately 120 L/min). Healthy subjects will maintain the same MVV flow rate throughout the maneuver. Subjects who have pulmonary disease will show decreased absolute values, and often the MVV will decrease significantly as the maneuver progresses because of fatigue of the respiratory muscles, increased work of breathing, or air trapping.

volume greater than the VT but less than the VC on each breath. The test is usually conducted for a specific interval, usually 10, 12, or 15 seconds. The volume expired (or inspired) may be measured by a suitable spirometer; it is important that the spirometer have an adequate frequency response (see Chapter 11). The volume may be read from a volume-time spirogram (Fig. 3-9), or from a recording of accumulated volume. Manual calculation requires measurement and summing of each individual deflection, which can be quite time-consuming. By incorporating a one-way valve in the breathing circuit, either the volume exhaled or inhaled can be isolated, but if a volume-displacement spirometer is used, it must have sufficient volume to accumulate the gas for the 10- to 15-second interval. Most spirometers have volume ranges of 7 to 10 L, and are not suitable for collecting the accumulated volume even for 10 seconds. Some older systems use a mechanical pen system that records only expired volume versus time, allowing the total volume to be read directly from the tracing, similar to the computer-generated graphic in Fig. 3-9. The absolute volume of gas moved as determined by any of these methods is extrapolated from 10, 12, or 15 seconds to 1 minute and the result recorded as a flow rate, in liters per minute, as follows:

$$MVV = \frac{Vol_x}{X} \times 60$$

where

Vol_x = Volume inspired or expired in X seconds, in liters
X = Duration of the maneuver in seconds (usually 10, 12, or 15)
60 = Factor for extrapolation from seconds to minutes

The volumes must be corrected to BTPS.

Significance

The MVV is a test of the entire respiratory system. It is influenced by the status of the respiratory muscles, the compliance of the lung-thorax system, the condition of the ventilatory control mechanisms, and the resistance offered by the airways and tissues. MVV values of healthy young men average between 150 and 200 L/min. Values are slightly lower in healthy women and decrease with age in both men and women. The MVV is quite variable in a healthy population; normal values may vary by as much as 30% from the mean, so that only large reductions in MVV are usually considered significant.

The MVV is typically decreased markedly in subjects with moderate or severe obstructive disease, due to increased airway resistance and/or hyperinflation. The MVV maneuver exaggerates air trapping and air flow limitation. Volume-time tracings made with a volume-displacement device may show a shift in the tracing if gas is shifted from the spirometer to the lungs because of air trapping. The MVV also places a load on the respiratory muscles. Because both inspiratory and expiratory muscles are used in the MVV maneuver, weakness or decreased endurance of either system may result in low values. Similarly, poor coordination of the respiratory muscles because of a neurologic deficit may also cause low MVV values. A markedly reduced MVV is correlated with postoperative risk; subjects who have low preoperative MVV values have an increased incidence of complications when the respiratory system is compromised by thoracic or upper abdominal surgery.

Maximum voluntary ventilation may be helpful in estimating the level of ventilation that can be expected during exercise testing. Subjects who have moderate or severe obstruction and who have MVV values much less than 50 L/min usually exhibit ventilatory limitation during exercise. Maximal ventilation during exercise is normally less than 70% to 80% of the MVV. In subjects who have obstruction, the maximal ventilation during exertion may approach the MVV, although it is typically reduced.

MVV may be within normal limits in some subjects who have restrictive pulmonary disease, since limitation of lung or thoracic expansion may not interfere with flow. Subjects who have lung restriction often compensate by performing the MVV maneuver with low VT and high breathing rates.

The MVV maneuver is largely dependent on subject effort and cooperation. Low MVV values should always be weighed to ascertain whether the reduction is a result of obstruction, muscular weakness, inadequate ventilatory control, or poor subject performance. An indirect index of subject effort on the MVV maneuver may be obtained by multiplying the $FEV_{1.0}$ by a factor of 35. For example, a subject who has an $FEV_{1.0}$ of 2.0 L might be expected to move about 70 L/min (35 × 2.0 L) during the MVV test. If the measured MVV is much less than 70 L/min, then subject effort may be suspect. If the MVV exceeds 70 L/min by a large volume, the $FEV_{1.0}$ may be erroneous. Criteria for acceptability of the MVV maneuver are outlined in Chapter 11.

COMPLIANCE

Description

Compliance is the volume change per unit of pressure change. Compliance of the lungs (CL), of the thorax (CT), or of the lungs-thorax system (CLT) may be measured. Compliance is recorded in liters or milliliters per centimeter of water. The elastic recoil pressure is the force generated by the lungs or thorax at a particular lung volume; it is recorded in centimeters of water (cm H_2O) and the reported value is usually measured at TLC.

Technique

The compliance of the lungs-thorax system (CLT) may be measured as a unit; if compliance of the lungs (CL) alone is determined as described in the following paragraph, the thoracic compliance (CT) can be calculated by subtraction.

The CLT is measured by inflating the lungs of a subject in a sealed chamber by reducing the pressure around the thorax, as in an "iron lung;" a volume-pressure curve is then plotted. The subject may likewise be intubated with an endotracheal tube and have the lungs inflated by positive pressure. The pressure changes at various volumes above the end-expiratory level are then plotted to obtain a pressure-volume curve. This technique normally requires that the subject be anesthetized.

A similar technique is sometimes used with patients receiving mechanically-supported ventilation with positive pressure. By inflating the lung-thorax system with different volumes and recording the pressure during periods of no flow, usually by occluding the expiration valve of the ventilator, a pressure-volume curve can be constructed.

Both of these techniques, in anesthetized subjects and in subjects receiving mechanically-supported ventilation, may be influenced by the position of the subject or by any contribution from the respiratory muscles.

Alternatively, a subject may be allowed to breath tidally from a spirometer before and after weights are added. The pressures used to calculate compliance are the system pressures when different weights are added. The volumes used are the changes in the end-expiratory levels from the spirogram that occur in response to the different pressures. Each of the techniques for measuring CLT presents difficulties, which limits their usefulness for clinical studies.

Measurement of CL is accomplished by passing a catheter with a 10 cm long balloon attached to the end into the esophagus to midthorax level and then connecting it to a suitable pressure transducer. Serial pressure measurements are then recorded at various volumes and plotted (Fig. 3-10). Normally, the subject inspires to TLC before the measurements, to standardize the lung volume history; CL changes slightly after a full inspiration. Then the subject inspires again, and pressure and volume points are measured at points of zero flow; the subject may hold the breath with the glottis open, or flow may be interrupted by means of a shutter. If the latter technique is used, mouth pressure should be subtracted from esophageal pressure to obtain the recoil pressure of the lungs. Similar measurements are recorded during the subsequent expiration.

The CL is usually taken from the slope of the pressure-volume curve over the segment from FRC to FRC + 0.5 L. Because of the effects of a previous deep inspiration on the measured compliance, measurements are usually recorded from the deflation half of the curve. Maximum elastic recoil pressure is recorded as the most negative pressure attained at the maximum lung volume, normally TLC.

The optimal method of presenting compliance data is to plot the entire pressure curve (i.e., inflation and deflation) against either absolute lung volume or percent of TLC.

CT can be derived as follows if CLT and CL are known:

$$\frac{1}{C_{LT}} - \frac{1}{C_L} = \frac{1}{C_T}$$

Significance

Measurements of compliance determine the elasticity of the lungs, the thorax, and the combination of the two. The average CL in a normal adult is approximately 0.2 L/cm H_2O. The CT has been measured as 0.2 L/cm H_2O in normal adults. In series, the total compliance is calculated using the following equation:

$$\frac{1}{C_L} + \frac{1}{C_T} = \frac{1}{C_{LT}}$$

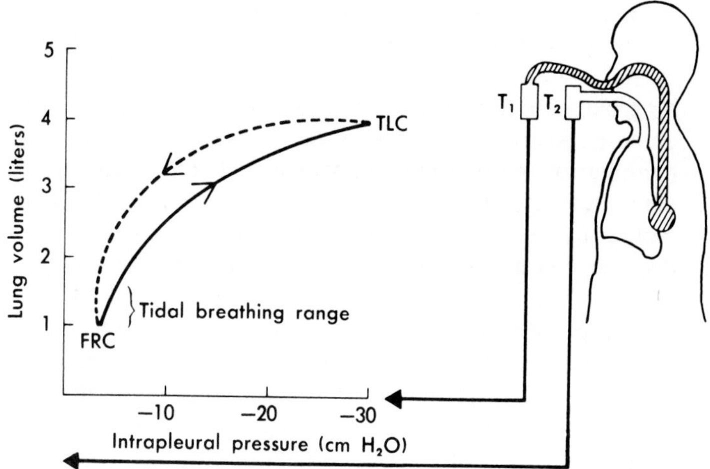

Fig. 3-10 Measurement of pulmonary compliance (CL) using the esophageal balloon technique. Determination of CL requires measurement of intrapleural pressure during periods of no flow at various lung volumes. Transducer T_1 is connected to an esophageal balloon containing a small amount of air and monitors changes in intrapleural pressure (ΔP). Transducer T_2 is actually a flow transducer (pneumotachometer) and is used to measure inspired or expired gas volumes (ΔV). Static CL is the slope of the line defined by:

$$\frac{\Delta V \text{ (in liters)}}{\Delta P \text{ (in cm } H_2O)}$$

and is normally recorded from the tidal breathing range (FRC + 500 ml). CL varies with the lung volume history, as illustrated by the steeper *expiratory* pressure-volume curve. Compliance measurements are often performed with the subject in the body plethysmograph to facilitate determination of absolute lung volumes.

or substituting the usual values:

$$\frac{1}{0.2} + \frac{1}{0.2} = 10$$

where the reciprocal of 10 is the total compliance, or CLT:

$$\frac{1}{10} \text{ or } 0.1 \text{ L/cm } H_2O$$

The total compliance, or CLT, is less than either of its two components because the forces act in series, resulting in the counterbalancing forces of the lung parenchyma and the thorax.

CL varies with the volume of the lungs at the end-expiratory level (i.e., the FRC). To compare the compliance of diseased lungs with that of normal lungs, the FRC in each case should be known. This is sometimes reported as the compliance/FRC ratio. CL is normally decreased in diseases that result in congestion of the pulmonary vasculature or airways, such as edema, atelectasis, pneumonia, or loss of surfactant. Diseases that alter the lung parenchyma, such as pulmonary fibrosis, silicosis, asbestosis, or sarcoidosis, also result in lower than normal compliance. These decreases in compliance may be the result of a pathologic reduction of FRC. When compliance is severely decreased from any cause, clinical findings typically include increased work of breathing and dyspnea on exertion. CL normally decreases with age, presumably because of the changes in the connective tissues of the lung.

Emphysema is often accompanied by an increase in compliance, as elastic tissue is lost with the destruction of alveolar septa. As a result of the decreased elastic recoil of the lungs, the balance of forces between the lungs and thorax is altered, with the lungs containing a larger volume at end-expiration. Compliance of the chest wall (CT) may also be modified in obstructive diseases because of the chronic hyperinflation; subjects who have severe air trapping typically have abnormal breathing patterns and markedly increased work of breathing.

CT may be decreased as a result of thoracic disease, such as kyphoscoliosis, or because of abdominal disorders, such as obesity. In moderate or severe cases of thoracic deformity, gas exchange may be compromised, particularly during exertion.

A specialized application of the compliance measurement is to determine its dependence on breathing frequency. Obstructive disease processes in small airways (i.e., airways less than 2 mm in diameter) may cause different regions of the lungs to ventilate asynchronously. This phenomenon can be detected by measurement of compliance at rapid breathing rates, usually 80 to 100/min. Compliance measured during breathing is called dynamic compliance (Cdyn). Healthy persons produce similar values for both compliance under static conditions (Cst) and dynamic conditions. The frequency dependence of compliance is expressed as the ratio of Cdyn/Cst × 100. Ratio values of less than 80%, at rates of 80-100/min are consistent with small airways obstruction. Frequency dependence is a very sensitive indicator of obstruction in smaller airways and may be present in persons who have asthma or bronchitis and whose conventional test (i.e., $FEV_{1.0}$, $FEF_{25\%-75\%}$, and airway resistance) values are within normal limits (Fig. 3-11).

AIRWAY RESISTANCE (Raw) AND CONDUCTANCE (Gaw and SGaw)

Description

Airway resistance (Raw) is the pressure difference developed per unit flow, measured as the difference in pressure between the mouth (i.e., atmospheric pressure) and that in the alveoli, related to gas flow at the mouth. This pressure difference is created primarily by the friction of gas molecules coming in contact with the conducting airways. Raw is recorded in centi-

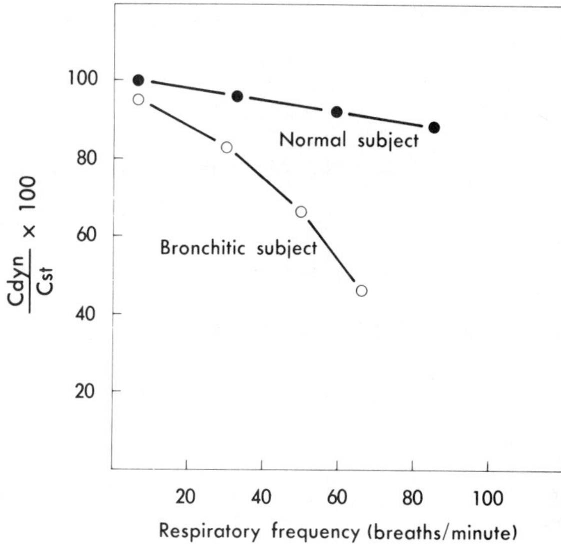

Fig. 3-11 Frequency dependence of compliance. Dynamic compliance (Cdyn) as a percentage of static compliance (Cst) for a normal patient (solid circles) and a bronchitic patient (open circles) is plotted at increasing respiratory frequencies. Increased resistance in the smaller airways (i.e., less than 2 mm in diameter) causes uneven distribution of gas, with most gas going to those lung units having normal resistance. At times of zero flow at the mouth, gas may still be moving within the lungs from one region to another (the *pendelluft* phenomenon). Because some regions are out of phase with others, gas distribution becomes more uneven as breathing frequency increases and causes a fall in the ratio of Cdyn to Cst.

meters of water per liter per second (cm H_2O/L/sec).

Conductance (Gaw) is the flow generated per unit of pressure drop in the airway. It is the reciprocal of Raw (i.e., 1/Raw) and is recorded in liters per second per centimeter of water (L/sec/cm H_2O).

Specific conductance (SGaw) is the conductance per liter of lung volume. SGaw is reported in liters per second per centimeter of water per liter of lung volume (L/sec/cm H_2O/L).

Technique

Raw is the ratio of alveolar pressure (P_A) to air flow ($\dot{V}$). Gas flow at the mouth can be measured easily with a pneumotachograph, and P_A is measured in the body plethysmograph (Fig. 3-12). For gas to flow into the lungs during inspiration, P_A must fall below atmospheric pressure; the opposite occurs during expiration. Changes in $\dot{V}$ are plotted simultaneously against plethysmograph pressure changes (which are proportional to alveolar volume changes) on a storage oscilloscope, or stored by computer. The subject

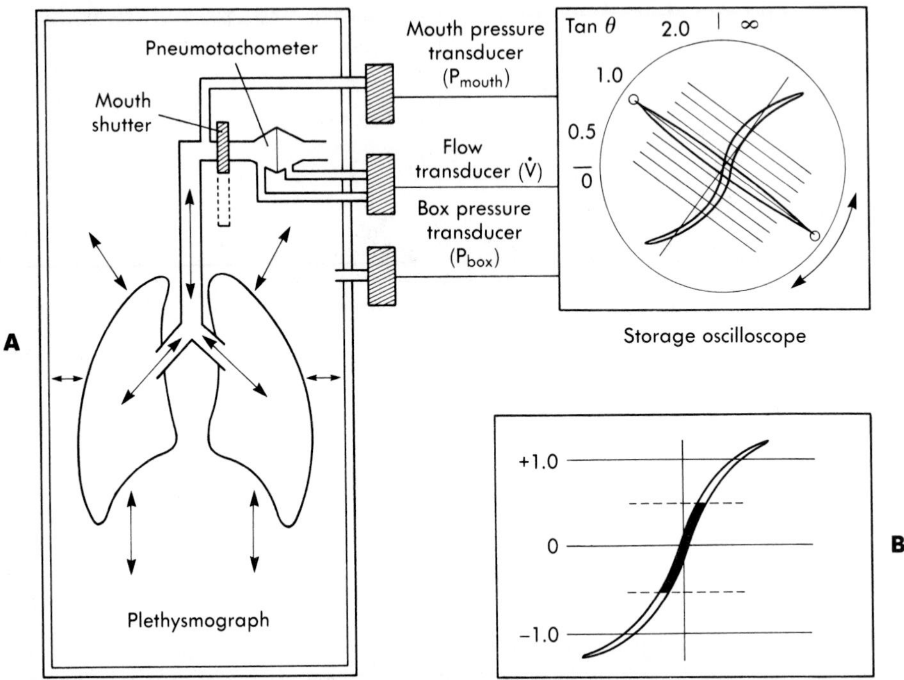

Fig. 3-12 Measurement of airway resistance (Raw) using the body plethysmograph. **A,** Diagrammatic representation of the measurement of Raw:

$$\text{Raw} = \frac{\text{Atmospheric pressure} - \text{Alveolar pressure}}{\text{Flow}}$$

Flow ($\dot{V}$) is measured directly by means of the pneumotachometer. As the patient pants with the shutter open, flow is plotted against box pressure ($\dot{V}/P_{box}$) as an *S*-shaped curve on the oscilloscope. A shutter occludes the airway momentarily, usually at end-expiration, and a sloping line representing the ratio of mouth pressure to box pressure (P_{mouth}/P_{box}) is recorded in a manner similar to that used for measurement of VTG. In this example, the flow tracing (shutter open) and volume tracing (shutter closed) are superimposed. The P_{mouth}/P_{box} tangent is measured as for the VTG. **B**, The flow tangent is measured from the steep portion of the flow tracing, from about −0.5 L/sec to +0.5 L/sec. Airway resistance is then calculated as the ratio of these two tangents using appropriate calibration factors (see text and Appendix).

pants with a small VT and a rate of 1 to 2 breaths/second. This produces an *S*-shaped pressure-flow curve (see Fig. 3-12). A tangent is measured through the zero flow point of this curve, with points at +0.5 L/sec and −0.5 L/sec flow defining the ends of the tangent. The slope of this line is $\dot{V}$/PP, where $\dot{V}$ is air flow and PP is the plethysmograph pressure.

Immediately after this measurement, an electronic shutter at the mouthpiece is closed, and changes in plethysmograph pressure are plotted against airway pressure at the mouth, as for measurement of the VTG. Since there is no air flow into or out of the lungs, mouth pressure approximates P_A. The slope of this line is P_A/P_P, where P_A equals alveolar pressure. This step serves to calibrate changes in P_A to changes in P_P for each subject.

Raw is then calculated by taking the ratio of these two slopes:

$$\text{Raw} = \frac{P_A/P_P}{\dot{V}/P_P} \times \frac{\text{mouth cal}}{\text{flow cal}}$$

where

$\dot{V}$ = Air flow
P_A = Alveolar pressure
P_P = Plethysmographic pressure, which is measured with the shutter open and closed
mouth cal = Calibration factor for the mouth pressure transducer
flow cal = Calibration factor for the flow pressure transducer

Calibration factors for the flow and mouth pressure transducers are included in the previous equation. (See example calculations in the Appendix.) Panting eliminates a number of artifacts from the tracing and allows measurements to be made at or near FRC. Corrections for the resistance of the mouthpiece and flow meter are usually made. Gaw can be calculated as the reciprocal of Raw.

Lung volume determinations can be made easily at the same time, using the plethysmographic method (see Chapter 1). The Raw and Gaw may be expressed per liter of lung volume, specific resistance and specific conductance (SRaw and SGaw, respectively). Expressing Raw and Gaw in this way allows comparisons between subjects who have different lung volumes, and in the same subject when lung volume increases or decreases.

Significance

Normal values of Raw in adults, panting and using a plethysmograph, range from 0.6 to 2.4 cm H_2O/L/sec. Gaw normally varies as the reciprocal between 0.42 and 1.67 L/sec/cm H_2O. Measurements are normally standardized at flow rates of 0.5 L/sec, as described previously.

Resistance in the normal adult is distributed across the airways as follows:

Nose, mouth, and upper airway ≅ 50%
Trachea and bronchi ≅ 30%
Small airways ≅ 20%

Because the small airways (i.e., airways less than 2 mm in diameter) contribute only about one-fifth of the total resistance to flow, significant obstruction can occur in them with relatively little increase in Raw. Lesions obstructing the larger airways may cause a significant increase in Raw, and are often accompanied by an increased work of breathing, along with symptoms such as dyspnea on exertion. Raw may be increased in asthma during an acute episode by as much as three times the normal values. Raw is increased in advanced emphysema because of airway narrowing and collapse in some of the larger airways, as well as in the more distal bronchioles. Other obstructive diseases, such as bronchitis, may cause increases in Raw proportionate to the degree of obstruction in medium and small airways.

Measurement of Raw may be useful in distinguishing between restrictive and obstructive diseases. Because Raw is decreased at increased lung volume, it is often advantageous to ascertain the FRC (i.e., the V_{TG} as noted previously) at the time of the Raw measurements. To use Gaw or Raw for comparative study, these values are often expressed per unit of lung volume (i.e., converted to SGaw and Sraw values). SGaw is particularly useful for assessing changes in airway caliber following bronchodilator therapy or inhalation challenge.

The test is objective insofar as the subject cannot influence results by degree of effort, and thus may be useful for determining airway status in patients who are unable or unwilling to exert maximum effort. Acceptable performance of the panting maneuvers in the plethysmograph does require a certain degree of subject coordination, and not all subjects may be able to perform these maneuvers. Subjects who have moderate or severe obstruction may produce pressure-flow curves during panting from which the accurate measurement of slopes is quite difficult, whether done manually or by computer.

In addition to resistance caused by $\dot{V}$ through the conducting tubes, some of the total pulmonary resistance results from the friction caused by the displacement of the lungs, rib cage, and diaphragm. Normally, this "tissue" resistance is only about one-fifth of the total resistance, and therefore total pulmonary resistance is approximately 20% greater than the measured Raw.

MAXIMAL INSPIRATORY PRESSURE (MIP) AND MAXIMAL EXPIRATORY PRESSURE (MEP)

Description

The maximal inspiratory pressure (MIP) is the greatest subatmospheric pressure that can be developed during inspiration against an occluded airway. MIP is normally measured at RV. The maximal expiratory pressure (MEP) is the highest pressure that can be developed during a forceful expiratory effort against an occluded airway. MEP is usually measured at TLC. Both MIP and MEP are recorded in either cm H_2O or mm Hg.

Technique

The subject is connected to a three-way valve or shutter apparatus, with a flanged mouthpiece and nose clip in place. The airway is occluded by switching the valve to one port that is blocked or by closing the shutter. In either method, a small leak is introduced between the occlusion and the mouth to negate any influence of the cheek muscles. The leak, usually a large-bore needle or similar opening, allows a small amount of gas to enter the oral cavity, but does not significantly influence the lung volume or pressure measurement. To measure MIP, the subject is instructed to expire maximally to RV. It is helpful to monitor expiratory flow, or have the subject signal when maximal expiration has been achieved. Then, with the airway occluded, the subject inspires and maintains the inspiration for 1 to 3 seconds. The maximal subatmospheric pressure may be measured using a manometer, aneroid-type gauge, or pressure transducer. The pressure-monitoring device should be linear and capable of recording pressures from -10 cm H_2O to approximately -200 cm H_2O. The most negative value from at least three efforts is reported. The first second of each maneuver is discarded since it may include transient pressure changes that occur initially with the maneuver. The MEP is recorded similarly, except that the subject inspires to TLC and then expires maximally against the occluded airway for 1 to 3 seconds. Longer efforts should be avoided because of the possibility of reduction of cardiac output by the high thoracic pressures (i.e., Valsalva maneuver). Because MEP is typically larger than MIP, the pressure-monitoring device should be able to accommodate the higher pressure developed. The best of three MEP efforts is reported, again disregarding any initial pressure transients. These tests require subject cooperation, and low values may reflect lack of understanding or insufficient effort.

Significance

The MIP primarily measures inspiratory muscle strength. The normal adult can generate inspiratory pressures in excess of -60 cm H_2O. For prediction regressions, see the Appendix. Decreased MIP is seen in subjects with neuromuscular disease or diseases involving the diaphragm, intercostals, or accessory muscles. MIP may also be decreased in patients who have hyperinflation, such as in emphysema, or in patients who have chest wall or spinal deformities. MIP is often used to assess subject response to training of the strength of the respiratory muscles. MIP, as a measure of respiratory muscle strength, may be used in conjunction with MSVC (see Chapter 2) in the assessment of respiratory muscle function (see also Chapter 8, Critical Care Monitoring).

The MEP measures the pressure generated during maximal expiration. It depends on the function of the accessory muscles of respiration and the abdominal muscles, as well as the elastic recoil of the lungs and thorax. Normal adults can generate MEP values in excess of 80 to 100 cm H_2O; adult males may develop pressures greater than 200 cm H_2O. MEP may be decreased in neuromuscular disorders, particularly those that result in generalized muscle weakness. Reduced MEP may be related to increased RV and may accompany decreased expiratory flow rates on simple spirometry or flow-volume maneuvers. Decreased MEP is associated with inability to cough effectively, and may complicate chronic bronchitis, cystic fibrosis, or other diseases that result in mucus hypersecretion.

SELF-ASSESSMENT QUESTIONS

1. A subject has an $FEV_{1.0}$ of 1.91 liters (52% of the predicted value). Which of the following might result in this low value:
   I. Small airways obstruction
   II. Poor effort at the start-of-test
   III. Restriction due to fibrosis
   IV. An FVC larger than predicted
   a. I, II, III, IV
   b. I, III, IV
   c. I, II, III
   d. II, IV

2. A subject has these results from simple spirometry:

	Measured	Predicted
FVC (L BTPS)	3.1	4.0
$FEV_{1.0}$ (L BTPS)	0.9	3.1

   These findings are consistent with:
   a. Combined obstruction and restriction
   b. A restrictive disease process
   c. Normal lung function
   d. Incorrectly selected predicted values

3. A subject has an $FEV_{3\%}$ of 80%. This is consistent with:
   a. Normal airway function
   b. Obstructive disease
   c. Restrictive disease
   d. Reversible airway obstruction

4. A subject performs MEFV curves using a spirometer that meets American Thoracic Society requirements; the following results are reported:

		Measured	Predicted
FVC	(L BTPS)	2.4	4.6
$FEV_{1.0}$	(L BTPS)	2.2	3.5
$FEV_{1\%}$		92%	76%
$FEF_{25\text{-}75\%}$	(L/sec BTPS)	3.9	3.3

   These results are consistent with:
   a. Normal pulmonary function
   b. Moderate obstructive disease
   c. Early small airways obstruction
   d. Restrictive lung disease

5. A subject performs an MVV maneuver for 12 seconds; the total volume expired in this interval is 20 L (BTPS). If the subject's predicted MVV is 100 L/min (BTPS), what percent of the predicted value did this subject perform?
   MVV (percent of predicted) = ______________________%

6. A subject has his CL measured using the esophageal balloon technique; a compliance of 0.050 L/cm H_2O is reported. This finding is consistent with which of the following disease entities?
   I. Pulmonary vascular congestion
   II. Emphysema
   III. Asthma
   IV. Pulmonary fibrosis
   a. I, III, IV
   b. I, IV
   c. II, III
   d. II only

7. An asthmatic subject has her Raw measured according to the standard procedure using a body plethysmograph; a diagnosis of asthmatic bronchitis is suspected from her clinical history. Which of the following measurements are consistent with this diagnosis:
   a. 0.71 cm H_2O
   b. 1.55 cm H_2O
   c. 2.25 cm H_2O
   d. 3.99 cm H_2O
   e. b, c, and d

8. A subject has spirometry performed, and the following results are reported:

	Measured	**Predicted**
FVC	3.42	3.70
$FEV_{1.0}$	1.60	2.92
MVV	101	105

   These findings are most consistent with which of the following interpretations:
   a. Moderate obstructive disease
   b. Moderate restrictive disease
   c. Normal spirometry
   d. Invalid $FEV_{1.0}$

9. The flow over the latter two-thirds of the expiratory limb of the MEFV:
   I. Is determined by the elastic recoil properties of the lung
   II. Is determined by the resistance to flow in the small airways (i.e., airways less than 2 mm in diameter)
   III. Is independent of subject effort
   IV. Is termed the $\dot{V}_{max\ 75\%}$
   a. I, II, III, IV
   b. I, II, III
   c. II, IV
   d. III only

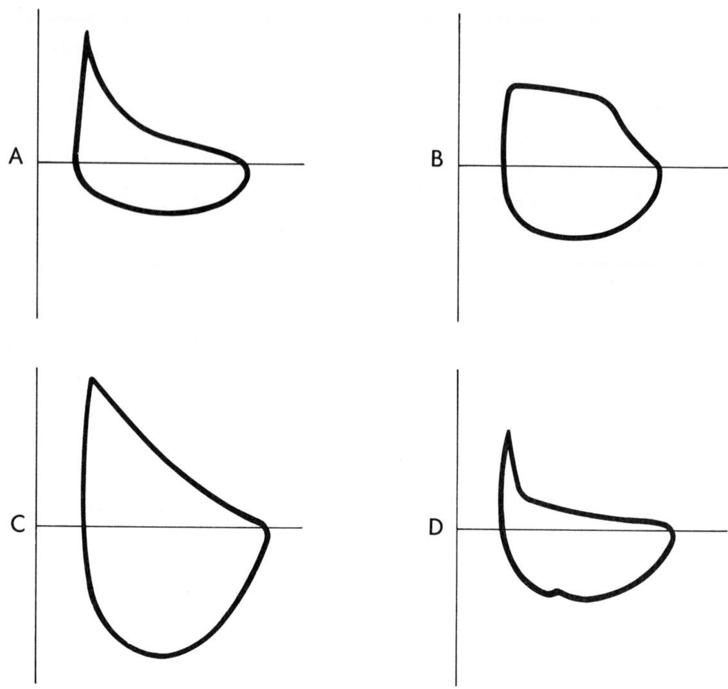

10. Which of the above flow-volume curves are consistent with fixed extrathoracic obstruction:

11. A subject performs MEFV maneuvers breathing air and then again breathing an 80% He-20% O_2 mixture. When the curves are superimposed, they coincide at approximately the same point as the $\dot{V}_{max\ 50}$. This finding is consistent with:
    a. Obstruction of small airways
    b. An improperly performed MEFV maneuver
    c. Large airway obstruction
    d. A restrictive disease process

12. A subject who has myasthenia gravis performs MIP and MEP maneuvers to assess respiratory muscle function; the following values are reported:

	Measured
MIP (cm H_2O)	−110
MEP (cm H_2O)	+179

These findings are consistent with:
    a. Normal respiratory muscle function
    b. Normal inspiratory and abnormal expiratory muscle function
    c. Abnormal inspiratory and normal expiratory muscle function
    d. Abnormal inspiratory and expiratory muscle function

SELECTED BIBLIOGRAPHY

General references

Bates DV, Macklem PT, and Christie RV: Respiratory function in disease, ed 2, Philadelphia, 1971, WB Saunders Co.

Kanner RE and Morris AH, editors: Clinical pulmonary function testing, ed 2, Salt Lake City, 1984, Intermountain Thoracic Society.

Forster RE: The lung: clinical physiology and pulmonary function tests, ed 3, Chicago, 1986, Year Book Medical Publishers, Inc.

Flow-volume curves

Acres J and Kryger M: Clinical significance of pulmonary function tests: upper airway obstruction, Chest 80:207, 1981.

Bass H: The flow volume loop: normal standards and abnormalities in chronic obstructive pulmonary disease, Chest 63:171, 1973.

Despas PJ, Leroux M, and Macklem PT: Site of airway obstruction in asthma as determined by measuring flow breathing air and a helium-oxygen mixture, J Clin Invest 51:3235, 1972.

Gelb AF and Klein E: The volume of isoflow and increase in maximal flow at 50 percent of forced vital capacity during helium-oxygen breathing as tests of small airway, Chest 71:396, 1977.

Hyatt RE and Black LF: The flow volume curve, Am Rev Respir Dis 107:191, 1973.

Knudson RJ et al: The maximal expiratory flow-volume curve: normal standards, variability and effects of age, Am Rev Respir Dis 113:587, 1976.

Knudson RJ et al: Changes in the normal maximal expiratory flow-volume curve with growth and aging, Am Rev Respir Dis 127:725, 1983.

Miller RD and Hyatt RE: Evaluation of obstructing lesions of the trachea and larynx by flow volume loops, Am Rev Respir Dis 108:475, 1973.

Maximal respiratory pressures

Arora NS and Rochester DF: Respiratory muscle strength and maximal voluntary ventilation in undernourished patients, Am Rev Respir Dis 126:5, 1982.

Block LF and Hyatt RE: Maximal static respiratory pressure in generalized neuromuscular disease, Am Rev Respir Dis 103:641, 1971.

Gilbert R, Auchincloss JH Jr, and Bleb S: Measurement of maximum inspiratory pressures during routing spirometry, Lung 155:23, 1978.

Compliance and airway resistance

Baydur A et al: A simple method for assessing the validity of the esophageal balloon technique, Am Rev Respir Dis 126:788, 1982.

Behrakis PK et al: Lung mechanics in sitting and horizontal body positions, Chest 83:643, 1983.

Dubois AB, Bothello SV, and Comroe JH: A new method for measuring airway resistance in man using a body plethysmograph: values in normal subjects and in patients with respiratory disease, J Clin Invest 35:327, 1956.

Gillespie DJ: Comparison of intraesophageal balloon pressure measurements with a nasogastric-esophageal balloon system in volunteers, Am Rev Respir Dis 126:583, 1982.

Woolcock AJ, Vincent NJ, and Macklem PT: Frequency dependence of compliance as a test for obstruction in the small airways, J Clin Invest 48:1099, 1969.

Spirometry

Knudson RJ and Lebowitz MD: Maximal midexpiratory flow ($FEF_{25\%-75\%}$): normal limits and assessment of sensitivity, Am Rev Respir Dis 117:609, 1978.

Kuperman AS and Riker JB: The predicted normal maximal midexpiratory flow, Am Rev Respir Dis 107:231, 1973.

Leuallen EC and Fowler WS: Maximal midexpiratory flow, Am Rev Tuberculosis 72:783, 1955.

Morris JF, Koski A, and Johnson LC: Spirometric standards for healthy nonsmoking adults, Am Rev Respir Dis 107:57, 1971.

Sackner MA, et al: Assessment of time-volume and flow-volume components of forced vital capacity, Chest, 82:272, 1982.

Smith AA and Gaensler EA: Timing of forced expiratory volume in one second, Am Rev Respir Dis 112:882, 1975.

Townsend MC, DuChene AG, and Fallat RJ: The effects of underrecording forced expirations on spirometric lung function indexes, Am Rev Respir Dis 126:734, 1982.

4

Gas Distribution Tests

SINGLE-BREATH NITROGEN WASHOUT (SBN_2), CLOSING VOLUME (CV), AND CLOSING CAPACITY (CC)

Description

The single-breath nitrogen washout test (SBN_2), also referred to as the SBO_2 and Fowler's test, measures the distribution of ventilation by analyzing change in N_2 concentration during expiration of the vital capacity (VC) following a single breath of 100% O_2. The evenness of distribution is assessed by two parameters: the $\Delta\%N_{2_{750\text{-}1250}}$, and the slope of Phase III, both described further in the following Technique section. Each of these indices is recorded as percent change per unit of lung volume.

Closing volume (CV) is that portion of the VC that can be expired from the lungs following the onset of airway closure. CV is usually expressed as a percentage of the VC. A related measurement, closing capacity (CC), is the sum of the CV and RV (Chapter 1). CC is expressed as a percentage of the TLC.

Technique

The subject expires to RV, then inspires a measured breath of 100% O_2, usually from a reservoir or demand flow system. Without holding the breath, the subject expires slowly and evenly, at a flow rate of 0.3 to 0.5 L/sec. An N_2 analyzer monitors the N_2 concentration of the expired gas while a spirometer measures the exhaled volume. The volume is plotted against N_2 concentration on a suitable graph (Fig. 4-1). This washout curve can be divided into four phases:

Phase I is extreme upper airway gas, from the anatomic dead space, consisting of 100% O_2.

Phase II is mixed V_D gas in which the relative concentrations of O_2 and N_2 change abruptly as the V_D volume is expired.

Phase III is a plateau caused by the exhalation of alveolar gas, in which relative O_2 and N_2 concentrations change slowly and evenly.

Phase IV is marked by an abrupt increase in the concentration of N_2 that continues until RV is reached.

The initial 750 ml of expired gas contains mostly dead space gas from Phases I and II and is not used in the analysis of distribution of ventilation.

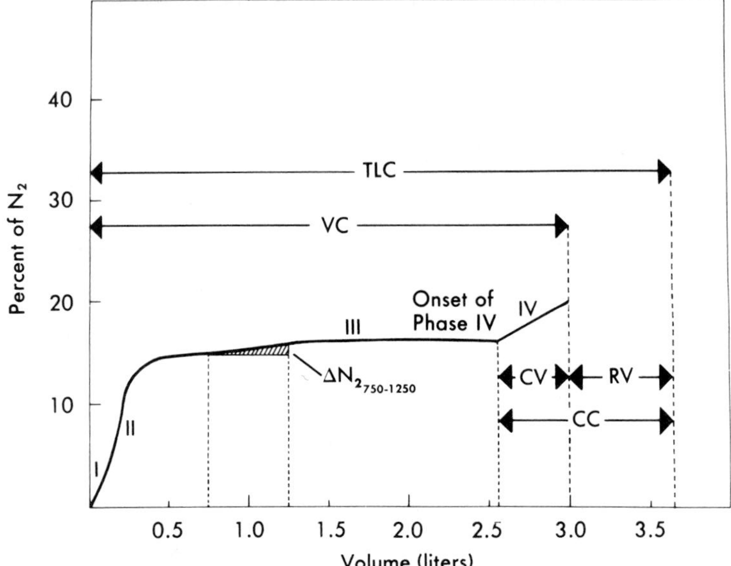

Fig. 4-1 Single-breath nitrogen elimination (SBN_2)—A plot of the increasing N_2 concentration on expiration following a single vital capacity breath of 100% O_2. The curve is divided into four phases: *Phase I* is the extreme beginning of the expiration when only O_2 is being exhaled. *Phase II* shows an abrupt rise in N_2 concentration as mixed bronchial and alveolar air is expired. *Phase III* is the alveolar gas plateau, and N_2 concentration changes slowly as long as ventilation is uniformly distributed. *Phase IV* is an abrupt increase in N_2 concentration as basal airways close and a larger proportion of gas comes from the N_2-rich lung apices. Several useful parameters are derived from the SBN_2 tracing. Anatomic dead space can be calculated (see Chapter 2). The $\Delta\%N_{2_{750\text{-}1250}}$ and slope of Phase III are indices of the evenness of ventilation distribution. CV can be read directly from the onset of Phase IV until RV is reached; VC can also be read directly. RV, TLC, and CC can be calculated if the area under the curve is determined either by planimetry or electronic integration (see text).

The difference in N_2 concentration between the 750 ml and 1250 ml points is called the delta N_2 ($\Delta\%N_{2_{750\text{-}1250}}$).

The slope of Phase III is the change in N_2 concentration from the point at which 30% of the VC remains to the onset of Phase IV, and is recorded as $\Delta\%N_2$ per liter of lung volume.

The volume expired from the onset of Phase IV to the termination of the breath is called the closing volume (CV). The CV may be added to the RV, if the RV has been determined, and expressed as the CC. CV is normally recorded as a percentage of the VC:

$$CV/VC \times 100$$

Closing capacity (CC) is recorded as a percentage of the TLC:

$$CC/TLC \times 100$$

TLC can be determined using the SBN_2 test by measuring the area under the washout curve, either by electronic integration or planimetry, using a dilution equation to calculate RV, then adding the RV to the measured VC. RV is calculated as follows:

$$RV = VC \times \frac{F\bar{E}_{N_2}}{FA_{N_2} - F\bar{E}_{N_2}}$$

where

$F\bar{E}_{N_2}$ = Mean expired N_2 concentration determined by a planimeter or electronic integration of the area under the curve

FA_{N_2} = N_2 concentration in the lungs at the beginning of inspiration, approximately 0.75 to 0.79

This method is accurate only in subjects who do not have significant obstructive disease or dead space-producing disease.

Significance

$\Delta\%N_{2_{750\text{-}1250}}$. The normal $\Delta\%N_{2_{750\text{-}1250}}$ is 1.5% or less in healthy young adults and up to approximately 3% higher in healthy older adults. Increases in $\Delta\%N_{2_{750\text{-}1250}}$ are found in the presence of diseases characterized by uneven distribution of gas during inspiration and unequal emptying rates during expiration. In subjects who have severe emphysema, $\Delta\%N_{2_{750\text{-}1250}}$ may exceed 10%.

Slope of Phase III. A best-fit line drawn through the Phase III segment of the tracing, from the point at which 30% of the VC remains above RV to the onset of Phase IV, is used to determine the slope of Phase III. This slope is used as an index of gas distribution, in a manner similar to the $\Delta\%N_{2_{750\text{-}1250}}$. Values in healthy young adults range from 0.5% to 1.0% N_2/L of lung volume, with wide variability. Very slow expiratory flow rates may cause oscillations in the tracing of Phase III, making the accurate measurement of $\Delta\%N_{2_{750\text{-}1250}}$ difficult. These oscillations are attributed to changes in alveolar N_2 concentrations as blood pulses through the pulmonary capillaries during cardiac systole. Increasing the expiratory flow rate slightly eliminates this common artifact. Subjects whose VC values are low may have difficulty exhaling enough gas to make the $\Delta\%N_{2_{750\text{-}1250}}$ meaningful.

CV and CC. Phase IV of the SBN_2 test can be explained by the fact that, after a maximal expiration by a subject sitting upright, more RV gas remains at the apices of the lungs than at the bases, resulting from the effects of gravity. When a test gas, such as O_2, is inspired, the apices receive the gas occupying the subject's dead space, then the test gas goes preferentially to the bases of the lungs. Gas concentrations in the lungs become widely different, because the apices contain RV gas and dead space gas, largely N_2, while the bases contain predominantly test gas, O_2 in this case. Compression of the airways during the subsequent expiration causes airways to narrow, and then close, as lung volume approaches RV. Dependent airways close first because of gravity and the weight of the lung in subjects sitting upright. As airways at the bases of the lung close, proportionately more gas comes from the apices, the concentration of N_2 rises, and Phase IV begins.

The onset of Phase IV indicates the lung volume at which airway closure begins and is sensitive to changes in the caliber of the small airways. In healthy young adults, closing volume occurs near the end of the vital capacity, after 80% to 90% of the VC has been expired. The CC in healthy young adults usually occurs at about 30% of the TLC, again with wide variations. Increases in CV and CC, indicating earlier onset of airway closure, may occur because of increase in age, restrictive processes in which the FRC becomes less than the CV, smoking and other causes of early obstructive disease of small airways, and congestive heart failure in which the caliber of the small airways is compromised by edema.

Subjects who have moderate or severe obstructive disease may display no sharp inflection separating Phases III and IV of the SBN_2 because of grossly uneven distribution of gas in the lungs. Subjects who have airway obstruction typically produce $\Delta\%N_{2_{750\text{-}1250}}$ values and slopes of Phase III that are greater than normal.

CV and CC measurements may be in error if the subject does not perform a true VC maneuver. The inspired and expired VC values should be within 5% of each other, and the VC during the SBN_2 test also should be within 5% of the FVC or SVC. Expiratory flow should be maintained between 0.3 and 0.5 L/sec. In some individuals who have no pulmonary disease, the onset of Phase IV cannot be accurately determined. Because of the variability in both the CV and CC, the mean of three tests is most often reported. Because of its poor reproducibility, the CV test is not widely used. Although it appears to be a sensitive indicator of abnormalities in the small airways, particularly in smokers, an increased CV/VC ratio is not highly predictive of which individuals will develop chronic airways obstruction. To calculate normal values for CV and CC according to age and sex, see the Appendix.

N_2 WASHOUT TEST (7-MINUTE)

Description

The N_2 washout test measures the concentration of N_2 in alveolar gas at the end of 7 minutes of breathing 100% O_2. The N_2 washout test value is recorded as a percentage of alveolar N_2.

Technique

The simplest method of calculating the degree of N_2 washout from the lungs is by having the subject breathe 100% O_2 for 7 minutes, then measuring the N_2 concentration of a sample of alveolar gas collected at the end of a forced expiration. The distribution of ventilation determines whether the concentration of N_2 has been reduced to a low level within 7 minutes. Alternatively, the duration of O_2 breathing to reduce the $\%N_2$ to less than 1% can be used as an index of gas distribution.

A more quantitative test is that in which the washout of N_2 by O_2 is graphed or displayed breath-by-breath using rapid analysis of expired gas. Normally, the percent of N_2 or its logarithm is plotted against the expired volume or number of breaths. The end-expiratory points of the typical washout curve are exponential and appear as a straight line when the percent of N_2 is graphed on semilog paper (Fig. 4-2).

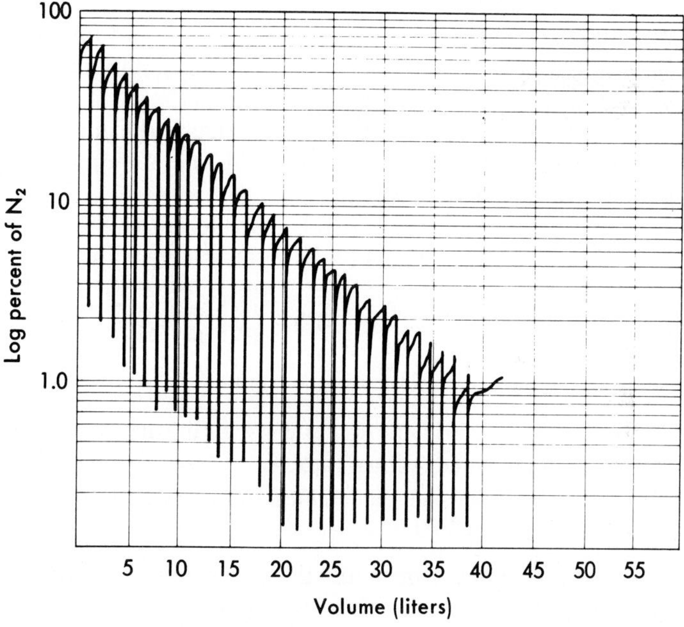

Fig. 4-2 Nitrogen washout test (7-minute). The N_2 concentration versus expired volume is plotted on semilog paper (Y axis is logarithmic). The elimination of N_2 from the lungs by O_2 breathing occurs exponentially. A single-chamber lung being washed out in this fashion would produce a J-shaped curve; the percent of N_2 is plotted on semilog paper, resulting in a straight line. Lungs with normal distribution of ventilation produce an approximately straight line; lungs with deranged distribution tend to show a rapid washout initially and progressive slowing as the test proceeds. This begins as a steep curve, with more and more flattening toward the end. The slope of the washout curve is determined mainly by the rate, V_T, FRC, and dead space. The inspired gas distribution index (IDI) offers a more quantitative analysis of the distribution characteristics (see text). The test normally lasts 7 minutes, or until the alveolar N_2 concentration has been reduced to less than 1% or until an expired volume limit has been reached (i.e., 60 liters). The log $\%N_2$ may also be plotted against time or number of breaths.

Significance

The normal value for the concentration of N_2 in alveolar gas after 7 minutes of O_2 breathing is less than 2.5%. The results of a 7-minute N_2 washout test are of little value without consideration of the V_T, V_D, and FRC of the individual subject during the test. Large increases in $\dot{V}_E$ (i.e., increased V_T or rate) can lower the percent of N_2 in the alveoli to near normal levels within the 7-minute limit even though there is marked unevenness of gas distribution. Persons who have no pulmonary disease wash N_2 out of their lungs with 3 to 4 minutes of O_2 breathing. Washout times longer than 3 to 4 minutes are usually consistent with poor distribution, increased FRC, reduced alveolar ventilation, or a combination of these.

The graphic method of displaying breath-by-breath washout provides a means of quantifying the evenness of ventilation. The slope of the washout curve is determined by the FRC, V_T, V_D, and frequency of breathing. If the N_2 is washed out of the lungs evenly, the curve will appear as a straight line on semilog paper, regardless of the slope (see Fig. 4-2). Because the lung is not a perfectly symmetrical organ, the curve is typically slightly concave. The deviation from a straight line is indicative of the extent to which ventilation is uneven.

Data from the washout can be used to derive the index of distribution of inspired gas (IDI) (Fig. 4-3). The IDI is determined as follows:

$$\text{IDI} = \frac{V_{A_{total}}}{\text{FRC (k)}}$$

where

$V_{A_{total}}$ = Alveolar volume accumulated during the entire test
FRC = Functional residual capacity
k = Constant such that an ideal single-compartment lung will have an IDI equal to 1.00

This technique eliminates the dependence on the V_T, f, and V_D as determinants of the slope of the washout curve. Total V_A can be calculated as follows:

$$V_{A_{total}} = V_{total} - f(V_D)$$

where

V_{total} = Total volume expired during test
V_D = Respiratory dead space
f = Number of breaths

In a single-chambered lung, the IDI would equal 1.000. In healthy individuals, the IDI is about 1.80 ± 0.2. Subjects who have obstructive diseases have mean IDI values of 3.40 ± 0.9. Thus, the IDI is a quantitative expression of the gas distribution as analyzed by the multiple-breath N_2 technique.

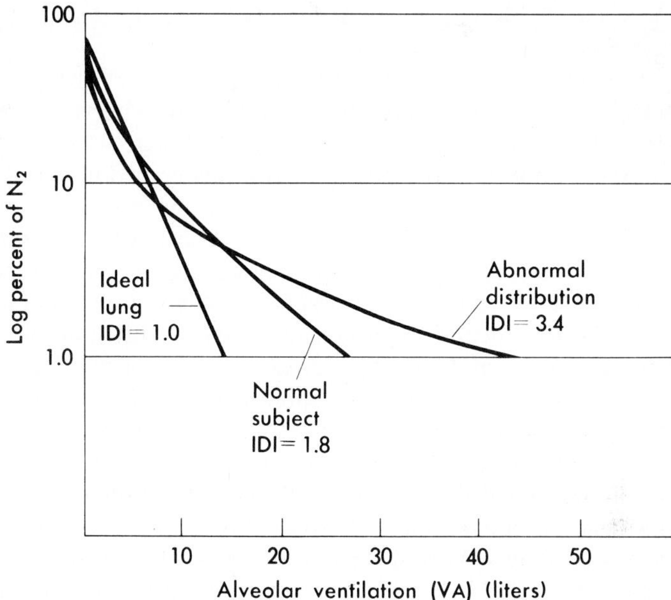

Fig. 4-3 Inspired gas distribution index (IDI). Illustrated is a plot of the logarithm of N_2 concentration versus the VA. The IDI is derived thus:

$$IDI = \frac{VA_{total}}{FRC\ (k)}$$

where

k = Constant equal to the natural log of 72

By definition, IDI for an ideal, single-chambered lung is 1.0. Plotting log $\%N_2$ concentration against VA instead of total expired volume eliminates dependence on rate, VT, and dead space as determinants of the shape of the washout curve and allows a quantitative measurement of the evenness of distribution. (From Application Note AN729, San Diego, Hewlett-Packard Co.)

Uneven distribution is characteristic of all obstructive disease patterns, with patients who have emphysema often showing the greatest degree of maldistribution. Patients having bronchitis and asthma show similar unevenness of ventilation, particularly during acute exacerbations. The effect of uneven distribution of ventilation is largely dependent on the matching of ventilation and perfusion. Uneven ventilation often results in blood gas abnormalities, specifically hypoxemia (see Chapter 6). Some subjects who have marked maldistribution, such as those who have emphysema, may have rather even matching of ventilation and perfusion if the disease process destroys pulmonary capillaries along with the other alveolar structures.

As a result, blood gas values may be relatively normal with little or no hypoxemia.

Normal washout values often are produced by subjects who have pure restrictive patterns, especially subjects who hyperventilate as a result of restriction. However, tumors and other space-occupying lesions may impinge upon the airways and cause regional differences in ventilation. Thoracic deformities, such as kyphoscoliosis and pectus excavatum, may also cause marked unevenness in the distribution of ventilation. The 7-minute washout test may appear abnormal in the presence of many of these types of restrictive disorders. Ventilation and perfusion lung scans offer the best means of assessing regional gas distribution and blood flow.

Both the simple multiple-breath N_2 test and the IDI are independent of subject effort, although the subject must maintain an adequate seal on the mouthpiece of the apparatus to prevent contamination of the test gas (O_2). Leaks in the breathing circuit or in the N_2 sampling device usually result in room air being mixed with the washed-out gas. This almost always results in prolonged washout times or inability to reduce the alveolar N_2 to less than 2.5%, even in normal lungs. Leaks are usually identifiable by abrupt increases in the N_2 concentration during the maneuver.

LUNG SCANS (^{133}Xe)

Description

Lung scans using ^{133}Xenon (^{133}Xe), as well as techniques employing inhalation of ^{81m}Krypton and ^{127}Xe, measure the regional distribution of ventilation.

Technique

1. The subject, usually in a sitting position, inhales either a V_T or a VC breath from a reservoir that contains a measured dose of ^{133}Xe (10 to 20 mCi). The subject then holds the breath for 10 to 20 seconds, during which scintiphotos are made over the lung fields to demonstrate areas of poor ventilation (Fig. 4-4).
2. Then, the subject is allowed to rebreathe the gas mixture containing the ^{133}Xe for 3 to 5 minutes, during which serial scintiphotos are made to demonstrate the rapidity and evenness of equilibration of the ^{133}Xe. Addition of O_2 and removal of CO_2 are required, since this is a closed circuit similar to that used in the He dilution FRC determination. Because the rebreathing period is usually short, the circuit may be flushed with 100% O_2 to provide adequate O_2 during the maneuver. If the reservoir bag is of sufficient volume ($\cong$10 L), addition of O_2 may be unnecessary. However, 100% O_2 breathing in subjects who have poorly ventilated lung units, even for a short interval, may cause some absorption atelectasis, causing greater unevenness of ventilation than might normally be seen.
3. During the final step, the subject is returned to breathing air to

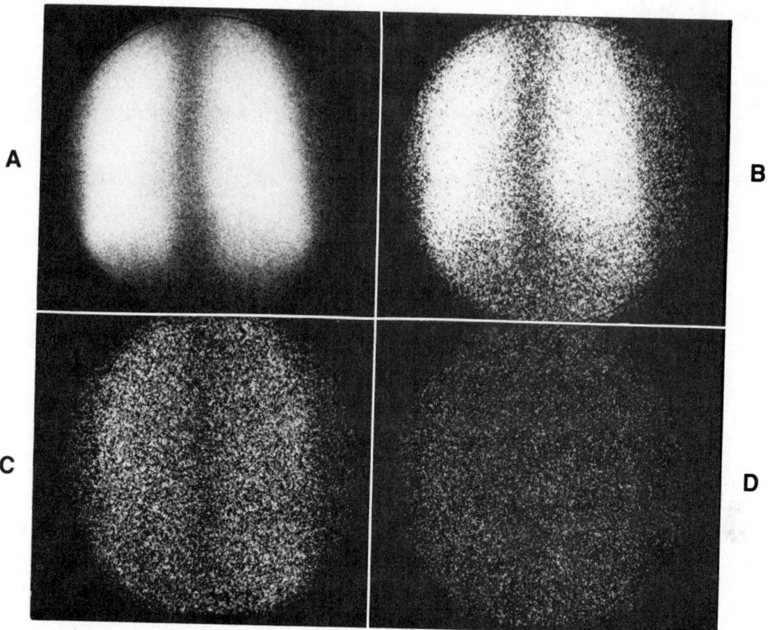

Fig. 4-4 ^{133}Xe ventilation lung scan showing posterior-anterior views of normal lung fields. **A,** Wash-in or equilibration after rebreathing radioactive Xe. **B,** 30 seconds after washout begins, with the patient breathing room air. **C,** 1 minute after breathing room air. **D,** 3 minutes after breathing air: only background radiation remains. (Courtesy Nuclear Medicine Department, St. Louis University Hospital, St. Louis)

cause the ^{133}Xe to be washed out. Serial scintiphotos indicate those areas that have trapped the ^{133}Xe during the equilibration phase. Ratios of counts from various lung zones can be used to compare the relative degree of ventilation of each lung zone. This normally requires discrete counters or computerized segregation of counts from the various lung zones.

Significance

^{133}Xe is ideal for identifying regional ventilation disorders. It has a half-life of 5.27 days and requires sophisticated monitoring equipment, but it is not metabolized by the body and tends to remain in the gas phase. The three steps used in ^{133}Xe studies, as described previously, can be done individually or as a series, and are helpful diagnostically in cases of pronounced regional differences in ventilation.

Regional distribution of inspired gas is dependent on the volume of air in the lungs before the breath and the volume of the breath itself. Differences in regional ventilation can be quantified by calculating the concentration of ^{133}Xe in each lung zone by means of external counters placed over the chest. The fractional concentration of ^{133}Xe during the initial breath can be derived by comparing radiation counts during an initial breath of ^{133}Xe to counts at the same lung volume after rebreathing, when the concentration of ^{133}Xe is equal in both the lung and the breathing circuit. This fractional concentration can then be stated as a ventilation index, expressing it as a percentage of the simultaneous mean concentration of ^{133}Xe in the lungs. The concentration of ^{133}Xe is expressed per unit of lung volume, and similar data from different subjects can be compared. Of more practical value, although less quantitative, is direct visual examination of the scintiphotos to determine the size and pattern of the ventilation defect.

^{133}Xe scans in healthy persons sitting upright show proportionately greater ventilation at the bases of the lungs than in the apices because gravity causes most perfusion to be directed to the lower two-thirds of the lungs, ventilation is closely matched to blood flow in healthy individuals. Despite the smaller alveolar size in the lower lung zones, due to gravity and hydrostatic pressure, tidal ventilation is directed to those areas of gravity-dependent blood flow, so that a major portion of lung units have ventilation/perfusion ($\dot{V}/\dot{Q}$) ratios of 0.8 to 1.0.

Technical problems with ventilation lung scans may involve the breathing circuitry, with leaks causing inaccurate measurements and escape of radioactive gas. Most systems, however, enclose the reservoir and the majority of the breathing circuit in a shielded container. The subject must be instructed carefully, and must keep nose clips in place during the procedure to prevent inadvertent loss of the radioactive gas.

The distribution of pulmonary blood flow may be demonstrated by intravenous injection of radioactive particles of technetium (Tc). Macroaggregated albumin (MAA) labeled with ^{99m}Tc (^{99m}Tc-MAA) or human albumin microspheres (HAM) labeled with ^{99m}Tc (^{99m}Tc-HAM) are commonly used. The particles, which measure 30 to 40 microns, are injected by a venous route, then they mix with blood passing through the right side of the heart and lodge in the pulmonary arterioles. Their distribution matches the pulmonary blood flow at the time of injection. Scintiphotos are normally made of six views: anterior, posterior, left lateral, right lateral, left posterior oblique, and right posterior oblique (Fig. 4-5). These particles normally break up, pass through the pulmonary capillaries, and are removed in the liver and spleen. When the usual dosage is used, only one of every 1000 arterioles is occluded and no functional abnormalities can be demonstrated following injection.

Perfusion lung scanning may be contraindicated in subjects who have severe pulmonary hypertension because of their reduced vascular bed, and in individuals who have anatomic right-to-left shunts, because the particles pass unchanged through the lungs for embolization in the brain, kidney, heart, or other organs.

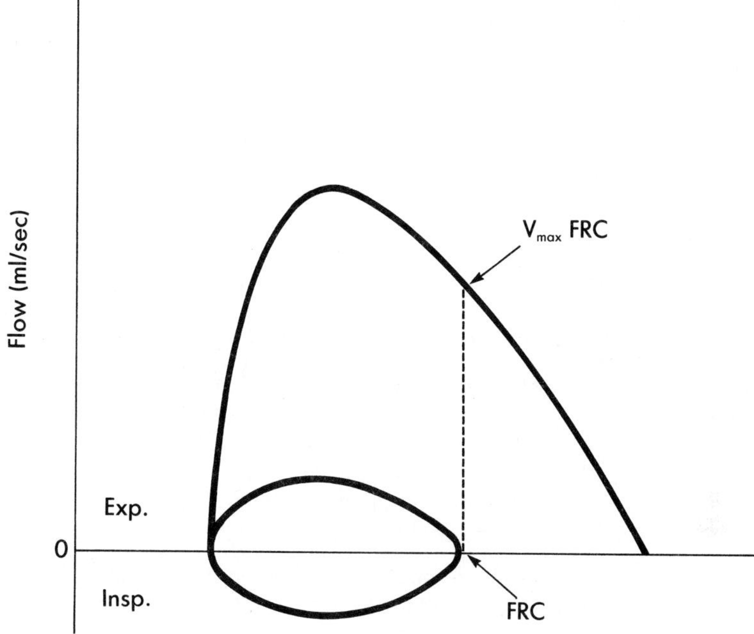

Fig. 4-5. ^{99m}Tc-HAM perfusion lung scan—normal perfusion lung scan using human albumin microspheres (HAM) tagged with radioactive technetium (Tc). **A,** posterior; **B,** left posterior oblique; **C,** right posterior oblique; **D,** left lateral; **E,** right lateral; **F,** anterior. (Courtesy Nuclear Medicine Department, St. Louis University Hospital, St. Louis)

Perfusion scanning is routinely combined with ventilation scans of the lung to evaluate subjects who have obstructive airways disease or suspected pulmonary emboli. Perfusion scanning may be computer enhanced to provide projection of the $\dot{V}/\dot{Q}$ characteristics of various lung segments.

SELF-ASSESSMENT QUESTIONS

1. The evenness of distribution of ventilation within the lungs is assessed by which of the following parameters:
   a. Duration of Phase I of the SBN_2
   b. Slope of Phase III of the SBN_2
   c. $\Delta\%N_{2_{750\text{-}1250}}$
   d. All of the above
   e. b and c only

2. A subject performs an SBN_2 maneuver. Interpretation includes "early onset of Phase IV"; this interpretation is consistent with:
   a. Poor effort during the last half of the maneuver

b. Increased anatomic dead space
c. Pulmonary stenosis
d. Small airway obstruction

3. A subject performs simple spirometry and an SBN_2 maneuver, with the following results:

	Measured	Predicted
FVC (L BTPS)	4.3	4.0
$FEV_{1.0}$ (L BTPS)	3.4	3.1
$FEV_{1\%}$ (%)	79	78
Slope of Phase III (%/L)	2.0	0.66

These findings are consistent with:
a. Normal function in older healthy adults
b. Large airway obstruction
c. Moderately advanced restrictive disease
d. Abnormal distribution of ventilation

4. A subject performs the 7-minute N_2 washout procedure; after 7 minutes, the $\%N_2$ displayed on the graph of the washout is 3.7%. This is consistent with:
a. Severe obstructive lung disease
b. Severe restrictive disease
c. Increased intrapulmonary shunting
d. Normal distribution of ventilation

5. Radioactive xenon is well-suited for assessing regional ventilation because:
a. It is quickly metabolized in the liver
b. It decays completely in about 45 mintues
c. It is relatively insoluble so it remains in the gas phase
d. All of the above

6. In subjects who have obstructive lung disease, breathing air after rebreathing ^{133}Xe will show:
a. ^{133}Xe trapped in poorly ventilated regions
b. A rapid washout of ^{133}Xe from poorly ventilated regions
c. Better ventilation at the bases of the lungs
d. Areas with the greatest pulmonary blood flow

7. Perfusion lung scanning is performed using:
a. ^{81m}Krypton gas
b. ^{99m}Tc macroaggregated albumin
c. ^{99m}Tc human albumin microspheres
d. All of the above
e. b and c only

8. Ventilation and perfusion scans of healthy persons sitting upright show:
   a. $\dot{V}/\dot{Q}$ ratios of 4.0 to 5.0 throughout the lung
   b. $\dot{V}/\dot{Q}$ ratios of 0.8 to 1.0 in most lung units
   c. Most gas exchange occuring at the apices of the lungs
   d. Little or no gas exchange in the middle lung sections

9. A 7-minute nitrogen washout test is plotted on semilog paper; after about the first minute of O_2 breathing, the N_2 concentration begins to show a steady rise of about 4% per minute. This could be best explained by:
   a. A leak in either the breathing or analyzer circuit
   b. Uneven ventilation due to small airways obstruction
   c. Pulmonary blood flow in excess of ventilation
   d. Severe air trapping

10. Which of the following might be abnormal in a subject who has early small airways obstruction:
    I. CV/VC ratio
    II. Slope of Phase III
    III. 7-minute N_2 washout
    IV. Viso$\dot{V}$ (Volume of isoflow)
    a. I, II, III, IV   c. I, III, IV
    b. I, II, IV   d. II, IV

SELECTED BIBLIOGRAPHY

General references

Bouhuys A: Distribution of inspired gas in the lungs. In Fenn WO and Rahn H, editors: Handbook of physiology—respiration I, Washington, DC, 1964, American Physiological Society.

Comroe JH and Fowler WS: Lung function studies VI: detection of uneven alveolar ventilation during a single breath of oxygen, Am J Med 10:408, 1951.

Darling RC, Cournand A, and Richards DW: Studies of intrapulmonary mixture of gases. V. Forms of inadequate ventilation in normal and emphysematous lungs analyzed by means of breathing pure oxygen, J Clin Invest 23:55, 1944.

Fowler WS: Lung function studies III: uneven pulmonary ventilation in normal subjects and in patients with pulmonary disease, J Appl Physiol 2:283, 1949.

Hathirat S, Renzetti AD, and Mitchell M: Intrapulmonary gas distribution: a comparison of the helium mixing time and nitrogen single breath test in normal and diseased subjects, Am Rev Respir Dis 102:750, 1970.

Shinokazi T, et al: Theory of a digital nitrogen washout computer, J Appl Physiol 21:202, 1966.

Closing volume

Abboud R and Morton J: Comparison of maximal mid-expiratory flow, flow-volume curves, and nitrogen closing volumes in patients with mild airway obstruction, Am Rev Respir Dis 111:405, 1975.

Becklake MR and Permutt S: Evaluation of tests of lung function for "screening" for early detection of chronic obstructive lung disease. In Maclem PT and Permutt S, editors: The lung in transition between health and disease, New York, 1979, Marcel Dekker, Inc.

Berend N, Glanville AR, and Grunstein MM: Determinants of the slope of phase III of the single breath nitrogen test, Bull Eur Physiopathol Respir 20:521, 1984.

Buist AS and Ross BB: Predicted values for closing volumes using a modified single breath nitrogen test, Am Rev Respir Dis 107:744, 1973.

Cormier Y and Belanger J: The role of gas exchange in phase IV of the single breath nitrogen test, Am Rev Respir Dis 125:396, 1982.

MacFadden ER, Holmes B, and Kiker R: Variability of closing volume measurements in normal man, Am Rev Respir Dis 111:135, 1975.

Make B and Lapp NL: Factors influencing the measurement of closing volume, Am Rev Respir Dis 111:749, 1975.

Martin R and Macklem PT: Suggested standardization procedures for closing volume determinations (nitrogen method), Division Health and Disease, National Heart, Lung and Blood Institute, 1973.

McCarthy DS, et al: Measurement of closing volume as a simple and sensitive test for early detection of small airway disease, Am J Med 52:747, 1972.

Lung scans

Bernier DR, Zangman JK, and Wells LD: Nuclear medicine technology and techniques, ed 2, St. Louis: 1988, The Mosby Co.

Dolfuss RE, Milic-Emili J, and Bates DV: Regional ventilation of the lung studied with boluses of 133 Xenon, Respir Physiol 2:234, 1967.

Secker-Walker RH and Siegal BA: The use of nuclear medicine in the diagnosis of lung disease, Radiol Clin North Am 11:215, 1973.

5

Diffusion Tests

CARBON MONOXIDE DIFFUSING CAPACITY (DL_{CO})

Description

Carbon monoxide (CO) diffusing capacity (DL_{CO} or D_{CO}) measures the transfer of a diffusion-limited gas (CO) across the alveolocapillary membrane. The DL_{CO} is reported in milliliters of CO per minute per millimeter of mercury at 0°C, 760 mm Hg, dry, (i.e., STPD).

Technique

Carbon monoxide (CO) combines with hemoglobin (Hb) about 210 times more readily than O_2 does, but otherwise it acts similarly to O_2. In the presence of normal amounts of Hb and normal ventilatory function, the primary limiting factor to diffusion of CO is the status of the alveolocapillary membrane. Small amounts of CO in inspired gas produce measurable changes in the concentration of inspired versus expired gas. Because there is little or no CO in pulmonary capillary blood, the pressure gradient causing diffusion is basically the alveolar pressure of CO (PA_{CO}).

There are several methods for determining the DL_{CO} (Table 5-1), all of which use the general equation:

$$DL_{CO} = \frac{\dot{V}CO}{PA_{CO} - Pc_{CO}}$$

where

$\dot{V}CO$ = Milliliters of CO transferred per minute (STPD)

PA_{CO} = Mean alveolar partial pressure of CO

Pc_{CO} = Mean capillary partial pressure of CO, usually assumed to be zero

Diffusing capacity is essentially a measure of conductance of CO across the alveolocapillary membranes, that is, milliliters of gas per minute per unit of driving pressure. An additional method of quantifying diffusing capacity, fractional uptake of CO, simply relates the inspired and expired CO concentrations during normal breathing.

Modified Krogh technique—single-breath ($DL_{CO}SB$). The subject inspires a VC breath from a spirometer or reservoir (Fig. 5-1) containing a gas mixture of 0.3% CO, 10% He, 21% O_2, and the remainder N_2, then

Table 5-1 Advantages and disadvantages of testing methods

Method	Technique	Advantages	Disadvantages	Application
$DL_{CO}SB$ (breath-hold)	He and CO analysis relatively simple; 10 seconds breath-hold	Easy calculations, simple; fast; no COHb back pressure; can be automated	Sensitive to distribution of ventilation and $\dot{V}/\dot{Q}$; "nonphysiologic;" not practical for exercise	Screening and clinical application; good standardization
$DL_{CO}SS_1$ (Filey technique)	CO, CO_2, O_2 analysis; arterial blood sample; relatively simple	Most accurate steady-state method; good for exercise testing	Arterial puncture and blood gas analysis; sensitive to uneven $\dot{V}/\dot{Q}$	Clinical application; exercise studies
$DL_{CO}SS_2$ (end-tidal CO)	End-tidal sample, FU_{CO} simultaneously; CO analysis only	No arterial puncture or breath-hold; easy calculation	COHb back pressure; V_T must be maintained high; very sensitive to $\dot{V}/\dot{Q}$;	Fast, easy screening and clinical method; not used for exercise studies
$DL_{CO}SS_3$ (assumed V_D)	CO analysis (slow or fast); large V_T improves accuracy	Relatively simple calculations; good for exercise study	Large error if V_T is too small; sensitive to COHb	Screening and clinical applications; exercise studies
$DL_{CO}SS_4$ (mixed venous P_{CO_2}	CO, CO_2 analysis; rebreathing required	No arterial puncture; easy calculations; slow CO analyzer acceptable	Sensitive to COHb; rebreathing must be closely controlled	Not yet widely used clinically
$DL_{CO}RB$ (rebreathing)	He and CO analysis (rapid); rebreathing required	Less sensitive to V_A than $DL_{CO}SB$; less sensitive to $\dot{V}/\dot{Q}$ abnormalities	Complex calculations; rapid CO and He analyzers required; sensitive to COHb	Clinically applicable; provides most accurate DL_{CO}
$DL_{CO}SS_{He}$ (equilibration washout)	CO, He analysis rapid; sequencing required	Eliminates V_A, $\dot{V}/\dot{Q}$, and distribution problems	Complex calculations (computerized)	Research applications
FU_{CO} (fractional CO uptake)	CO analysis; may be done with $DL_{CO}SS_2$	Simple; CO analysis of inspired and expired gas only	Sensitive to $\dot{V}_E$, $\dot{V}/\dot{Q}$, and V_D/V_T	Screening or correlation to $DL_{CO}SS_2$
$1/Dm + 1/\theta Vc$ (membrane and red blood cell resistance)	$DL_{CO}SB$ repeated before and after O_2 breathing	Differentiates membrane from red blood cell components; calculates VC	Complex calculations; estimates of alveolar P_{O_2} critical	Research with limited clinical applications

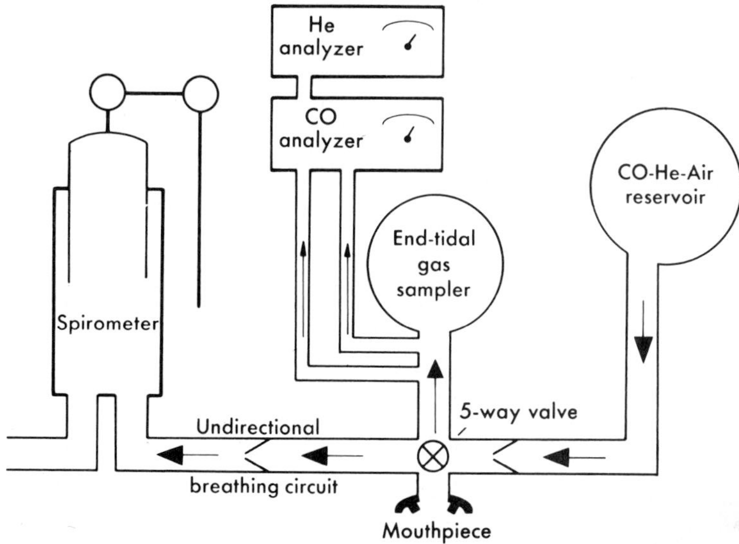

Fig. 5-1 DL_{CO} apparatus. The basic equipment for performing the DL_{CO} test (specifically the $DL_{CO}SB$) is illustrated. Included is a CO-He-air reservoir, which may be a large-volume bag, a sealed spirometer, or a demand valve system connected directly to a tank of special gas mixture. A multidirectional valve, which may be automatic or manual, allows rapid switching of the breathing gases and directs exhaled gas to the end-tidal sampler or spirometer, or both. A method of measuring the inspired volume is also required, and is usually accomplished by using a bag-in-box or similar apparatus for the diffusion mixture reservoir. A spirometer or pneumotachometer is required to measure the exhaled volume to determine the volume of dead space to be washed out. Some systems connect the spirometer to the bag-in-box apparatus to measure both inspired and expired volumes. He and CO analyzers are used to analyze the end-tidal sample, as well as to determine inspired gas concentrations from the CO-He-air reservoir. Most automated systems include electronic timing of the maneuver, automatic switching of the valve, and direct sampling of the end-tidal gas.

holds the breath for approximately 10 seconds. The subject then expires, and a sample of alveolar gas is collected in a small volume bag (≅500 ml), after a suitable washout volume (750 ml to 1000 ml) is discarded (Fig. 5-2). The sample is analyzed to obtain the fractional CO and He concentrations in alveolar gas after a given time interval (T), FA_{CO_T} and FA_{He}, respectively. The concentration of CO in the alveolar gas at the beginning of the breath-hold, with T equal to zero (FA_{CO_0}), is computed as follows:

$$FA_{CO_0} = FI_{CO} \times \frac{FA_{He}}{FI_{He}}$$

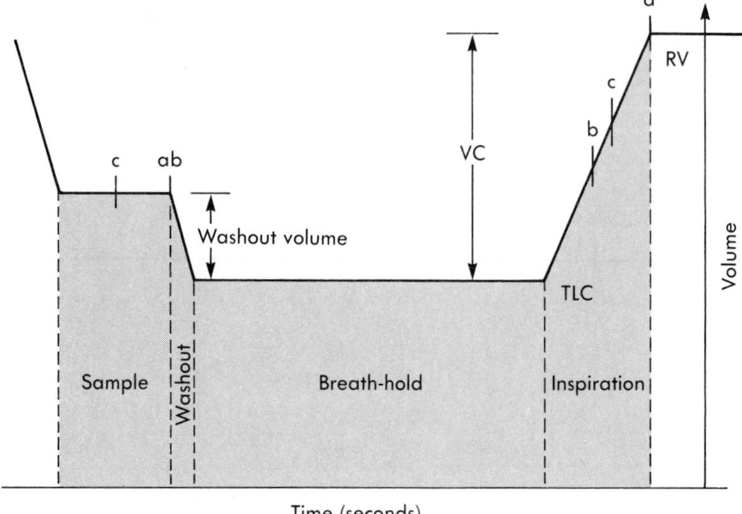

Fig. 5-2 Typical $DL_{CO}SB$ maneuver tracing. A tracing of the single-breath DL_{CO} maneuver proceeding from right to left: the subject starts from RV, inspires a VC breath rapidly to TLC, then breath-holds for approximately 10 seconds. At the end of the breath-hold, the subject exhales a fixed washout volume (usually 0.750 to 1.0 liter), then a sample of alveolar gas is taken (usually 0.5 to 1.0 liter); any remaining volume is exhaled. Various timing methods are illustrated. Method *a,* Ogilvie, considers diffusion to occur from the beginning of inspiration to the beginning of alveolar sampling; method *b,* ESP, considers diffusion to occur from the midpoint of inspiration to the beginning of alveolar sampling; method *c,* Jones, measures diffusion from two thirds of the inspired VC to the midpoint of the alveolar sample.

where

FA_{CO_0} = Fraction of CO at the beginning of the breath-hold (time = 0)
FI_{CO} = Fraction of CO in the reservoir (usually 0.003)
FA_{He} = Fraction of He in alveolar gas in the end-tidal sample
FI_{He} = Fraction of He in inspired gas (known)

The $DL_{CO}SB$ is then calculated as follows:

$$DL_{CO}SB = \frac{V_A \times 60}{(P_B - 47) \times (T)} \times \operatorname{Ln} \frac{FA_{CO_0}}{FA_{CO_T}}$$

where

V_A = Alveolar volume (STPD)
60 = Correction from seconds to minutes
P_B = Barometric pressure
47 = Water vapor pressure (PH_2O) at 37°C

T = Breath-hold interval (usually 10 seconds)
Ln = Natural logarithm
$F_{A_{CO_0}}$ = Fraction of CO in alveolar gas at the beginning of the breath-hold, before diffusion
$F_{A_{CO_T}}$ = Fraction of CO in alveolar gas at the end of diffusion

V_A may be calculated from the single-breath dilution of He as follows:

$$V_A = \frac{V_I}{F_{A_{He}}/F_{I_{He}}} \times \text{STPD correction factor}$$

where

V_I = Volume of test gas inspired (Fig. 5-2)
$F_{A_{HE}}$ = Fraction of He in alveolar gas
$F_{I_{HE}}$ = Fraction of He in inspired gas (known)

A simplification of the above single-breath method is widely employed. If both the He and CO analyzers are calibrated to read full scale (100% or 1.000) when sampling the diffusion mixture, and the analyzers are set to zero appropriately, the $F_{A_{He}}$ obtained from the end-tidal sample equals the $F_{A_{CO_0}}$. The assumption here is that both He and CO are diluted equally during inspiration. The logarithmic ratio of CO disappearance from the alveoli can then be expressed as follows:

$$Ln = \frac{F_{A_{He}}}{F_{A_{CO_T}}}$$

where

$F_{A_{He}}$ = Fraction of He in the alveolar sample, equal to $F_{A_{CO_0}}$
$F_{A_{CO_T}}$ = Fraction of CO in the alveolar sample after the breath-hold

This technique avoids the necessity of analyzing the absolute concentrations of the two gases, but requires that both analyzers be linear. Because analysis of CO is often done using infrared analyzers (see Chapter 9), and their output is nonlinear, care must be taken to ensure that corrected CO readings are used in the computation. This correction is easily accomplished either electronically or via software in automated systems. Corrections must be made for anatomic V_D and inspired dead space in the valve, and for expired dead space in the sample bag. All lung volumes must be corrected from ATPS to STPD for the $D_{L_{CO}}$ calculations; however, the V_A, when used to calculate the ratio of diffusing capacity to lung volume (D_L/V_A), is normally expressed in BTPS units. Two or more tests are usually averaged, with 4 minutes of delay between repeated maneuvers to allow for washout of the test gas from the lungs. Corrections for abnormal Hb concentrations should be applied, and corrections for carboxyhemoglobin (COHb) in the subject's blood and the effects of altitude may be necessary. Subjects should be asked to refrain from smoking for 24 hours before the test to reduce the CO back pressure in the blood.

Filey technique—steady state ($DL_{CO}SS_1$). The subject breathes a gas mixture of 0.1% to 0.2% CO in air for 5 to 6 minutes. During the final 2 minutes, expired gas is collected in a Douglas bag and an arterial blood sample is drawn. The exhaled volume is measured and the expired gas is analyzed for CO, CO_2, and O_2. The arterial blood is analyzed to determine PCO_2. Steady-state diffusing capacity is calculated using the following equation:

$$DL_{CO}SS_1 = \frac{\dot{V}_{CO}}{PA_{CO}}$$

where

$\dot{V}_{CO}$ = Volume of CO transferred in milliliters per minute (STPD)
PA_{CO} = Mean alveolar partial pressure of CO

$\dot{V}_{CO}$ is determined from an analysis of the fractional inspired and expired CO (FI_{CO} and FE_{CO} respectively), the $\dot{V}E$, and the fractional inspired N_2 and the fractional expired N_2 (FI_{N_2}), which is known, (FE_{N_2}), which is determined indirectly from the fractions of O_2, CO_2, and H_2O vapor in the exhaled gas as follows:

$$\dot{V}_{CO} = \dot{V}E(FI_{CO}\frac{FE_{N_2}}{FI_{N_2}} - FE_{CO})$$

The PA_{CO} is determined using a form of the Bohr equation, as follows:

$$PA_{CO} = PB - 47\,\frac{(FE_{CO} - rFI_{CO})}{1 - r}$$

where

$$r = \frac{Pa_{CO_2} - PE_{CO_2}}{PE_{CO_2}}$$

where

Pa_{CO_2} = Partial pressure of arterial CO_2
PE_{CO_2} = Partial pressure of expired CO_2

Estimating PA_{CO} in this way avoids the necessity of obtaining a direct alveolar sample.

End-tidal CO determination ($DL_{CO}SS_2$). The $DL_{CO}SS_2$ method is basically the same as the $DL_{CO}SS_1$, in that the $\dot{V}_{CO}$ is derived similarly. PA_{CO}, however, is determined by taking the average end-tidal CO tension (PET_{CO}) from instantaneous analysis of multiple breaths. The end-tidal value is assumed to equal the mean PA_{CO}.

Assumed VD technique ($DL_{CO}SS_3$). The $DL_{CO}SS_3$ method is similar to the $DL_{CO}SS_1$. $\dot{V}_{CO}$ is determined as in $DL_{CO}SS_1$, but the PA_{CO} is measured differently. The fraction of CO in alveolar gas (FA_{CO}), which can be used to derive PA_{CO} when PB is known, is computed as follows:

$$F_{A_{CO}} = \frac{V_T(F_{E_{CO}}) - V_D(F_{I_{CO}})}{V_T - V_D}$$

where

V_T = Tidal volume
V_D = Dead space volume
$F_{E_{CO}}$ = Fraction of expired CO
$F_{I_{CO}}$ = Fraction of inspired CO

V_T is measured by averaging multiple breaths. V_D is often assumed to be equal to 1 milliliter per pound of body weight. The mechanical V_D of the breathing circuit is subtracted.

Mixed venous P_{CO_2} technique ($D_{L_{CO}}SS_4$). $\dot{V}_{CO}$ is obtained as in $D_{L_{CO}}SS_1$. The $P_{A_{CO}}$ is calculated by estimating the partial pressure of mixed venous CO_2 ($P\bar{v}_{CO_2}$) from an equilibration technique, then determining the $P_{A_{CO_2}}$ from the $P\bar{v}_{CO_2}$ and the normal gradient. Once the $P_{A_{CO_2}}$ is derived, an equation similar to that used to determine $P_{A_{CO}}$ in the $D_{L_{CO}}SS_1$ technique can be employed. Using mixed venous P_{CO_2} avoids the necessity of arterial puncture.

Rebreathing technique ($D_{L_{CO}}RB$). The subject rebreathes from a reservoir containing a mixture of 0.3% CO, 10% He, and the remainder air for 30 to 60 seconds at a rate of about 30 breaths per minute. After this interval, measurements of the final CO, He, and O_2 concentrations in the reservoir are made. An equation similar to that used for the single-breath technique is used (see $D_{L_{CO}}SB$):

$$D_{L_{CO}}RB = \frac{V_S \times 60}{(P_B - 47)(T2 - T1)} \times \mathrm{Ln}\,\frac{F_{A_{CO_{T1}}}}{F_{A_{CO_{T2}}}}$$

where

V_S = Volume of the lung reservoir system (initial volume $\times$ $F_{I_{He}}/F_{A_{He}}$)
60 = Correction from seconds to minutes
P_B = Barometric pressure
47 = Water vapor pressure (P_{H_2O}) at 37°C
T2 − T1 = Rebreathing interval
Ln = Natural logarithm
$F_{A_{CO_{T1}}}$ = Fraction of CO in alveolar gas before diffusion
$F_{A_{CO_{T2}}}$ = Fraction of CO in alveolar gas at the end of diffusion

Equilibration—washout method ($D_{L_{CO}}SS_{He}$). The subject rebreathes from a reservoir containing 0.3% CO, 10% He, and the remainder air until equilibrium is reached. Then the subject again breathes room air, and the washouts of both CO and He are recorded by a rapid gas analyzer. During the washout, CO is removed at a rapid rate by diffusion as well as by ventilation, while He is removed more slowly by ventilation alone. The difference in washout rates is caused by the rate of CO diffusion. An equation similar to the $DL_{CO}SB$ equation is used to calculate $DL_{CO}SS_{He}$; a logarithmic expression of the ratio of final He concentration to initial He concentration is included as a factor along with the CO concentration ratio. Representation of these washout curves in real time normally requires computerization.

Fractional CO uptake (FU_{CO}). The subject first inspires a mixture of 0.1% CO in air from a reservoir to establish a steady-state breathing pattern, then expires into a spirometer or reservoir, from which an average expired CO sample is analyzed. The FU_{CO} is expressed as:

$$FU_{CO} = \frac{FI_{CO} - FE_{CO}}{FI_{CO}}$$

where

FI_{CO} = Fraction of inspired CO
FE_{CO} = Fraction of expired CO

The resultant fraction may be multiplied by 100 and expressed as a percentage. The level of $\dot{V}E$ is critical for a valid determination of FU_{CO} and should be monitored closely.

Membrane diffusion coefficient (Dm) and capillary blood volume (Qc). The subject performs two $DL_{CO}SB$ tests, each at a different level of alveolar P_{O_2}. The first $DL_{CO}SB$ is performed as outlined previously. The subject then breathes a high concentration of O_2, with the balance being N_2, for approximately 5 minutes, and then immediately exhales to RV and performs the second $DL_{CO}SB$ maneuver. The DL_{CO} values are calculated for both the air and O_2 breathing maneuvers. The total resistance caused by the alveolocapillary membrane (Dm) and the resistance caused by the rate of chemical combination with Hb and transfer into the red blood cell (θQc) is calculated according to the following equation:

$$1/DL_{CO} = 1/Dm + 1/\theta Qc$$

where

$1/DL_{CO}$ = Reciprocal of diffusing capacity, or resistance
$1/Dm$ = Alveolocapillary membrane resistance
$1/\theta Qc$ = Resistance caused by the red blood cell membrane and rate of reaction with Hb
θ = Transfer rate of CO per milliliter of capillary blood
Qc = Capillary blood volume

Because CO and O_2 compete for binding sites on Hb, measurement of diffusion of CO at different levels of PO_2 can be used to distinguish resistance caused by the alveolocapillary membrane from resistance caused by the red blood cell membrane and Hb reaction rate. Qc is presumed to remain the same for both tests, but θ varies in response to changes in PO_2.

By plotting θ at two points against $1/D_{L_{CO}}$ and extrapolating back to zero, as if no O_2 were present, the resistance caused by the alveolocapillary membrane can be calculated.

Significance

The average $D_{L_{CO}}$ value for resting subjects using the single-breath method is 25 ml CO/min/mm Hg (STPD). Regression equations for calculation of normal values are included in the Appendix. Values derived using steady-state methods are usually slightly less than values obtained using the single-breath method in healthy subjects, but may vary by as much as 30%. Females have slightly lower normal values, presumably in correlation with smaller normal lung volumes. $D_{L_{CO}}$ values can increase two to three times in healthy individuals during exercise. Diffusing capacity is generally decreased in alveolar fibrosis associated with sarcoidosis, asbestosis, beryl-liosis, O_2 toxicity, or silicosis. These states are sometimes categorized as "diffusion defects," although they are probably more closely related to the loss of lung volume, alveolar surface area, or capillary bed. Restrictive disease patterns typically result in reductions in $D_{L_{CO}}$. Diffusion capacity is decreased by parenchymal loss or replacement, space-occupying lesions, pulmonary edema, and lung resection. Many drugs cause reductions in $D_{L_{CO}}$ because of their effects on the alveolocapillary membranes; diffusing capacity is sometimes used to monitor drug toxicity.

$D_{L_{CO}}$ is decreased in emphysema because of the decrease in surface area, loss of capillary bed, increased distance from the terminal bronchiole to the alveolocapillary membrane, and mismatching of ventilation and blood flow. Other obstructive processes, such as bronchitis and asthma, may not reduce the diffusing capacity unless they result in markedly abnormal ventilation/perfusion ($\dot{V}/\dot{Q}$) patterns. Abnormalities in Hb, either in concentration or structure, may result in spurious $D_{L_{CO}}$ values. Therefore, $D_{L_{CO}}$ values are usually corrected as described in the following material.

Table 5-1 compares some of the advantages and disadvantages of the different $D_{L_{CO}}$ testing methods discussed in this chapter.

The $D_{L_{CO}}SB$ is the most widely used method because of its relative simplicity and noninvasive nature. The rapidity with which repeated maneuvers can be performed also lends to its popularity. Many automated systems use the $D_{L_{CO}}SB$, thus contributing a certain degree of standardization to the methodology. There is, however, a large variability in reported results between laboratories. This variability has been attributed to differing testing techniques, problems in the gas analysis involved in the test, and differences in computations. In addition, because breath-holding at TLC is not a physiologic maneuver, and the measured value of $D_{L_{CO}}$ varies with lung volume while holding the breath, the $D_{L_{CO}}SB$ may not be an entirely accurate description of diffusing capacity. The $D_{L_{CO}}SB$ is not practical for use during exercise, and some subjects have difficulty expiring fully, inspiring fully, or breath-holding. The American Thoracic Society has published guidelines to improve standardization of the single-breath maneuver. See Chapter 11 for criteria for acceptability for DL_{CO} maneuvers.

The steady-state methods, ($DL_{CO}SS_{1\ to\ 4}$), use various techniques to estimate PA_{CO}. $DL_{CO}SS_1$ probably has the broadest application of the steady-state methods, and the availability of arterial blood gas analysis has enabled more common usage. The $DL_{CO}SS_2$ is gaining in popularity because of the availability of fast response CO analyzers (Chapter 9) and is often done in combination with the FU_{CO}. The $DL_{CO}SS_3$ is commonly used for measurement of diffusion capacity during exercise, since small differences in the assumed VD become less significant when the VT increases. All of the steady-state methods can be applied to exercise testing.

The rebreathing method is more complicated in terms of the calculations involved but offers the advantage of a normal breathing pattern without arterial puncture. $DL_{CO}RB$ is less sensitive to $\dot{V}/\dot{Q}$ abnormalities and uneven ventilation distribution than either the $DL_{CO}SB$ or the steady-state methods. The rebreathing method and the steady-state methods may suffer from some inaccuracy because of a buildup of COHb in the capillary blood and the resultant back pressure. Capillary PCO is routinely assumed to be zero, but the actual alveolocapillary gradient at the time of testing can be estimated, though with some difficulty.

$DL_{CO}SS_{He}$ is the most sophisticated technique. It is relatively insensitive to $\dot{V}/\dot{Q}$ and ventilation abnormalities. However, it requires computerization, and is probably limited to research applications.

Measurement of the membrane and red blood cell components of diffusion resistance has revealed that each component accounts for approximately half of the total resistance. Difficulty in quantifying the partial pressure of O_2 in the lungs (i.e., in the pulmonary capillaries) restricts the use of the membrane-diffusing capacity determination.

Since DL_{CO} is directly related to VA, expression of this relationship is often useful in differentiating disease processes in which there may be decreased DL_{CO} as a direct result of loss of lung volume (i.e., restrictive diseases) from those in which decreased DL_{CO} is caused by uneven $\dot{V}/\dot{Q}$ or uneven distribution of inspired gas (i.e., obstructive diseases). As an index, the measured DL_{CO} may be divided by the lung volume at which the measurement was made to obtain an expression of diffusing capacity per unit of lung volume (VL). This is recorded as the DL/VL or DL/VA and may be accomplished easily, since the VA must be calculated to derive the DL_{CO}. In healthy subjects, the DL/VL is approximately 4 to 5 (i.e., 4 to 5 ml of CO transferred per minute, per liter of lung volume). In obstruction, loss of DL_{CO} without reduction in lung volume results in a low ratio. In restriction, the loss of DL_{CO} parallels the loss of lung volume and the ratio is preserved.

Numerous other factors can influence the observed DL_{CO}:

1. Hematocrit (Hct) and Hb—Decreased Hct and Hb reduce the DL_{CO}, while increased Hb and Hct elevate the DL_{CO}); the DL_{CO} may

be corrected if the subject's Hb is known. CO uptake varies approximately 7% for each gram of Hb; the measured DL_{CO} may be adjusted so that the value reported is standardized to an Hb of approximately 14.6 gm%. The adjustment factor may be calculated as follows:

$$\text{Hb correction} = \frac{10.22 + \text{Hb}}{1.7 \times \text{Hb}}$$

The DL_{CO} may then be corrected:

$$\text{Hb adjusted } DL_{CO} = \text{Hb correction} \times \text{observed } DL_{CO}$$

It should be noted that when this correction is applied, the DL_{CO} will be reduced for Hb values greater than 14.6, and increased for Hb values less than 14.6. Both the corrected and uncorrected values should be reported.

2. Alveolar P_{CO_2}—increased P_{CO_2} raises DL_{CO} because the alveolar P_{O_2} is necessarily decreased; significant increases in the alveolar P_{CO_2} lower the alveolar P_{O_2}.
3. COHb—Elevated carboxyhemoglobin (COHb) levels, as found in smokers, reduce DL_{CO}; smokers may have COHb levels of 5% to 10% or even greater, causing significant CO back pressure, as well as an anemia-like effect. In practice, each 1% increase in the COHb level in the blood causes an approximate 1% decrease in the measured DL_{CO}. The DL_{CO} may be adjusted, as follows:

   $$\text{COHb adjusted } DL_{CO} = \text{Measured } DL_{CO} \times (1.00 + [\%\text{COHb}/100])$$

   CO back pressure corrections can also be made by estimating the partial pressure of CO in the pulmonary capillaries and correcting the FA_{CO_0} and the FA_{CO_T}.
4. Pulmonary capillary blood volume—Increased Qc increases DL_{CO}.
5. Body position—Supine position increases DL_{CO}; changes in body position affect the distribution of capillary blood flow.
6. Altitude—Increasing altitude and a constant fractional concentration of O_2 will result in increasing DL_{CO}. Adjustments for differences in altitude may be applied by correcting either the PA_{O_2} or the PI_{O_2}. For a PA_{O_2} of 120 mm Hg:

   $$\text{Altitude adjusted } DL_{CO} = \text{measured } DL_{CO} \times (1.0 + 0.0035[PA_{O_2} - 120])$$

   For a PI_{O_2} of 150 mm Hg (sea level):

   $$\text{Altitude adjusted } DL_{CO} = \text{measured } DL_{CO} \times (1.0 + 0.0031[PI_{O_2} - 150])$$

Several technical considerations may affect the measurement of the DL_{CO} (particularly the $DL_{CO}SB$). Calculation of VA from He dilution during the single-breath maneuver may result in an underestimate of the lung volume in subjects who have moderate or severe obstruction. Low estimated V_A values result in low DL_{CO} values. Some clinicians prefer to use a previously determined lung volume to estimate V_A. RV, as measured by one of the foreign gas techniques, or by plethysmography, can be added to the inspired volume to derive V_A. However, V_A calculated in this way is typically larger in subjects who have obstruction than V_A calculated using the single-breath dilution technique, resulting in a larger estimated DL_{CO} value. This approach may not be valid since the single-breath He dilution value (FA_{He}) is also used to derive the logarithmic ratio that describes the disappearance of CO from the alveoli. Some laboratories report DL_{CO} calculated by both methods.

Various methods of measuring the breath-holding time may also lead to differing DL_{CO} values (see Fig. 5-2). Most systems measure breath-holding time using one of three methods: 1. Ogilvie method—From the beginning of inspiration (V_I) to the beginning of alveolar sampling. 2. Epidemiology Standardization Project (ESP) method—From the mid-point of inspiration (½ of the V_I) to the beginning of alveolar sampling. 3. Jones method—From the ⅔ point of inspiration to the mid-point of the alveolar sample.

Theoretically, the breath-holding time is considered the time during which diffusion occurs. However, because some gas transfer may take place early in inspiration, DL_{CO} may be greater if timing starts at the mid-V_I point, as when the ESP method is used. Similarly, some diffusion may occur during alveolar sampling. If the timing period is extended into the alveolar sampling phase, using the Jones method, the actual time of breath-holding is increased and the additional diffusion accounted for. The exact timing method may become significant if the predicted values used for comparison were generated by one of the other methods. Rapid inspiration and rapid expiration to the alveolar sampling phase reduce the differences resulting from the timing methods.

The volume of gas discarded before collecting the alveolar sample may affect the measured DL_{CO}. Most automated systems allow variable washout volumes, with 0.75 L to 1.0 L being most commonly used. Washout volume may need to be reduced when the subject's VC is less than 2.0 L. In subjects who have obstructive disease, reducing the washout volume may result in an increased volume of dead space gas being added to the alveolar sample. Since dead space gas resembles the diffusion mixture, DL_{CO} tends to be underestimated.

Alveolar sampling technique also affects the measurement of DL_{CO}. If alveolar gas is collected for longer than 3 seconds, DL_{CO} will increase if the Ogilvie timing method is used. A sample volume of 0.5 to 1.0 liters is commonly used; subjects with VC values of less than 2.0 L may require a smaller volume, just as with the washout volume. If only a very small sample is obtained, the gas may not accurately reflect the alveolar concentrations of CO and He, particularly in the presence of $\dot{V}/\dot{Q}$ abnormalities. Continuous analysis of the expirate using a mass spectrometer allows better identification of alveolar gas, but this method is not yet practical for clinical use. Other procedural considerations related to the acceptability and reproducibility of the $DL_{CO}SB$ are included in Chapter 11.

SELF-ASSESSMENT QUESTIONS

1. Carbon monoxide is used to measure diffusion instead of oxygen because:
   a. It does not react with hemoglobin
   b. It diffuses more slowly than O_2
   c. There is little or no CO in capillary blood
   d. All of the above

2. In the $DL_{CO}SB$ method, helium is used to:
   a. Estimate the FA_{CO_0}
   b. Measure dead space, VD
   c. Measure alveolar volume, VA
   d. All of the above
   e. a and c only

3. Which of the following DL_{CO} methods requires an arterial blood gas to allow calculation of the PACO?
   a. $DL_{CO}SB$
   b. $DL_{CO}SS_1$
   c. $DL_{CO}SS_2$
   d. All of the above
   e. a and c only

4. The membrane diffusion coefficient (resistance to diffusion by the alveolocapillary membrane) is estimated by:
   a. The $DL_{CO}SS_{He}$ method
   b. Dividing the DL_{CO} by the PA_{O_2}
   c. Performing the $DL_{CO}SB$ test at two different levels of alveolar O_2 tension
   d. Subtracting $FA_{CO_{T1}}$ from $FA_{CO_{T2}}$ obtained from the $DL_{CO}RB$

5. The average $DL_{CO}SB$ for healthy adults is approximately 25 ml CO/min/mm Hg; the DL_{CO} by the steady-state methods is usually:
   a. Slightly less
   b. Slightly higher
   c. Two to three times that of the $DL_{CO}SB$
   d. Equal to the $DL_{CO}SB$

6. DL_{CO} may be decreased in emphysema due to:
   I. Increased distance from terminal bronchiole to aveolocapillary membrane
   II. Decreased surface area

III. Loss of pulmonary capillary bed
IV. Ventilation/perfusion abnormalities
a. I, II, III, IV
b. II, III, IV
c. II, IV
d. III only

7. Which of the following factors might account for a decreased DL_{CO} in the absence of pulmonary disease?
I. Measurements made at altitude
II. Decreased hemoglobin (anemia)
III. Increased capillary blood volume
IV. Elevated carboxyhemoglobin (COHb)
a. I, II, III, IV
b. I, III, IV
c. II, III, IV
d. II and IV only

8. A subject who smokes has a COHb of 10% and a DL_{CO} of 12; if the observed value were adjusted for the increased CO level, the "corrected" DL_{CO} would be:
a. Slightly higher
b. Slightly lower
c. About the same
d. Cannot be determined without Hb concentration

9. If VA is calculated from a multiple-breath lung volume technique and then used to compute DL_{CO} in a subject who has severe obstruction, the resulting DL_{CO} will be ________ ________ the DL_{CO} calculated from a single-breath dilution of He.
a. Equal to
b. Larger than
c. Smaller than
d. Either a or c

10. Differences in the calculation of $DL_{CO}SB$ due to the timing of the breath-hold period may be minimized by:
a. Having the subject practice breath-holding before testing
b. Measuring breath-hold from the mid-point of inspiration
c. Having the subject inspire and expire rapidly
d. Limiting the breath-hold to less than 9 seconds

SELECTED BIBLIOGRAPHY

General references

Bates DV, Macklem PT, and Christie RV: Respiratory function in disease, Philadelphia, 1971, WB Saunders Co.

Cotes JE: Lung function assessment and application in medicine, ed 4, Boston, 1979, Blackwell Scientific Publications, Inc.

Ferris BG, editor: Epidemiology standardization project: recommended standardized procedure for pulmonary function testing, Am Rev Respir Dis 118(suppl 2:55):1, 1978.

Forster RE: Diffusion of gases, In Fenn WO and Rahn H, editors: Handbook of physiology—respiration I, Washington, DC, 1964, American Physiological Society.

McNeill RS, Rankin J, and Forster RE: The diffusing capacity of the pulmonary membrane and the pulmonary capillary blood volume in cardiopulmonary disease, Clin Sci 17:465, 1958.

Morris AH, et al: Clinical pulmonary function testing, ed 2, Salt Lake City, 1984, Intermountain Thoracic Society.

Symonds G, Renzetti AD Jr, and Mitchell MM: The diffusing capacity in pulmonary emphysema, Am Rev Respir Dis 109:391, 1974.

West JB: Pulmonary pathophysiology: the essentials, ed 3, Baltimore, 1987, Williams & Wilkins.

$DL_{CO}SB$

Cotes JE, et al: Iron-deficiency anaemia: its effects on transfer factor for the lung (diffusing capacity) and ventilation and cardiac frequency during submaximal exercise, Clin Sci 42:325, 1972.

Crapo RO and Morris AH: Standardized single breath normal values for carbon monoxide diffusing capacity, Am Rev Respir Dis 123:185, 1981.

Dinakara P, et al: The effect of anemia on pulmonary diffusing capacity with derivation of a correction equation, Am Rev Respir Dis 102:965, 1970.

Gaensler EA and Smith AA: Attachment for automated single breath diffusing capacity measurement, Chest 63:136, 1973.

Graham BL, Mink JT, and Cotton DJ: Overestimation of the single breath carbon monoxide diffusing capacity in patients with air-flow obstruction, Am Rev Respir Dis 129:403, 1984.

Kanner RE and Crapo RO: The relationship between alveolar oxygen tension and the single breath carbon monoxide diffusing capacity, Am Rev Respir Dis 133:676, 1986.

Leech JA, et al: Diffusing capacity for carbon monoxide: the effects of different durations of breath-hold time and alveolar volume and of carbon monoxide back pressure on calculated results, Am Rev Respir Dis 132:1127, 1985.

Mohsenifar Z and Tashkin DP: Effect of carboxyhemoglobin on the single breath diffusing capacity: derivation of an empirical correction factor, Respiration 37:185, 1979.

Ogilvie CM, et al: A standardized breath-holding technique for the clinical measurement of the diffusing capacity of the lung for carbon monoxide, J Clin Invest 36:1, 1957.

$DL_{CO}SS$

Filey GF, Macintosh DJ, and Wright GW: Carbon monoxide uptake and pulmonary diffusing capacity in normal subjects at rest and during exercise, J Clin Invest 33:530, 1954.

6

Blood Gas Analysis, Capnography, and Related Tests

BLOOD pH

Description

The pH is the negative logarithm of the hydrogen ion (H^+) concentration in the blood, used as a positive number. The pH of water (7.00) is the center of the pH scale, while the physiologic range of blood pH is usually from 7.00 to 8.00.

Technique

Blood pH is measured by exposing the specimen to a glass electrode under anaerobic conditions (see Fig. 9-19). Normally, pH measurements are made at 37°C. The pH of arterial blood is related to the Pa_{CO_2} using the Henderson-Hasselbalch equation:

$$pH = pK + \log \frac{[HCO_3^-]}{[CO_2]}$$

where

pK = Negative log of dissociation constant for carbonic acid (6.1)
$[HCO_3^-]$ = Molar concentration of serum bicarbonate
$[CO_2]$ = Molar concentration of CO_2

The Pa_{CO_2}, which is measured directly by the CO_2 electrode, may be multiplied by 0.03, the solubility coefficient for CO_2, to express the Pa_{CO_2} in milliequivalent per liter (mEq/L). The equation then may be written:

$$pH = 6.1 + \log \frac{[HCO_3^-]}{0.03(Pa_{CO_2})}$$

Because the pH and P_{CO_2} are measured by the blood gas analyzer, the bicarbonate can be easily calculated. Most blood gas analyzers perform this calculation along with others to derive values such as total CO_2 (i.e., dissolved CO_2 plus HCO_3^-) and standard bicarbonate (i.e., HCO_3^- corrected to a Pa_{CO_2} of 40 mm Hg). If the Hb is measured or estimated, the base excess can be calculated. The base excess is the difference between the actual buffering capacity of the blood and the normal buffer base at a pH of 7.40, approximately 48 mEq/L; the main buffers are the HCO_3^- and the Hb. Guidelines for quality control of blood gas analysis are included in Chapter 11.

Significance

The pH of arterial blood in healthy adults averages 7.40, with a normal range of 7.35 to 7.45. Arterial pH below 7.35 constitutes acidemia; a pH above 7.45 constitutes alkalemia. A change of 0.3 pH units represents a twofold change in H^+ concentration. When the pH falls from 7.40 to 7.10, with no change in P_{CO_2}, the concentration of hydrogen ions has doubled. Conversely, if the concentration of H^+ is halved, the pH rises from 7.40 to 7.70, assuming the P_{CO_2} remains at 40 mm Hg. Changes of this magnitude represent marked abnormalities in the acid-base status of the blood, and are almost always accompanied by clinical symptoms, such as cardiac arrhythmias.

Acid-base disorders arising from respiratory origins are related to the P_{CO_2} and its transport in the form of carbonic acid (see P_{CO_2}, later in this chapter). If the pH value is outside of the normal range and the P_{CO_2} is not consistent with the observed disorder (i.e., acidemia or alkalemia), the condition is termed nonrespiratory or metabolic (Table 6-1). The HCO_3^-, although it is a calculated value (as described above), is a useful indicator of the relationship between the pH and P_{CO_2}. In the presence of acidemia (i.e., pH < 7.35) and a normal CO_2 tension (i.e., P_{CO_2} = 35 to 45 mm Hg), the HCO_3^- will be low and a nonrespiratory acidosis is present. If the P_{CO_2} is less than 35, ventilatory compensation for the acidemia is likely to be occurring, and the status would be considered partially compensated nonrespiratory (i.e., metabolic) acidosis. Complete compensation has occurred if the pH has returned to within the normal range but both the HCO_3^- and P_{CO_2} remain low.

In the presence of alkalemia (i.e., pH > 7.45) and a normal P_{CO_2} (i.e., P_{CO_2} = 35 to 45 mm Hg), the bicarbonate will be increased and a nonrespiratory (i.e., metabolic) alkalosis is present. If ventilatory compensation occurs, the P_{CO_2} will be slightly elevated. However, decreased ventilation is necessary to allow the CO_2 to rise, and may interfere with oxygenation. For this reason, the Pa_{CO_2} seldom rises above 50 to 55 mm Hg in compensation for a nonrespiratory (i.e., metabolic) alkalosis, and compensation may never be complete if the alkalosis is severe.

Combined respiratory and nonrespiratory acid-base disorders are characterized by abnormalities of both the P_{CO_2} and HCO_3^-. In combined acidosis, the P_{CO_2} is elevated (i.e., $P_{CO_2} > 45$ mm Hg) and the HCO_3^- is low (i.e., $HCO_3^- < 22$ mEq/L). In combined alkalosis the HCO_3^- is high (i.e., $HCO_3^- > 26$ mEq/L) and the P_{CO_2} is low (i.e., $P_{CO_2} < 35$ mm Hg).

Technical problems encountered in the measurement of pH include contamination of the measuring electrode by protein or blood products

Table 6-1 Acid-base status

Status	pH	P_{CO_2}	HCO_3^-
Simple disorders			
Metabolic acidosis	Low	Normal	Low
Metabolic alkalosis	High	Normal	High
Respiratory acidosis	Low	High	Normal
Respiratory alkalosis	High	Low	Normal
Compensated disorders			
Compensated respiratory acidosis, or metabolic alkalosis	Normal*	High	High
Compensated metabolic acidosis, or respiratory alkalosis	Normal*	Low	Low
Combined disorders			
Metabolic/respiratory acidosis	Low	High	Low
Metabolic/respiratory alkalosis	High	Low	High

*Compensation cannot return values to within normal limits in severe acid-base disturbances. In addition, a normal pH may result in instances where there are respiratory and metabolic disturbances that occur together but are not compensatory.

and depletion of the potassium chloride (KCl) bridge. Excessive liquid heparin in the specimen does not alter the pH because of the buffering capacity of whole blood; changes in gas tensions caused by dilution may occur. Arterial blood is normally used for pH determinations. Venous blood pH may be useful in detecting grossly abnormal acid-base disorders if an arterial sample cannot be obtained.

CARBON DIOXIDE TENSION (P_{CO_2})

Description

The P_{CO_2} is a measure of the partial pressure exerted by CO_2 in solution in the blood. The measurement is expressed in millimeters of mercury (mm Hg or torr), or in kilopascals (kPa), used in the International System of Units (1 mm Hg = 0.133 kPa).

Technique

The P_{CO_2} is measured by submitting blood to a modified pH electrode (i.e., a Severinghaus electrode) that is contained in a jacket with a Teflon membrane at its tip (see Chapter 9). Inside the jacket is a bicarbonate buffer; as CO_2 diffuses through the membrane, it combines with water to form carbonic acid (H_2CO_3). The H_2CO_3 dissociates into H^+ and HCO_3^-, thereby changing the pH of the bicarbonate buffer. The change in pH is measured by the electrode and is proportional to the P_{CO_2}. The blood must be anticoagulated and kept in an anaerobic state in an ice-water bath until analysis. The PCO_2 may also be estimated using a transcutaneous electrode. Guidelines for quality control of blood gas analysis are included in Chapter 11.

Significance

The arterial CO_2 tension (Pa_{CO_2}) of a healthy adult is approximately 40 mm Hg, and may range from 35 to 45 mm Hg. The PCO_2 of venous or mixed venous blood is seldom used clinically. The Pa_{CO_2} is inversely proportional to the alveolar ventilation ($\dot{V}A$) (see Chapter 2). When $\dot{V}A$ is decreased so that CO_2 is being produced more rapidly than it is excreted by the lungs, the Pa_{CO_2} increases, the pH falls as the subject becomes acidotic, and the condition is called hypoventilation, or respiratory acidosis. Conversely, when CO_2 is being removed by $\dot{V}A$ more rapidly than it is produced by the tissues, the Pa_{CO_2} falls, the pH rises as the subject becomes alkalotic, and the condition is called hyperventilation, or respiratory alkalosis.

In the presence of increased dead space (i.e., ventilation without perfusion) such as occurs with pulmonary embolization, high $\dot{V}E$ may be required to provide adequate $\dot{V}A$ and keep the Pa_{CO_2} within normal limits. The Pa_{CO_2} may be normal, or even reduced, in the presence of significant pulmonary disease. Subjects who have localized disorders such as lobar pneumonia may increase their $\dot{V}E$, causing more $\dot{V}A$ in functioning lung units, thus compensating for those units not participating in gas exchange. Hypoxemia is a common cause of hyperventilation, and may be seen in subjects who have asthma, emphysema, bronchitis, or foreign body obstruction. Anxiety or central nervous system disorders may also cause hyperventilation.

Increased Pa_{CO_2} (i.e., hypercapnia) is commonly found in subjects who have advanced obstructive or restrictive disease. These individuals are characterized by markedly abnormal ventilation/perfusion ($\dot{V}/\dot{Q}$) patterns and the inability to maintain adequate $\dot{V}A$. Not all subjects who have advanced pulmonary disease retain CO_2; those who do become hypercapnic often have low ventilatory response to CO_2. Their response to the increased work of breathing imposed by the obstructive or restrictive disease is to allow the CO_2 level to rise rather than to increase ventilation. The respiratory acidosis that results from the increased CO_2 tension is managed by renal compensation (see Table 6-1). Elevated Pa_{CO_2} is also seen in subjects who hypoventilate as a result of central nervous system or neuromuscular disorders. Whether CO_2 retention is the result of primary lung disease, central nervous system dysfunction, or neuromuscular disease, the pH is maintained as close to normal as possible by an increase in the HCO_3^- level in the blood. The kidneys retain and produce bicarbonate to match the increased Pa_{CO_2}. This response may completely compensate for mildly elevated Pa_{CO_2}, but seldom can produce a normal pH when the Pa_{CO_2} is greater than 65 mm Hg. When the disorder responsible for the increased Pa_{CO_2} is acute, such as foreign body aspiration, little or no renal compensation may be observed.

Hypoxemia is always present in subjects who retain CO_2 while breathing air; as alveolar CO_2 increases, alveolar O_2 decreases. If the cause of the hypercapnia is primary lung disease, either obstructive or restrictive, the hypoxemia may be more severe because of $\dot{V}/\dot{Q}$ abnormalities. O_2 therapy is commonly used in these subjects, and changes in the P_{CO_2} during breathing of supplementary O_2 must be carefully evaluated. Some subjects who have chronic hypoxemia have a decreased ventilatory response to CO_2, as noted above. O_2 administered to these individuals may cause a reduction of the hypoxic stimulus to ventilation, resulting in a further elevation of the Pa_{CO_2}. O_2 therapy must be titrated to produce acceptable Pa_{O_2} values, usually 55 to 60 mm Hg, without hypercapnia and acidosis.

Technical problems related to the measurement of P_{CO_2} usually relate to the function of the electrode. A damaged or improperly functioning membrane, due to protein contamination or blood clots, may reduce the response time of the electrode, making both calibration and measurements inaccurate. Depletion of the bicarbonate electrolyte buffer within the electrode may also reduce accuracy and cause unacceptable drift. Measurement of end-tidal CO_2 tension ($P_{ET_{CO_2}}$) is sometimes used to track the Pa_{CO_2} (see Capnography section).

OXYGEN TENSION (P_{O_2})

Description

Oxygen tension, or P_{O_2}, is a measurement of the partial pressure exerted by O_2 dissolved in the blood. It is recorded in millimeters of mercury (mm Hg or torr), or in kilopascals, (kPa), used in the International System of Units (1 mm Hg = 0.133 kPa).

Technique

The P_{O_2}, either arterial or mixed venous, is measured by exposing whole blood, obtained anaerobically, to a platinum electrode covered with a thin polypropylene membrane (i.e., a Clark electrode). O_2 molecules are reduced at the platinum cathode after diffusing through the membrane (see Chapter 9). Arterial samples are usually obtained from either the radial or brachial artery. (Before a radial artery puncture, the adequacy of collateral circulation to the subject's hand via the ulnar artery should be established by means of the modified Allen's test. With both the radial and ulnar arteries occluded, the subject is instructed to make a fist, then open the hand and relax the fingers. The ulnar artery is released while the radial artery remains occluded; the hand should be reperfused rapidly within 5 to 10 seconds if the ulnar supply is adequate. If perfusion is inadequate, an alternate site should be used.

Mixed venous samples are drawn from a pulmonary artery catheter after withdrawing a volume greater than the volume of the catheter to ensure that the sample is not diluted by the flush solution present in the catheter. Venous samples from peripheral veins are not useful for assessing oxygenation since the blood reflects only the metabolism of the area drained by that particular vein.

The blood is usually collected in a heparinized syringe and sealed from the atmosphere immediately. Specimens may be collected in either glass or plastic syringes. Small changes in Po_2 may occur when plastic syringes are used, because of the partial pressure of O_2 dissolved in the plastic. Slower changes in the Po_2 may occur because of diffusion of gas through the walls or plunger tip of the plastic syringe. Glass syringes should have tightly fitting, matched plungers to avoid leakage of gas. Differences in Po_2 caused by syringe material are usually not significant in most clinical situations, provided the specimen is handled properly. If the sample has a high Po_2 (i.e., $Po_2 > 150$ mm Hg) or if precise Po_2 measurements are to be made, as in a shunt determination, a glass syringe may be preferable. The sample should be stored in ice water if analysis is not to be done immediately. Specimens with O_2 tensions in the normal physiologic range (i.e., 50 to 150 mm Hg) show minimal changes in Po_2 in 1 to 2 hours. Changes in specimens held at room temperature are related to the metabolism of the cells in the blood, particularly white blood cells and platelets. In all cases, specimens with high Po_2 values (i.e., $Po_2 > 150$ mm Hg) are most susceptible to alterations because of gas leakage or temperature, because small changes in O_2 content result in large changes in O_2 tension. Capillary samples are useful in infants when arterial puncture is impractical. The area for collection should be heated by warm compress, lanced, and blood allowed to fill the required volume of heparinized capillary tube(s). Squeezing the tissue should be avoided since predominately venous blood will be obtained. The capillary tubes should be carefully sealed to avoid bubbles. Guidelines for quality control of blood gas analyzers and for the safe handling of blood specimens are included in Chapter 11.

Significance

The Pa_{O_2} of a healthy young adult at sea level varies from 85 to 100 mm Hg and decreases slightly with age. The Pa_{O_2} can be increased by a person whose lung function is normal by hyperventilation to values as high as 120 mm Hg. Healthy persons breathing 100% O_2 may exhibit Pa_{O_2} values higher than 600 mm Hg. The alveolar Po_2 for any particular inspired O_2 fraction can be calculated as described in the Shunt Calculation section. Decreased Pa_{O_2} can result from hypoventilation, diffusion defects, ventilation/blood flow imbalances, and inadequate atmospheric O_2 (altitude).

Because the P_{O_2} is the pressure of dissolved O_2 in blood, it is not influenced by the amount of Hb present or whether the Hb is capable of binding O_2. Hypoxemia may occur even though the Pa_{O_2} is normal or elevated, as in O_2 breathing, if inadequate amounts or abnormal forms of Hb are present. Many automated blood gas analyzers allow *calculation* of the oxygen saturation (Sa_{O_2}) from the Pa_{O_2} and pH, assuming that the normal Hb reaction occurs. The ability of the Hb to bind O_2 at a particular pressure is quantified by the P_{50}, which specifies the partial pressure at which a specific Hb is 50% saturated. The P_{50} may be determined by tonometering (i.e., equilibrating) blood at several low O_2 tensions, then constructing a O_2Hb dissociation curve to estimate the partial pressure at 50% saturation. A second method allows estimation of the P_{50} by comparing the measured Sa_{O_2}, using a spectrophotometer (see below), to the expected saturation based on a P_{50} of 26.7. Calculated Sa_{O_2} values usually presume a P_{50} value of 26 to 27, although this may be quite different depending on the types of Hb and interfering substances present. A common example is the subject who has an elevated carboxyhemoglobin (COHb) because of smoking or smoke inhalation: the Pa_{O_2} may be within the normal range while the Sa_{O_2} is markedly decreased. Calculating Sa_{O_2} from Po_2 in this case would result in a dangerous overestimate of the O_2 content of the blood. Measured Sa_{O_2}, as described in the Oxygen Saturation section, is preferred to the calculated value.

The severity of impairment of arterial oxygenation is indicated by the Pa_{O_2} at rest. The Pa_{O_2} is a good index of the ability of the lungs to match pulmonary capillary blood flow with adequate ventilation. If ventilation matches perfusion, pulmonary capillary blood leaves the lungs with a Po_2 close to that of the alveoli. If ventilation is adequate and there is sufficient atmospheric O_2, pulmonary capillary blood is almost completely saturated. When either of these conditions is not met (i.e., poor ventilation or mismatching of gas and blood exists), pulmonary capillary blood has a reduced O_2 content; Pa_{O_2} is reduced in proportion to the number of lung units contributing blood with low O_2 content. Well-ventilated and well-perfused lung units cannot compensate for their poorly functioning counterparts, because pulmonary capillary blood leaving them is almost fully oxygenated already. Because of the shape of the O_2Hb dissociation curve, O_2 binding to Hb is almost complete at Pa_{O_2} values greater than 60 mm Hg (i.e., 90% saturation). As the Pa_{O_2} falls from 60 to 40 mm Hg, the saturation typically decreases from 90% to 75%, with symptoms of hypoxia (i.e., mental confusion and shortness of breath) increasing. The delivery of O_2 to the tissues, however, also depends on the Hb concentration and the cardiac output. Since most O_2 transported is bound to Hb, there must be an adequate supply (i.e., 12 to 15 gm/dl) of functional Hb. Adequate cardiac output (4 to 5 L/min) is necessary to deliver the oxygenated arterial blood to the tissues. Signs and symptoms of hypoxia may be present in spite of an adequate Pa_{O_2} because of severe anemia and/or reduced cardiac function.

The mixed venous O_2 tension ($P\bar{v}_{O_2}$) in healthy subjects at rest ranges from 37 to 43 mm Hg, with an average of 40 mm Hg. In healthy persons, the arterial O_2 content averages 20 ml/dl, and the mixed venous O_2 content averages 15 ml/dl, resulting in a content difference of 5 ml/dl (or vol%). While Pa_{O_2} varies with the inspired O_2 fraction and the matching of ventilation and perfusion, the $P\bar{v}_{O_2}$ changes in response to alterations in cardiac output and O_2 consumption at the tissue level. If cardiac output increases while O_2 consumption ($\dot{V}O_2$) remains constant, the difference in the O_2 contents of arterial and mixed venous blood ($C(a\text{-}\bar{v})_{O_2}$) decreases; conversely, if cardiac output falls without a change in O_2 consumption, the $C(a\text{-}\bar{v})_{O_2}$ increases. Increased cardiac output sometimes occurs in response to pulmonary shunting, allowing mixed venous oxygen content to rise and reduce the deleterious effect of the shunt. Critically ill subjects often display low $P\bar{v}_{O_2}$ values and increased $C(a\text{-}\bar{v})_{O_2}$ values as a result of poor cardiovascular performance. Alterations in the $P\bar{v}_{O_2}$ often occur even though the Pa_{O_2} may be within normal limits. $P\bar{v}_{O_2}$ values of less than 28 mm Hg in critically ill patients, usually accompanied by an increased (i.e., > 6 vol%) $C(a\text{-}\bar{v})_{O_2}$, suggest marked cardiovascular decompensation.

Resting subjects who have severe obstructive or restrictive diseases may show decreased Pa_{O_2} values, occasionally as low as 40 mm Hg. Subjects with less advanced pulmonary disease may show little decrease in Pa_{O_2} if hyperventilation is present, or if the disease process affects both $\dot{V}$ and $\dot{Q}$ in the same lung units. In subjects who have emphysema, the destruction of alveolar septa eliminates pulmonary capillaries as well, resulting in poor ventilation and equally poor blood flow. These subjects may have severe airways obstruction but little or no decrease in Pa_{O_2}. Subjects who have chronic bronchitis or asthma, particularly during acute exacerbations, may have moderate or severe resting hypoxemia because of $\dot{V}/\dot{Q}$ abnormalities. Analysis of Pa_{O_2} during exercise in subjects who have obstructive disease often shows a decrease in Pa_{O_2} commensurate with the extent of the disease process. Pa_{O_2} during exercise is correlated with the subject's DL_{CO} and $FEV_{1.0}$, but a wide range of variability exists. Subjects with markedly decreased DL_{CO} (i.e., less than about 50% of predicted DL_{CO}) typically show low Pa_{O_2} values at rest and during exercise, but the degree of arterial desaturation cannot be predicted from static pulmonary function measurements.

Pa_{O_2} may be decreased for nonpulmonary reasons, such as anatomic shunts (intracardiac) or neuromuscular hypoventilation. Tissue hypoxia can occur because of inadequate or nonfunctional Hb, or because of poor cardiac output. The Pa_{O_2} should be correlated with spirometry measurements (i.e., $FEV_{1.0}$ and $FEF_{25\%\text{-}75\%}$), DL_{CO}, ventilation (i.e., $\dot{V}E$, VT, and VD) and lung volume tests (i.e., VC, RV, and TLC) to distinguish pulmonary disease from nonpulmonary causes of inadequate oxygenation.

ARTERIAL AND MIXED VENOUS OXYGEN SATURATION (Sa_{O_2}, $S\bar{v}_{O_2}$)

Description

O_2 saturation measures the ratio of oxygenated Hb (O_2Hb) to either the total available Hb or to the functional Hb. This ratio of content to capacity is normally expressed as a percentage, but the values may differ slightly depending on the method of calculation:

1. *Oxyhemoglobin fraction of total Hb*

$$= \frac{O_2Hb}{O_2Hb + RHb + COHb + MetHb}$$

2. *Oxygen saturation of available Hb*

$$= \frac{O_2Hb}{O_2Hb + RHb}$$

where

RHb = Reduced hemoglobin concentration
COHb = Carboxyhemoglobin concentration
MetHb = Methemoglobin concentration

Measurement of O_2 saturation using multiple wavelength spectrophotometers usually employs method 1 above, while pulse oximeters normally use method 2.

Technique

O_2 saturation of Hb is commonly measured using one of several techniques. In the first technique, the O_2 content of arterial blood is measured volumetrically; then the blood is exposed to the atmosphere so the Hb may combine with atmospheric O_2; then, the content is measured again. Saturation is determined after corrections for dissolved O_2 are made. In the second technique, the O_2 saturation is measured spectrophotometrically by analyzing the ratio of O_2Hb to total Hb (method 1 above). The total Hb, O_2Hb, COHb, and MetHb are usually reported in conjunction with routine blood gas parameters. In the third method, saturation is obtained noninvasively by pulse oximetry using either the ear, finger, or other site (method 2 above). In the fourth technique, mixed venous O_2 saturation may be measured by a reflective spectrophotometer in an indwelling pulmonary artery catheter that includes fiberoptic bundles for "in vivo" measurements. Descriptions of both the spectrophotometric and pulse oximeters are included in Chapter 9. Guidelines for quality control of blood gas analysis are included in Chapter 11.

Measurement of percent saturation allows calculation of the O_2 content of either arterial or mixed venous blood (Ca_{O_2} and $C\bar{v}_{O_2}$, respectively). The O_2 content is determined by the concentration of Hb and by the partial pressure of dissolved O_2; for arterial blood, it is described by the following equation:

$$Ca_{O_2} = (1.34 \times Hb \times Sa_{O_2}) + (.0031 \times Pa_{O_2})$$

where

1.34 = O_2 binding capacity of Hb in milliliters (some clinicians prefer 1.36 or 1.39 ml/gm)

Hb = Hemoglobin concentration, in grams per deciliter
Sa_{O_2} = O_2 saturation expressed as a fraction ($Sa_{O_2}/100$)
.0031 = Solubility coefficient for O_2, in ml/mm Hg
Pa_{O_2} = Partial pressure of O_2 in the specimen

The content derived by this calculation is expressed in milliliters of O_2 per 100 ml of blood (vol%). The halves of the equation (i.e., the terms in parentheses) define the volumes of O_2 transported bound to Hb and in the dissolved form. The same calculation can be applied to a mixed venous sample, by substituting the $S\bar{v}_{O_2}$ and $P\bar{v}_{O_2}$ for Sa_{O_2} and Pa_{O_2}, respectively.

Significance

The Sa_{O_2} for a healthy young adult with a Pa_{O_2} of 95 mm Hg is approximately 97%. Because the O_2Hb dissociation curve is relatively flat when the Pa_{O_2} is above 60 mm Hg (i.e., $Sa_{O_2} \geqq 90\%$), the saturation changes only slightly even when there is a marked change in Pa_{O_2}. The Pa_{O_2}, therefore, is a more sensitive indicator of oxygenation in lungs that do not have gross abnormalities. When the P_{O_2} falls below 60 mm Hg, the Sa_{O_2} decreases rapidly, with small decrements in Pa_{O_2} resulting in large decreases in saturation. As Sa_{O_2} falls below 90%, the O_2 content of the blood decreases proportionately. At saturations less than 85% (i.e., $Pa_{O_2} < 55$ mm Hg), symptoms of hypoxemia increase, and supplementary O_2 may be indicated.

Healthy persons have small amounts of Hb that cannot carry O_2. COHb is present in blood because of metabolism and environmental exposure, which is usually in the range of 0.5% to 2% of the total Hb. Sources of increased COHb include smoking (cigarettes, cigars, and pipes), smoke inhalation, improperly vented furnaces, and auto emissions. In smokers, the levels may be increased to between 3% and 15%, depending on the recent smoking history. Smoke inhalation or CO poisoning from other sources may also result in elevated COHb levels, sometimes as high as 50%. Since O_2Hb saturation falls as COHb rises, COHb levels greater than 15% almost always result in hypoxemia. CoHb absorbs light at wavelengths similar to O_2Hb so that the blood is bright red and cyanosis (which requires an increased concentration of reduced Hb) is absent. COHb interferes with O_2 transport in two ways: by binding competitively to the Hb and by shifting the O_2Hb curve to the left, so that less O_2 is unloaded from the Hb. It is important to note that the Po_2 in the blood may be normal in spite of an increased COHb. Calculation of the O_2 saturation based on the Po_2 and pH, as used in many automated blood gas analyzers, will result in erroneously high estimates of the saturation and O_2 carrying capacity of the blood. For this reason O_2Hb and COHb should be measured using blood oximetry whenever possible. COHb concentrations in blood decrease once the source of CO has been removed. Removal of CO from the blood depends on the minute ventilation, and may require several hours to reduce even moderate levels to normal. Breathing 100% O_2 speeds the washout of CO and is indicated whenever dangerously high levels of COHb are encountered.

MetHb results when the iron atoms of the Hb molecule are oxidized from Fe^{++} to Fe^{+++}; normally the MetHb level is less than 1.5% of the total Hb. High levels of MetHb can result from ingestion of or exposure to strong oxidizing agents. Both COHb and MetHb reduce the O_2 carrying capacity of the blood by reducing the available Hb and shifting the O_2Hb dissociation curve to the left.

The percent saturation of mixed venous blood ($S\bar{v}_{O_2}$) in healthy subjects is approximately 75%, with a $P\bar{v}_{O_2}$ of 40 mm Hg. Healthy subjects have a content difference, $C(a\text{-}\bar{v})O_2$, of 5 vol%, with arterial blood carrying about 20 vol% and mixed venous blood carrying about 15 vol%. Pulmonary disease patterns that cause arterial hypoxemia may reduce the $S\bar{v}_{O_2}$ if the O_2 uptake and cardiac output remain constant. Normally, however, cardiac output increases to combat arterial hypoxemia due to intrapulmonary shunting. Increased O_2 delivery to the tissues results in a reduced extraction of O_2 from the blood, so that the mixed venous blood returning to the lungs has a normal or even increased O_2 saturation. The shunted blood thus has a higher O_2 content, thereby reducing the shunt effect. $S\bar{v}_{O_2}$ may be reduced if the cardiac output is compromised, either with or without arterial hypoxemia. $S\bar{v}_{O_2}$ is useful in monitoring cardiac performance in the critical care setting. Patients who have good cardiovascular reserves can maintain a $S\bar{v}_{O_2}$ in the range of 70 to 75%. Patients whose $S\bar{v}_{O_2}$ values are in the 60% to 70% range have a limited ability to deliver more O_2 to the tissues. $S\bar{v}_{O_2}$ values less than 60% usually indicate cardiovascular decompensation and tissue hypoxemia. The indwelling reflective spectrophotometer allows continuous monitoring of this important parameter. $S\bar{v}_{O_2}$ also decreases during exercise. Despite increased cardiac output, O_2 extraction by the exercising muscles reduces the content of blood returning to the lungs.

Measurement of Sa_{O_2} by most pulse oximeters is based on the relative absorption of light at two wavelengths, and hence is limited to detection of two species of Hb. Absorption in the red and near-infrared portions of the visible spectrum allows measurement of the O_2Hb and reduced Hb, providing an estimate of the oxygen saturation of available hemoglobin (see Description section). These measurements may be confounded by the presence of abnormal Hb or dyes that absorb light at similar wavelengths. COHb, which has a red coloration, absorbs light at a similar wavelength as O_2Hb. In the presence of increased amounts of COHb, the pulse oximeter "sees" the COHb as O_2Hb and will overestimate oxygen saturation. MetHb tends to force the O_2Hb saturation estimate toward 85%, but the effect is small unless large concentrations of MetHb are present. In the presence of dyes such as methylene blue or indocyanine green, which are sometimes injected for blood flow studies, the Sa_{O_2} may be underestimated; that is, the pulse oximeter will read lower than the true saturation.

Other technical problems in estimating Sa_{O_2} using pulse oximetry include motion artifact, interference from external light sources, and altered perfusion at the probe location. Movement of the probe causes the pulse oximeter to mistake the motion for arterial pulsation. If the motion is consistent and of long enough duration, as in the case of shivering, the Sa_{O_2} tends to be forced toward 85% (see Oximeters, Chapter 9). Decreased perfusion at the site of the oximeter probe may also result in inaccurate estimates of Sa_{O_2}. Some potential causes of altered perfusion include hypotension, hypothermia, vasoconstrictor drugs, and redirection of blood flow during exercise.

CAPNOGRAPHY

Description

Capnography includes continuous, noninvasive monitoring of expired CO_2 and analysis of the single-breath CO_2 waveform. Continuous monitoring of expired CO_2 allows trending of changes in alveolar and dead space ventilation. Analysis of a single breath of expired CO_2 measures the uniformity of both ventilation and pulmonary blood flow. $P_{ET_{CO_2}}$ is reported in mm Hg. The slope of the alveolar phase of the waveform is recorded as a percentage.

Technique

Continuous monitoring of expired CO_2 is performed by sampling gas from the subject's proximal airway and submitting the gas to an infrared analyzer or to a mass spectrometer (see Chapter 9). The analyzer signal is then passed to either an oscilloscope, a recorder, or computerized data storage. The CO_2 waveforms may be displayed either individually (Fig. 6-1) or as a series of peaks to form a trend plot. $P_{ET_{CO_2}}$ may be read from the maxima of the waveforms or obtained by a simple peak detector and displayed digitally. Continuous CO_2 monitoring is most commonly used in subjects who have artificial airways, in the critical care setting. Pa_{CO_2} is often measured at intervals to establish the gradient with the $P_{ET_{CO_2}}$. Respiratory rate may be determined from the frequency of the pulsations in the CO_2 waveforms.

The change in CO_2 concentration of a single expiration may be recorded to obtain a washout curve (Fig. 6-2), as in the SBN_2 test. A rapid CO_2 analyzer is used and the washout curve is recorded, usually plotting expired CO_2 versus volume or time. The slope of the alveolar plateau is recorded as a percent change in CO_2 per liter of volume. The $P_{ET_{CO_2}}$ is also recorded from the maximal concentration at the end of the expiration.

Significance

In healthy individuals, the concentration of CO_2 in expired gas rises to a plateau as alveolar gas is expired and remains more or less constant. If all lung units emptied CO_2 at exactly the same rate, the concentration of CO_2 would remain constant. However, because lungs that have ventilation and blood flow imbalances empty CO_2 at varying rates, the CO_2 concentration

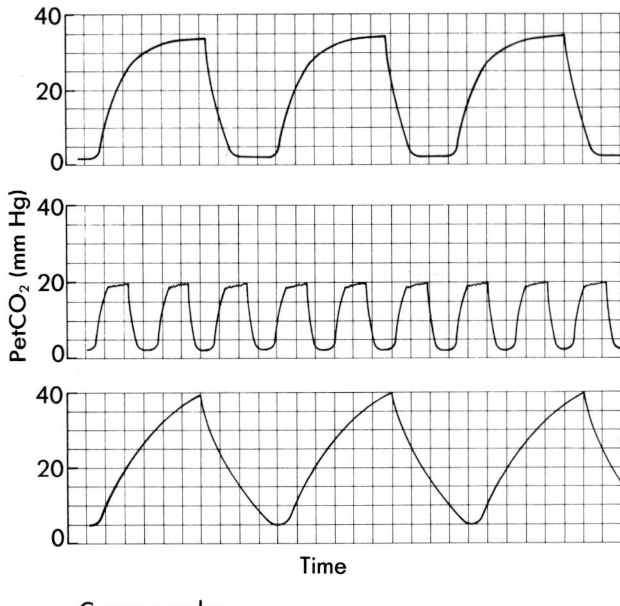

Fig. 6-1 Capnographic tracings. Expired CO_2 is plotted versus time in three subjects; in each example, expiration is marked by the rapid increase in CO_2 to a peak ($P_{ET_{CO_2}}$) followed by a return to baseline during inspiration. *Top:* a normal respiratory pattern with $P_{ET_{CO_2}}$ near 40 mm Hg and a relatively flat alveolar phase (see Fig. 6-2). *Middle:* a rapid respiratory rate and low $P_{ET_{CO_2}}$ (20 mm Hg), such as might be found in a subject who is hyperventilating; the expiratory waveform has a normal configuration. *Bottom:* an abnormal expired CO_2 waveform consistent with $\dot{V}/\dot{Q}$ abnormalities; no alveolar plateau is present.

rises as more and more of the breath is expired. The end-tidal CO_2 theoretically should not exceed the Pa_{CO_2}; in healthy subjects the $P_{ET_{CO_2}}$ is usually quite close to the Pa_{CO_2}. When $\dot{V}$ and $\dot{Q}$ become grossly uneven, as in many obstructive disease patterns, the CO_2 concentration at the end of the alveolar plateau may actually exceed the Pa_{CO_2}.

Continuous CO_2 analysis provides several useful parameters for monitoring critically ill patients, particularly those requiring ventilatory support. End-tidal CO_2 measurements allow trending of changes in Pa_{CO_2}, provided there is little or no change in the shape of the CO_2 waveform (i.e., indicating $\dot{V}/\dot{Q}$ abnormalities). Once a reference blood gas is obtained, $P_{ET_{CO_2}}$ can be used as a continuous and noninvasive monitor. Respiratory rate can be measured by analysis of the frequency of expired CO_2 waveforms; marked changes such as hyperpnea or apnea can be quickly detected. Analysis of the individual CO_2 waveforms, in conjunction with

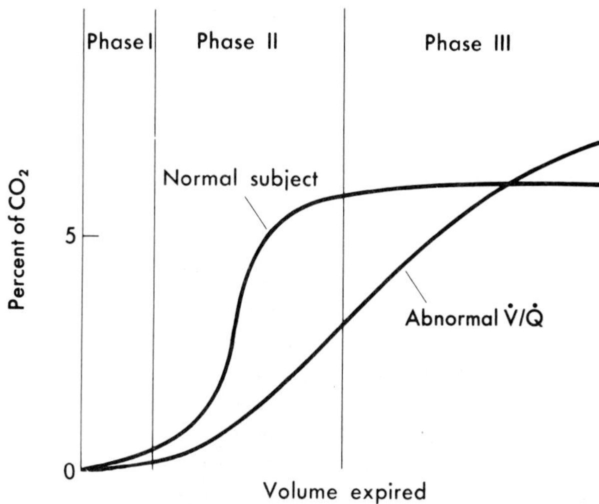

Fig. 6-2 CO_2 elimination. A plot of expired CO_2 concentration against expired volume yields a curve distinctly similar to a SBN_2 curve. Three phases can be defined: *Phase I* includes the expiration of upper airway dead space gas containing little CO_2. *Phase II* shows an abrupt rise in the percent of CO_2, as mixed bronchial and alveolar air is expired. *Phase III* shows the typical plateau as alveolar gas is monitored. Also illustrated is a waveform typical of abnormal ventilation/blood flow ratios. When different parts of the lungs have varying CO_2 concentrations and empty at dissimilar rates, the CO_2 elimination curve will show a constant rise during the entire expiration. The SBN_2 test (see Chapter 4) indicates abnormality of ventilation alone; the CO_2 waveform indicates abnormal matching of blood flow and ventilation because only perfused alveoli contribute CO_2 to the expirate. If ventilation shifts to match uneven blood flow, or vice versa, the elimination curve will assume more of an "S" shape.

the Pa_{CO_2}, may be helpful in identifying abrupt changes related to dead-space-producing disorders such as pulmonary embolization or reduced cardiac output. Problems related to ventilatory support devices can be detected; disconnection or leaks in breathing circuits can be quickly recognized. Increased mechanical dead space (i.e., gas rebreathed in the ventilator circuit) can be identified by a baseline CO_2 concentration greater than zero. Irregularities in the shape of the waveform often signal that the patient is "out of phase" with the ventilator.

The shape of a single CO_2 expiration curve (Fig. 6-2) is determined by the matching of $\dot{V}$ to $\dot{Q}$. Only those lung units that are both ventilated *and* perfused contribute CO_2 to the expirate. The CO_2 waveform in subjects who do not have lung disease shows a flat initial segment of pure anatomic dead space gas containing little or no CO_2. This is followed by a rapid increase in CO_2 tension as the gas composition becomes a mixture of dead space and alveolar gas. Finally, an "alveolar" plateau occurs in which gas composition changes only slightly because of different emptying rates of different lung units. The absolute concentration of CO_2 at the alveolar plateau depends on factors such as minute ventilation and CO_2 production. Dead-space-producing disease, such as pulmonary embolization or a marked decrease in cardiac output, may cause a profound decrease in the CO_2 concentration. In subjects who have pulmonary disease, most notably airways abnormalities, the phases of the CO_2 washout curve may not be clearly delineated. The alveolar plateau may show continuous up-sloping throughout expiration, making measurement of even $P_{ET_{CO_2}}$ misleading.

Technical problems involved in capnography include the necessity of accurate calibration and management of the gas sampling system itself. Calibration to a known gas standard, preferably two gas concentrations, is required if the system will be used to trend Pa_{CO_2}. Water condensate in the sampling tubing or connectors can change the gas flow rate, thereby altering the calibration. Saturation of a water absorber column, if one is used, can also lead to inaccurate readings. Long sampling lines or low sampling flow rates can cause damping of the CO_2 waveform, making use of the shape for the estimation of $P_{ET_{CO_2}}$ inaccurate.

SHUNT CALCULATION ($\dot{Q}_S/\dot{Q}_T$)

Description

Shunt calculation is a measurement of the portion of the cardiac output that traverses the pulmonary system without participating in gas exchange. It is expressed as a ratio of shunted blood ($\dot{Q}_S$) to total perfusion ($\dot{Q}_T$) and recorded as a percent of the total cardiac output, or sometimes as a fraction.

Technique

There are two techniques of measuring the shunt fraction. The first uses O_2 content differences:

$$\frac{\dot{Q}_S}{\dot{Q}_T} = \frac{Cc_{O_2} - Ca_{O_2}}{Cc_{O_2} - C\bar{v}_{O_2}}$$

where

Cc_{O_2} = O_2 content of end-capillary blood, normally estimated from the saturation associated with the calculated $P_{A_{O_2}}$

Ca_{O_2} = Arterial O_2 content, measured from an arterial sample (see Oxygen Saturation section)

$C\bar{v}_{O_2}$ = Mixed venous O_2 content, measured from a sample obtained from an indwelling pulmonary artery catheter

The denominator of this equation reflects potential arterialization of mixed venous blood, while the numerator reflects the actual arterialization.

In the second technique, the patient is allowed to breathe 100% O_2 for at least 20 minutes at atmospheric pressure so that all N_2 is washed out of the lungs and the Hb can become completely saturated. The percent shunt is then calculated as follows:

$$\frac{\dot{Q}s}{\dot{Q}T} = \frac{(PA_{O_2} - Pa_{O_2}) \times 0.0031}{C(a\text{-}\bar{v})_{O_2} + [(PA_{O_2} - Pa_{O_2}) \times 0.0031]}$$

where

PA_{O_2} = Alveolar O_2 tension
Pa_{O_2} = Arterial O_2 tension
$C(a\text{-}\bar{v})_{O_2}$ = Arteriovenous O_2 content difference
0.0031 = Conversion factor to volume % for O_2

PA_{O_2}, when the subject is breathing 100% O_2, can be estimated as follows:

$$PA_{O_2} = PB - PA_{H_2O} - PA_{CO_2}/0.8$$

where

PB = Barometric pressure
PA_{H_2O} = Partial pressure of water vapor at body temperature (47 mm Hg)
PA_{CO_2} = Alveolar CO_2 tension (estimated from arterial PCO_2)
0.8 = Respiratory exchange ratio

When using either method, the shunt fraction or ratio may be multiplied by 100 and the result reported as a percentage (i.e., 0.20 ratio × 100 equals a 20% shunt).

The second method of calculating the shunt is accurate only when the Hb is completely saturated; this normally requires a Pa_{O_2} of greater than 150 mm Hg. This is usually easily accomplished by breathing pure O_2. See the Appendix for a more detailed description of the technique. In situations in which breathing 100% O_2 does not raise the Pa_{O_2} high enough to completely saturate the Hb, the method using O_2 content differences (method #1 above) should be used.

Significance

Normally, less than 5% of the cardiac output is shunted through the pulmonary system. The accuracy of the shunt measurement using the second method described in previous paragraph depends on the accuracy of the PO_2 determinations, because in small shunts the Hb still becomes 100% saturated, and the difference between alveolar and arterial PO_2 values results simply from the amount of O_2 dissolved; this difference in the actual content of dissolved O_2 versus the amount that potentially could dissolve is the basis for the calculation.

The actual value for percent of shunt also depends largely on the $C(a\text{-}\bar{v})_{O_2}$ value used in the denominator of the equation. Because the $C(a\text{-}\bar{v})_{O_2}$ is determined not only by the status of the pulmonary system, but by the cardiac output and perfusion status, the value used in the equation should ideally be measured rather than estimated. Arterial content can be measured or calculated easily from a sample taken from a peripheral artery, but mixed venous content can only be measured accurately from a sample taken from the pulmonary artery. In subjects in whom the right side of the heart has not been catheterized, an estimated value must be used. $C(a-\bar{v})_{O_2}$ values between 4.5 and 5.0 vol% are reasonable in subjects who have good cardiac outputs and perfusion states. Values of 3.5 vol% are probably more realistic in individuals who are critically ill.

When the $C(a-\bar{v})_{O_2}$ cannot be reliably estimated or the Hb cannot be maximally saturated by breathing 100% oxygen, the alveolar-arterial O_2 gradient ($A\text{-}aD_{O_2}$) may be used as an index for matching of ventilation to blood flow. The $\dot{Q}S/\dot{Q}T$ does not directly provide absolute values for $\dot{Q}S$, but if the cardiac output ($\dot{Q}T$) is known, $\dot{Q}S$ can be determined simply.

An increased shunt fraction indicates low ventilation in relation to blood flow, often found in both obstructive and restrictive disease patterns. It should be noted, however, that even in advanced obstructive or severe restrictive diseases, blood flow may be decreased to the areas of poor ventilation by the lesions themselves, as in emphysema, or by compensatory mechanisms, such as pulmonary arteriole vasoconstriction. In these cases, there may be a minimal amount of shunting, even though severe ventilatory impairment exists. Perhaps most common is increased shunting caused by acute disease patterns such as atelectasis or aspiration of a foreign body. Diseases such as pneumonia or the adult respiratory distress syndrome (ARDS) usually result in a shunt-like effect because of the reduction of ventilation in proportion to blood flow in a large number of lung units.

Several technical considerations should be noted regarding the shunt measurement. The first method requires placement of a pulmonary artery catheter to obtain mixed venous O_2 content. The second method should also use measured $C(a-\bar{v})_{O_2}$; in addition, it requires inhalation of pure O_2 for 20 minutes, which may be contraindicated in subjects whose main respiratory drive is hypoxemia. Breathing pure O_2 washes N_2 out of the lungs completely. In subjects in whom certain lung units may be poorly ventilated, the washout of N_2 plus the removal of O_2 by the perfusing blood flow may reduce the size of alveoli to their critical limit and cause alveolar collapse. The net effect of this "nitrogen shunting" may be clinical shunt values that are falsely high, because a certain amount of shunting was induced by the testing procedure.

Measurement of the shunt fraction is often performed in conjunction with the determination of the VD/VT ratio (see Chapter 2) to assess both types of gas exchange abnormalities together.

SELF-ASSESSMENT QUESTIONS

1. Specimens for blood gas analysis should be placed in an ice-water bath:
   a. To slow down diffusion of gas through the container
   b. To inhibit clotting of the sample

c. To reduce cellular metabolism in the sample
d. To stabilize the pH of the sample

2. In addition to a normal Pa_{O_2}, adequate delivery of O_2 to the tissues depends on:
   a. Adequate functional Hb
   b. Normal amounts of dissolved O_2
   c. Hb saturation greater than 97%
   d. Adequate cardiac output
   e. a and d

3. Calculate the O_2 content, in milliliters of O_2 per 100 milliliters of blood, of a sample with the following blood gas measurements:

   Hb = 14.6 gm/dl
   Sa_{O_2} = 87% (0.87)
   Pa_{O_2} = 58 mm Hg
   Ca_{O_2} = ______________________ ml O_2/dl

4. Hyperventilation may be defined as:
   a. A minute ventilation greater than 10 L/min
   b. Respiratory rate greater than 30/min
   c. Decreased Pa_{CO_2} and alkalosis (respiratory)
   d. All of the above

5. A subject who smokes has his carboxyhemoglobin (COHb) measured as 12%; the highest O_2 saturation he could have would be:
   a. 94%
   b. 88%
   c. 85%
   d. 75%

6. Which of the following accurately describes the Pa_{CO_2}:
   I. It is often elevated in subjects with diffusion defects.
   II. It is inversely related to the alveolar ventilation.
   III. It may be low or normal in the presence of hypoxemia.
   IV. It may be elevated in the presence of hypoxemia.
   a. I, II, III
   b. I, II, IV
   c. II, III, IV
   d. II, III

7. A subject has the following arterial blood gas values:

pH	7.37
Pa_{CO_2}	62
Pa_{O_2}	55
HCO_3^-	35

These are best described as:
a. Normal acid-base status, moderate hypoxemia
b. Compensated metabolic alkalosis, moderate hypoxemia
c. Uncompensated respiratory acidosis with mild hypoxemia
d. Compensated respiratory acidosis, moderate hypoxemia

8. Continuous monitoring of exhaled CO_2 (capnography) may be used to follow trends in the Pa_{CO_2} provided that:
   a. The shape of the waveform remains constant
   b. A reference blood gas is obtained
   c. The respiratory rate remains constant
   d. All of the above
   e. a and b only

9. Measurement of O_2 saturation by pulse oximetry:
   a. Relates O_2Hb to the fraction of total Hb
   b. Relates O_2Hb to the available Hb
   c. Relates O_2Hb to the O_2 content (Ca_{O_2})
   d. Reduces O_2Hb to RHb

10. Which of the following accurately describes the calculation of percent shunt by the O_2 content difference method:
    I. The O_2 content of end-capillary blood must be estimated
    II. The subject must breathe 100% O_2 for 20 minutes
    III. A mixed venous blood sample is required
    IV. An arterial blood sample is required
    a. I, II, III, IV
    b. I, II, IV
    c. I, III, IV
    d. II, IV

SELECTED BIBLIOGRAPHY

General references

Comroe JH: Physiology of respiration, Chicago, 1965, Year Book Medical Publishers, Inc.

Morris AH, et al: Clinical pulmonary function testing, ed 2, Salt Lake City, 1984, Intermountain Thoracic Society.

Shapiro BA, et al: Clinical application of blood gases, ed 4, Chicago, 1989, Year Book Medical Publishers, Inc.

West JB: Pulmonary pathophysiology: the essentials, ed 3, Baltimore, 1987, Williams & Wilkins.

West JB: Respiratory physiology: the essentials, ed 3, Baltimore, 1985, Williams & Wilkins.

Blood gases

Barker SJ and Tremper KK: Pulse oximetry: applications and limitations. In Tremper KK and Barker SJ, editors: International anesthesiology clinics, Boston, 1987, Little, Brown and Co, Inc.

Harris EA, et al: The normal alveolar-arterial oxygen gradient in man, Clin Sci Molec Med 46:89, 1974.

Lichtman MA, Murphy MS, and Pogal M: The use of a single venous blood sample to assess oxygen binding to hemoglobin. Br J Haematol 32:89, 1976.

Severinghaus JW: Blood gas calculator, J Appl Physiol 21:1108, 1966.

Severinghaus JW: Simple, accurate equations for human blood O_2 dissociation computations, J Appl Physiol 46:599, 1979.

Siggard-Anderson O: Acid-base and blood gas parameters: arterial or capillary blood, Scand J Clin Lab Invest 21:289, 1968.

Shunt and capnography

Cane RD, et al: Minimizing errors in intrapulmonary shunt calculations, Crit Care Med 8:294, 1980.

Cheng EY, et al: Noninvasive respiratory monitoring of patients during weaning from mechanical respiratory support. Anesth Analg 65:S29, 1986.

Harrison RA, et al: Reassessment of the assumed a-v oxygen content difference in the shunt calculation, Anesth Analg 54:198, 1975.

Mellemgaard K: The alveolar-arterial oxygen difference: its size and components in normal man, Acta Physiol Scand 67:10, 1966.

Rahn H and Farhi LE: Ventilation, perfusion, and gas exchange: the VA/Q concept, In Fenn WO and Rahn H, editors: Handbook of physiology—respiration I, Washington, DC, 1964, American Physiological Society.

7

Exercise Testing

The efficiency of the cardiopulmonary system may be quite different during periods of increased metabolic demands than at rest. Therefore, tests designed to assess ventilation, gas exchange, and cardiovascular function during exercise can provide information not obtainable from tests of cardiopulmonary function performed at rest. Exercise testing allows evaluation of the heart and lungs under conditions of increased metabolic demand, so that abnormalities not readily defined in terms of decreased flows, volumes, or diffusing capacities may be quantitied. Limitations to work are not entirely predictable from any single resting measurement of pulmonary function, although estimates may be made from multiple parameters (i.e., $FEV_{1.0}$, DL_{CO}). To define work limitations, an exercise test is necessary. In all forms of exercise testing, measured parameters of cardiopulmonary function are assessed in relation to the work load (i.e., the level of exercise). Indications for performing exercise testing on subjects include dyspnea on exertion. Exercise testing can detect:

1. The presence and nature of ventilatory limitations to work.
2. The presence and nature of cardiovascular limitations to work.
3. The extent of conditioning or deconditioning.
4. The maximum tolerable work loads and safe levels of daily exercise.
5. The extent of disability for rehabilitation purposes.
6. O_2 desaturation and suitable levels of supplemental O_2 therapy.

Exercise testing may be indicated in apparently healthy individuals, particularly in adults older than 40, to ascertain fitness before engaging in vigorous physical activities such as running. Cardiopulmonary testing may be useful in assessing risk of postoperative complications, particularly in subjects undergoing thoracotomy. Chapter 12 includes examples of exercise studies (see Cases 7, 8, and 9).

WORK LOAD DETERMINATION AND EXERCISE PROTOCOLS

Exercise tests can be divided into two general categories, with regard to the protocols involved in performing the test: (1) progressive multistage tests and (2) steady-state tests.

Progressive multistage tests are designed to examine the effects of increasing work loads on various cardiopulmonary parameters without necessarily allowing a steady state to be achieved. Most often, this protocol is used to determine the work load at which the individual reaches maximum O_2 uptake, maximum ventilation, or maximum heart rate, and to trend the various exercise parameters measured. In a typical progressive multistage test, the work load of the exercising subject is increased at predetermined intervals, and all measurements are performed toward the end of each interval (see Table 7-1). Increments of work may be increased at intervals of 1 to 6 minutes, depending on the complexity of the measurements being made. The combination of intervals and work increments chosen should allow the subject to reach exhaustion or limitation by symptoms within a reasonable period, usually 8 to 10 minutes after a warm-up. With a device that allows continuous adjustment of the work load in small intervals (see the following discussion of the cycle ergometer), a "ramp," or continuously increasing work load, test may be performed. During multistage tests using short intervals (i.e., 1 to 3 minutes) or a ramp protocol, a steady state of gas exchange, ventilation, and cardiovascular response may not be attained; healthy subjects may reach a steady state in 2 to 3 minutes at low and moderate work loads. Attainment of a steady state, however, is not necessary if the primary objective of the evaluation is to determine the maximum values of various exercise parameters (i.e., O_2 uptake, heart rate (HR), or ventilation). Short exercise intervals also lessen muscle fatigue that may occur during prolonged tests, and may allow better delineation of gas exchange (i.e., $\dot{V}_{O_2}$ and $\dot{V}_{CO_2}$) kinetics. Incremental tests using intervals of 4 to 6 minutes at each work load may actually result in a steady state (i.e., relatively constant gas exchange, ventilation, and cardiovascular response), but should not be confused with steady-state tests, discussed in the next paragraph.

Steady-state tests are designed to assess parameters of cardiopulmonary function specifically under conditions of constant metabolic demand. Steady-state conditions are usually defined in terms of HR, O_2 consumption, or ventilation. This type of test is useful for assessing responses to a known work load and for evaluating the effectiveness of various therapies or pharmacologic agents on exercise ability. For example, a progressive multistage test may be performed initially to determine an individual's maximum tolerable work load; a steady-state test is then used to evaluate specific parameters at a submaximal level, such as at 50% and 75% of the highest O_2 uptake achieved. Work is performed for 5 to 8 minutes at the predetermined level to allow a steady state to develop; measurements are performed during the last 1 or 2 minutes of the period. Successive steady-state determinations at higher power outputs may be made continuously or spaced with short periods of light exercise or rest. A similar protocol may be used for evaluation of exercise-induced bronchospasm (see Chapter 8).

Two methods of varying exercise work load are commonly employed: the treadmill and the cycle ergometer (Figs. 7-1 and 7-2). The work load on the treadmill is adjusted by changing the speed of the walking surface, the slope of the surface, or both. The speed of the treadmill may be cali-

Table 7-1 Exercise protocols

Treadmill	Speed (MPH)/grade (%)	Interval	Comment
Bruce	1.7/10 2.5/12 3.4/14 4.2/16 5.0/18 5.5/20 6.0/22	3 min	Large work load increments; 1.7/0 and 1.7/5 may be used as preliminary stages for deconditioned subjects
Balke	3.3-3.4/0 increasing grade by 2.5% to exhaustion	1 min	Small work load increments; may use 3 MPH and 2-min intervals for deconditioned subjects, or reduce slope changes to 1%
Jones	1.0/0 2.0/0 2-3.5/2.5 increasing grade by 2.5% to exhaustion	1 min	Small work load increments and low starting work load
Cycle ergometer	**Work load**	**Interval**	**Comment**
Astrand	50 W (300 KPM) to exhaustion	4 min	Large work load increments and long intervals; 33W (200 KPM) may be used for females
"Ramp"	10 W/min to exhaustion	continuous	Requires electronically braked ergometer; different work rates may be used to alter ramp slope
Jones	16 W/min (100 KPM) to exhaustion	1 min	Smaller increments (50 KPM) may be used for deconditioned subjects
Other	**Description**	**Interval**	**Comment**
Master step test	Either constant or variable step height combined with increasing step rates	variable	Simple to perform; work load may be difficult to quantify
12-min walk	Distance covered in 12 min	12 min	Simple, useful in subjects with limited reserves or following rehabilitation

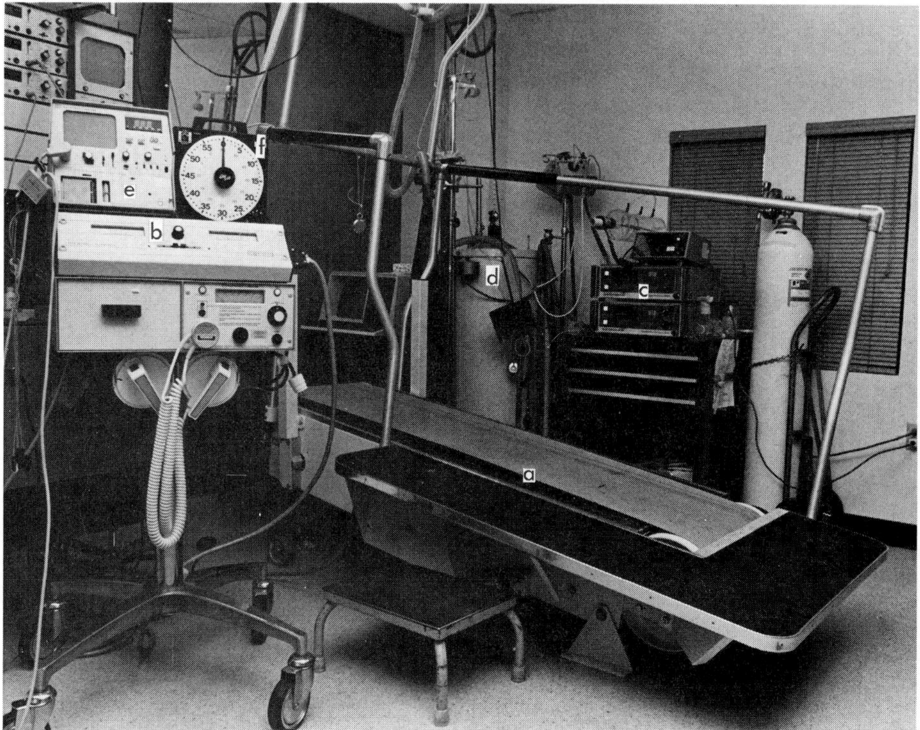

Fig. 7-1 Typical exercise laboratory setup. **A,** Motor-driven treadmill with adjustable slope and speed, side rails, and platform; **B,** treadmill controls with speed and slope indicators; **C,** gas analyzers (O_2 and CO_2); **D,** Tissot spirometer for ventilation measurements; **E,** cardiac monitor/recorder; **F,** electric timer.

brated in either miles per hour or in kilometers per hour; the slope is registered as "percent grade" on most devices. Percent grade refers to the relationship between the length of the walking surface and the elevation of one end above level. The primary advantages of the treadmill are that it elicits walking, jogging, or running, which are familiar forms of exercise; and that maximal levels of exercise can be easily attained, even in conditioned healthy subjects. However, the actual work performed during treadmill walking is a function of the weight of the subject, as well as a function of the slope and speed of the device. Subjects of different weights walking at the same speed and slope perform different work loads; different walking patterns, stride length, and grip on the handrails may also affect the actual amount of work being done.

The cycle ergometer allows the work load to be varied by adjustment of the resistance to pedaling and by the pedaling frequency, usually specified in revolutions per minute. The flywheel of a mechanical ergometer turns against a belt or strap, both ends of which are connected to a weighted physical balance; the diameter of the wheel is known, the resistance can be easily measured, and when the pedaling speed is determined, usually 50 to 90 RPM, the amount of work performed can be accurately calculated. One of the chief advantages of the cycle ergometer is that the work load can be changed rapidly and is independent of the weight of the subject. Other advantages include smaller size and better stability of the subject for gas collection, blood sampling, and blood pressure monitoring. Electronically-braked cycle ergometers (see Fig. 7-2) provide a smooth, rapid, and more reproducible means of changing exercise work load than do mechanical ergometers. Electronically-braked ergometers allow continuous adjustment of the work load independent of pedaling speed, so that the exercise level can be "ramped." The ramp test allows the subject to advance from low to high work loads quickly, and provides all the infor-

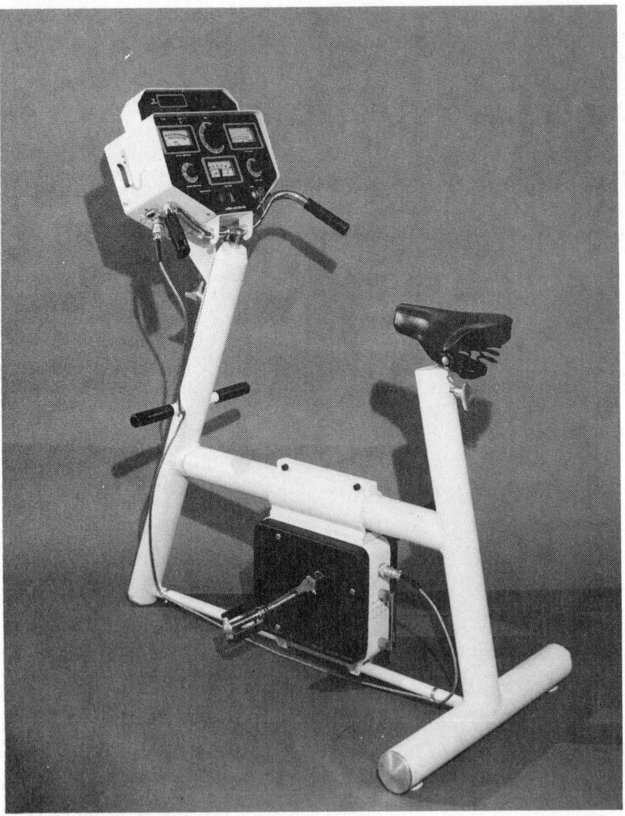

Fig. 7-2 Electronically braked cycle ergometer—A typical cycle ergometer with continuous adjustable electronic braking. Included are controls for adjusting the pedaling resistance, a timer, and analog meters for pedaling frequency (RPM) and external work load (watts). (Courtesy Warren E. Collins, Inc., Braintree, Mass.)

mation normally sought during a progressive maximal exercise test. A ramp protocol typically requires computerization for adjustment of the work load and rapid collection of physiologic data.

There are some differences in the work load performance obtained using the treadmill and the cycle ergometer, largely because of the muscle groups used. In most subjects, cycling does not produce as high a maximum O_2 consumption as walking on the treadmill (i.e., approximately 7% less). Ventilation and lactate production may be slightly greater on the cycle ergometer because of the different muscle groups used. These differences between the treadmill and cycle ergometer are not significant in most clinical situations, and the choice of device may be dictated by the subject's clinical condition.

Work load may be expressed quantitatively in several ways:

1. Work is normally expressed in kilopond-meters (KPM). One KPM equals the work of moving a 1 Kg mass a vertical distance of 1 M against the force of gravity.
2. Power is expressed in kilopond-meters per minute (i.e., work per unit of time) or in watts. One watt equals 6.12 KPM/min (100 watts $\cong$ 600 KPM/min).
3. Energy is expressed by O_2 consumption ($\dot{V}_{O_2}$), in liters or milliliters per minute (STPD), or in terms of multiples of the resting O_2 uptake (METS). Resting or baseline $\dot{V}_{O_2}$ can be measured as described in the following paragraphs or estimated as being 3.5 ml O_2/min/kg.

In exercise evaluation, it is particularly useful to relate the ventilatory, blood gas, and hemodynamic measurements to the $\dot{V}_{O_2}$ as the independent variable. This requires measurement of ventilation and analysis of expired gas during exercise.

VENTILATION DURING EXERCISE

Collection and analysis of expired gas during graded exercise testing provides a noninvasive means of obtaining the following parameters:

$\dot{V}E$	Minute ventilation
V_T	Tidal volume
f_b	Frequency of breathing; respiratory rate
$\dot{V}O_2$	Oxygen consumption; oxygen uptake
$\dot{V}CO_2$	Carbon dioxide production
RER	Respiratory exchange ratio
$\dot{V}E/\dot{V}O_2$	Ventilatory equivalent for O_2
$\dot{V}E/\dot{V}CO_2$	Ventilatory equivalent for CO_2

Exhaled gas may be collected by using a one-way breathing circuit and either a collection system (Fig. 7-3), a flow transducer (Fig. 7-4) with electronic integration of volumes (see Chapter 9), or a breath-by-breath system (Fig. 7-5). The volume-measuring devices should be routinely calibrated

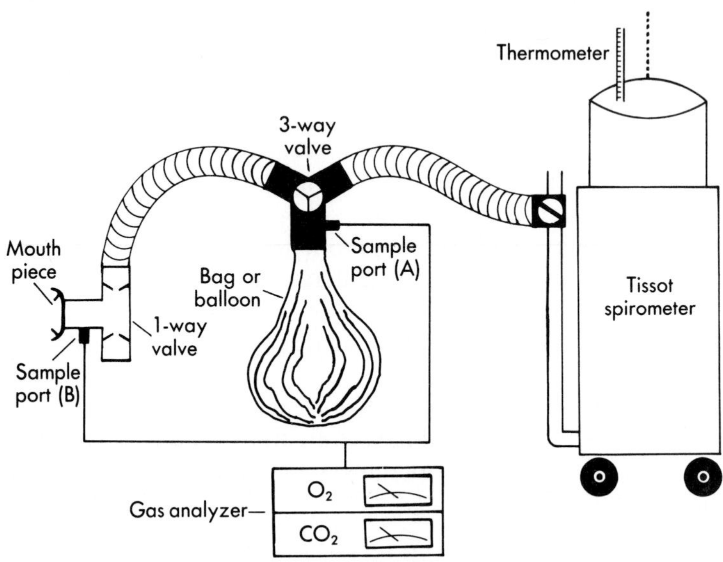

Fig. 7-3 System for collection and analysis of expired gas. The subject inspires from a one-way valve and expires through large-bore tubing into a Douglas bag, a meteorological balloon, or directly into a counterweighted Tissot spirometer. A three-way valve controls the breathing circuit. A sample may be collected over a timed interval into the bag or balloon; FE_{O_2} and FE_{CO_2} are determined by extracting a sample from *port A*. The volume in the bag/balloon may then be emptied into the Tissot spirometer for a volume measurement. The temperature of the gas in the spirometer is measured for conversion of gas volumes to BTPS and STPD. Alternatively, the volume may be collected directly into the Tissot spirometer, with a small sample collected in the bag/balloon for gas analysis; gas in the bag or balloon is then returned to the spirometer for the volume determination. Measurements may be obtained by sampling gas at *port B*, allowing for determination of end-tidal CO_2 and O_2, as well as the respiratory rate. A valve or solenoid may be used to sample alternatively between ports A and B, so that individual breaths and mixed expired gas can be analyzed.

before each procedure (see Chapter 11). Tissot spirometers usually remain accurate for extended periods if leaks are not present in tubing or valves. Pneumotachometers used to derive volumes should be checked by applying a known volume and/or flow signal, or by being connected in series with a spirometer of known accuracy. Gas analyzers should be calibrated and checked before each test procedure; some laboratories perform calibrations both before and after testing to detect instrument drift. Two-point calibrations, using gases that approximate the physiologic range to be tested, provide the best means of establishing the accuracy of the analyzers. Three-point calibration is necessary to check the linearity of the analyzers. For tests conducted without supplementary O_2, room air (i.e., 20.93% O_2 and 0.03% CO_2) and a gax mixture containing 12% to 16% O_2 with 5% to

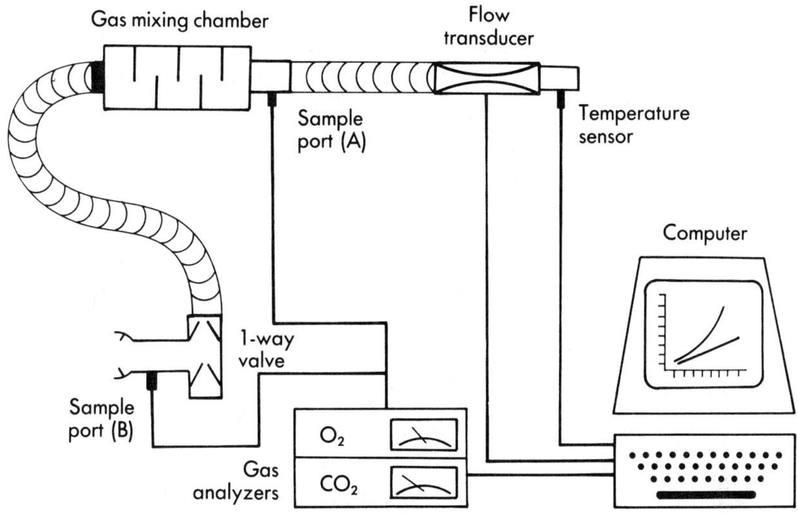

Fig. 7-4 Mixing chamber type system for analysis of expired gas. The subject inspires room air through a one-way valve and expires through large-bore tubing into a mixing chamber that has a volume of about 5 L. Baffles in the chamber cause the gas to be thoroughly mixed so that it is representative of mixed expired gas. A small volume is extracted at *sample port A* and directed to the O_2 and CO_2 analyzers for determination of the $F_{E_{O_2}}$ and $F_{E_{CO_2}}$. The expired gas then passes through a flow-sensing device, such as a pneumotachometer or turbine, from which volumes can be derived by integration. A temperature probe at the flow transducer provides data for conversion of the gas volume from ambient temperature to BTPS and STPD. Signals from the gas analyzers, flow transducer, and temperature sensor may be recorded directly on an analog recorder or converted to digital signals for processing by computer. Analysis of individual breaths of expired gas can be obtained by sampling at *port B.* This technique allows end-tidal CO_2 and O_2 concentrations, as well as respiratory rate, to be conveniently determined. A valve or solenoid can be used to sample alternatively between ports A and B, so that breath-by-breath and mixed expired samples can be analyzed.

7% CO_2 provide suitable gases for a two-point calibration. The one-way valve of the breathing circuit should have a low resistance (i.e., 1 to 2 cm H_2O at 100 L/min) and a small dead space. If a gas collection system (i.e., either a bag or Tissot spirometer) is being used, the subject should be allowed to breathe through the circuit with a nose clip in place long enough to wash out room air with expired gas. The exact washout volume, or time, depends on the volume of the collection system and whether it can be emptied before collecting gas. If the exhaled gas is collected directly in a Tissot spirometer, the spirometer should be washed out thoroughly before gas sampling is performed. Circuits employing a mixing chamber and flow-sensing device for volume measurements can usually be washed out quickly. Breath-by-breath systems (Fig. 7-5) normally require no washout, because fractional gas concentrations are sampled directly at the mouthpiece.

Depending on the protocol and equipment used, gas collection and analysis are performed for a specified interval toward the end of each exercise level. In steady-state protocols, collection is usually performed after 4 to 6 minutes at a constant work load. In progressive multistage protocols,

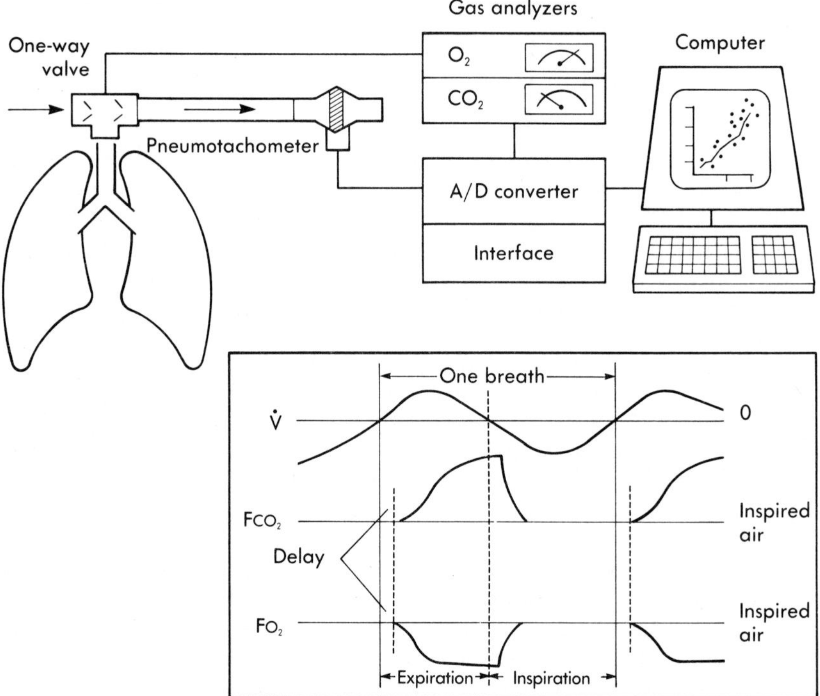

Fig. 7-5 Breath-by-breath system for determination of $\dot{V}O_2$, $\dot{V}CO_2$ and ventilation. The subject inspires room air through a one-way valve and expires through a pneumotachometer or similar flow-sensing device. Gas is continuously sampled at the subject's mouth for O_2 and CO_2. The flow signal and the signals from the gas analyzers are all integrated to derive volume, FE_{O_2}, and FE_{CO_2}, and to calculate $\dot{V}E$, $\dot{V}O_2$, $\dot{V}CO_2$, rate, and VT. To perform the necessary calculations and corrections, computerization is required. The insert shows the simultaneous recording of flow ($\dot{V}$) and fractional concentrations of O_2 and CO_2, (FO_2 and FCO_2, respectively). During expiration, FCO_2 rises and FO_2 falls. Because of the lag time required to transport gas from the mouthpiece to the analyzers, and because of the response time of the analyzers themselves, gas concentrations and flow are out of phase. By storing appropriate delay corrections (determined from calibrations) in the computer, the necessary signals can be matched up so that ventilatory and gas exchange parameters can be monitored and displayed on a breath-by-breath basis. In many applications, the breath-by-breath data is averaged over a short interval (10 to 60 seconds).

the appropriate sampling may be performed during the last minute of each stage. In breath-by-breath systems, sampling is normally done continuously, with data being displayed for each breath or values averaged over several breaths. Six raw data parameters are measured from each sample collected:

1. Volume expired, in liters
2. Temperature of the gas at the measuring device, in degrees Centigrade
3. Time of the collection, in seconds or minutes
4. Respiratory rate during the collection interval
5. Fraction of mixed expired O_2 ($F_{E_{O_2}}$)
6. Fraction of mixed expired CO_2 ($F_{E_{CO_2}}$)

These data can be recorded manually or by a multichannel recorder with appropriate analog signals. Similarly, the data may be entered into a computer either manually, or *on-line,* by means of an analog-to-digital (A/D) converter (see Chapter 10). On-line data reduction offers the advantage of immediate feedback of all measurements, as well as greater flexibility for using different exercise protocols (see Table 7-1). Breath-by-breath analysis requires that signals from the flow-sensing or volume-measuring transducer be integrated with the gas analyzer signals for $F_{E_{O_2}}$ and $F_{E_{CO_2}}$, and that any lag time, or phase delay, between the volume and gas analyzer signals be corrected (see Fig. 7-5). This can be done by computer if the appropriate delay times are measured, usually as part of calibration.

Minute ventilation ($\dot{V}_E$)

The $\dot{V}_E$ is the total volume of gas expired per minute by the exercising subject, expressed in liters, BTPS. A healthy adult at rest respires 5 to 10 L/min. During exercise, this value may increase to more than 200 L/min in trained subjects and commonly exceeds 100 L/min in healthy individuals (Figs. 7-6 and 7-7). The tremendous increase in ventilation provides adequate removal of CO_2, the primary product of exercising muscles, even at high work loads. $\dot{V}_E$ may be calculated using the following equation:

$$\dot{V}_E = \frac{\text{Volume expired} \times 60}{\text{Collection time, in seconds}} \times \text{BTPS factor}$$

Sample calculations and BTPS factors are contained in the Appendix.

Ventilation increases linearly with an increasing work load (i.e., $\dot{V}O_2$) at low and moderate levels of exercise. In healthy persons, this increase in ventilation during exercise follows the rise in $\dot{V}CO_2$. As higher levels of work are achieved (i.e., greater than about 60% of the $\dot{V}O_{2max}$), metabolic demand exceeds the capacity for energy production solely by aerobic pathways. To meet the increasing energy demands, anaerobic glycolysis assumes an increasing role. The main product of these reactions is lactate. As the blood lactate level rises, buffering occurs via the carbonic acid (H_2CO_3) pathway; the result is an increase in total $\dot{V}CO_2$. In healthy persons, ventilation

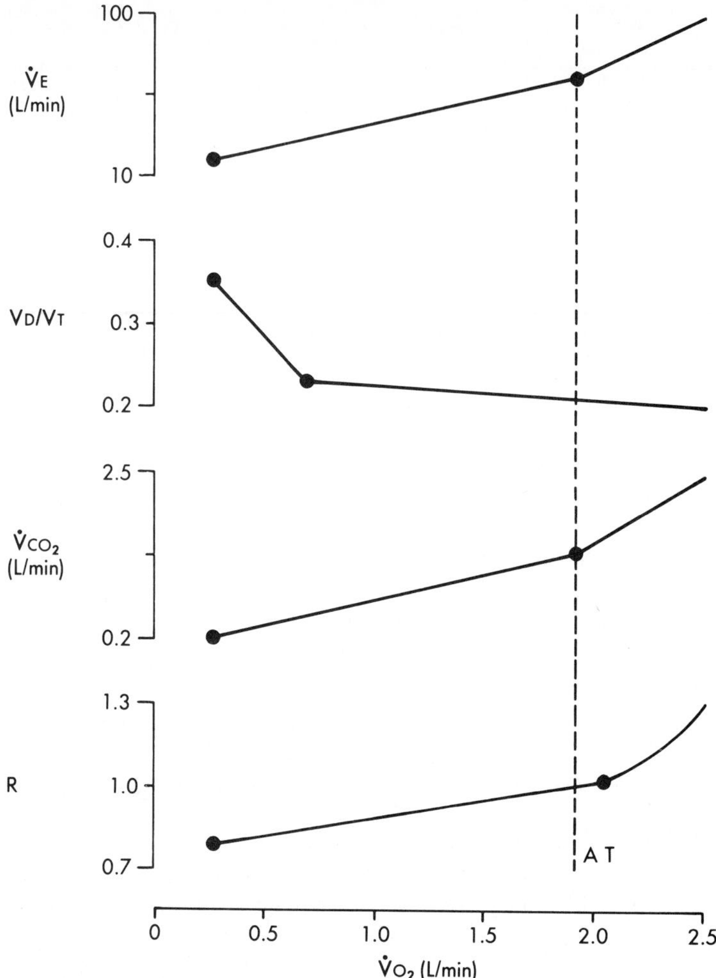

Fig. 7-6 Normal ventilation/gas exchange responses during exercise. Four parameters are plotted against $\dot{V}O_2$ as a measure of work rate, as they might appear in a healthy young adult. The dotted vertical line represents the anaerobic threshold (AT). $\dot{V}E$ increases linearly with work rate at low and moderate work loads up to the point of AT, as does $\dot{V}CO_2$. At higher levels, both $\dot{V}E$ and $\dot{V}CO_2$ increase at a faster rate as anaerobic metabolism (lactic acidosis) is buffered by HCO_3^- and CO_2 is produced. The ratio of $\dot{V}CO_2$ to $\dot{V}O_2$ (RER) follows a similar pattern. VD/VT, however, initially decreases rapidly as the VT increases; it then continues to fall, but at a slower rate.

increases simultaneously with increasing CO_2 production, facilitating CO_2 removal. Relating the $\dot{V}E_{max}$ achieved to resting measures of ventilatory function may provide indices of the role of ventilatory limitations to exercise. The dyspnea index is an example of a commonly-used technique of quantifying ventilation during exercise using a routine pulmonary function

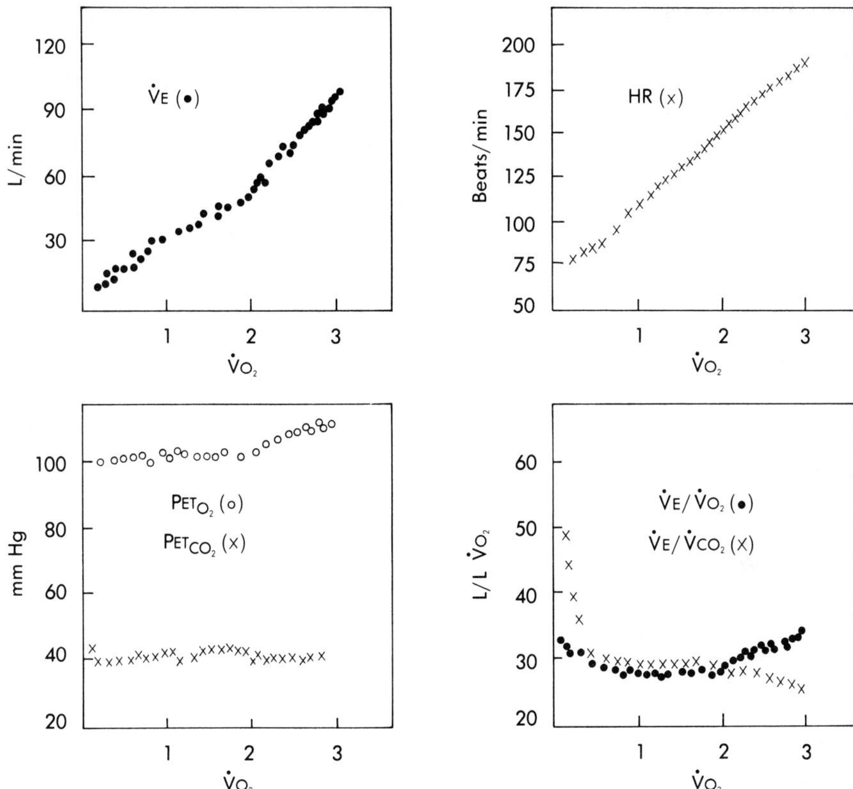

Fig. 7-7 Breath-by-breath exercise data—four plots of data obtained using a breath-by-breath technique, as in Fig. 7-5. Although data is recorded for each breath, the plots represent 30-second averages. All parameters are plotted against $\dot{V}O_2$ as the measure of work being performed. $\dot{V}E$ increases linearly up to about 2 L/min $\dot{V}O_2$; Heart rate (HR) increases linearly throughout the test. PET_{O_2} and PET_{CO_2} (end-tidal partial pressures of O_2 and CO_2, respectively) stay fairly constant up to approximately 2 L/min $\dot{V}O_2$, where the end-tidal O_2 begins to increase and the end-tidal CO_2 begins to fall. A similar pattern is in evidence on the plot of ventilatory equivalents for O_2 and CO_2 ($\dot{V}E/\dot{V}O_2$ and $\dot{V}E/\dot{V}CO_2$, respectively). A primary advantage of breath-by-breath analysis is that these plots may be viewed in "real time" as they occur, thus allowing modification of the testing protocol as required. The data in this example indicates the occurrence of anerobic threshold (AT) at approximately 2 L/min of $\dot{V}O_2$.

measurement, the maximal voluntary ventilation (MVV) (see Chapter 3). This index relates the $\dot{V}E$ achieved during a submaximal exercise level, usually 6 minutes at 0% grade and 2 MPH, to the MVV, and is calculated using this equation:

$$\text{Dyspnea index} = \frac{\dot{V}E \text{ during the last minute}}{\text{MVV}} \times 100$$

Values greater than 50% for this calculation are consistent with severe dyspnea. A valid MVV maneuver is essential to ensure that the dyspnea index is not overestimated. The MVV can be similarly related to the $\dot{V}E$ achieved at the highest work load attained, ($\dot{V}E_{max}$). The $\dot{V}E_{max}$ may approach the MVV if there is a primary ventilatory limitation to exercise, particularly when the MVV itself is reduced. The $\dot{V}E_{max}$ may also be compared to the $FEV_{1.0}$ multiplied by 35, because of the correlation between the MVV and the $FEV_{1.0} \times 35$. The $FEV_{1.0} \times 35$ provides a satisfactory estimate of the ventilation that can be maintained for 1 to 4 minutes, both by healthy subjects and in subjects who have moderate ventilatory impairment. In healthy subjects, maximal exercise will produce a $\dot{V}E$ that approaches 70% of the MVV, or similarly, 70% of the $FEV_{1.0} \times 35$. Subjects who have airways obstruction may actually achieve a $\dot{V}E$ during exercise that equals their MVV, albeit lower than the normal MVV range, indicating a ventilatory limitation. Individuals who have severe airway obstruction sometimes achieve a $\dot{V}E$ that exceeds the $FEV_{1.0} \times 35$, during maximal exercise. At high levels of ventilation (i.e., greater than 120 L/min in healthy persons), increases in O_2 uptake gained by further increases in ventilation serve mainly to supply O_2 to the respiratory muscles. The same phenomenon may occur at much lower levels of ventilation in subjects who have abnormal lung parenchyma or airways and increased work of breathing. Because of the enormous ventilatory reserve in the healthy person, exercise is seldom limited by ventilation, but rather by inability to further increase cardiac output or inability to extract more O_2 at the tissue level in the exercising muscles.

Tidal volume (VT) and respiratory rate (f, or f_b)

Tidal volume (VT) during exercise is usually derived by dividing the $\dot{V}E$ by the respiratory rate (f or f_b). Breath-by-breath systems may accumulate individual breaths, then report the average VT over a short interval or after a fixed number of breaths have been analyzed. In healthy subjects, VT increases at low and moderate work loads to account for the rise in ventilation, with only a small initial increase in f_b. This pattern continues until the VT approaches approximately 60% of VC. Further increases in total ventilation are accomplished by increasing the rate of breathing.

Subjects who have airway obstruction may be able to increase their $\dot{V}E$, but can not reach predicted values. If the VC is markedly reduced by the obstructive process, then there is little reserve to accommodate an increased VT. Subjects who have airway obstruction, when they have a relatively normal VC but increased resistance to flow, may increase their VT at a low f_b during exercise in an effort to minimize the work of breathing. This pattern continues until the VT reaches a plateau, as described previously, then the respiratory rate must be augmented to further increase $\dot{V}E$. Because of flow limitations, particularly during the expiratory phase, increases in respiratory rate must be accomplished by shortening the inspiratory portion of each breath. Reduction of the inspiratory time TI in relation to the total breath time (T_{total}) (i.e., T_I/T_{tot}) requires the inspiratory muscles to generate increasingly greater flows. The increased load placed on the muscles of inspiration typically results in dyspnea.

Unlike the pattern in obstruction, VT may remain relatively fixed in restrictive disease states, with increases in $\dot{V}E$ during exercise accomplished primarily by rapid respiratory rates. It is mechanically more efficient for subjects who have reduced volumes and "stiff" lungs to move small tidal volumes at fast rates to increase ventilation; flow limitation may be close to normal while the work of distending the lung is increased in restrictive patterns. The mechanism of increasing ventilation by primarily increasing flows places a load on the respiratory muscles, which, in combination with hypoxemia, often results in extreme shortness of breath.

OXYGEN CONSUMPTION ($\dot{V}O_2$), CO_2 PRODUCTION ($\dot{V}CO_2$), AND RESPIRATORY EXCHANGE RATIO (RER) IN EXERCISE

$\dot{V}O_2$ is the volume of O_2 taken up by the exercising (or resting) subject in liters, or milliliters, per minute, STPD. O_2 consumption is also commonly reported in milliliters per kilogram. $\dot{V}O_2$ is a result of the ventilation per minute and the rate of extraction from the gas breathed (i.e., the difference between the FI_{O_2} and the FE_{O_2}, see following paragraph). Healthy persons at rest have a $\dot{V}O_2$ of approximately 0.25 L/min, STPD, or about 3.5 ml O_2/min/Kg. During exercise, $\dot{V}O_2$ may increase to greater than 4.0 L/min, STPD in trained subjects. $\dot{V}O_2$ serves as the best single measure of the work load being performed; hence, exercise limitations caused by abnormalities of gas exchange or inappropriate cardiovascular responses may be quantified by relating specific parameters to the O_2 consumption. Figs. 7-6, 7-7, and 7-8 provide examples of ventilatory and cardiovascular measurements as they relate to the $\dot{V}O_2$ in healthy persons. Analyzing the trends of these parameters as the $\dot{V}O_2$ increases during exercise enables definition of the causes of work limitations in terms of pulmonary disease, cardiac disease, deconditioning, or a combination of these factors.

To calculate $\dot{V}O_2$ and $\dot{V}CO_2$, the fractional concentrations of O_2 and CO_2 in expired gas must be analyzed, using either a collection device (see Fig. 7-3), an appropriate mixing chamber (see Fig. 7-4), or a breath-by-breath analysis (see Fig. 7-5). In systems that accumulate a volume of gas (i.e., bag, balloon, Tissot, or mixing chamber), the water vapor is removed from the mixed expired sample by a calcium chloride drying tube. If the sample for analysis is removed before the volume determination is made, the $\dot{V}E$ should be corrected for the volume withdrawn, or the sample itself returned to the volume-measuring device. In breath-by-breath systems, fractional gas concentrations are sampled at the mouth using rapid gas analyzers and integrated with the expiratory flow signal to provide the volumes of O_2 and CO_2 exchanged for each breath.

$\dot{V}O_2$ is calculated from an accumulated gas volume using this equation:

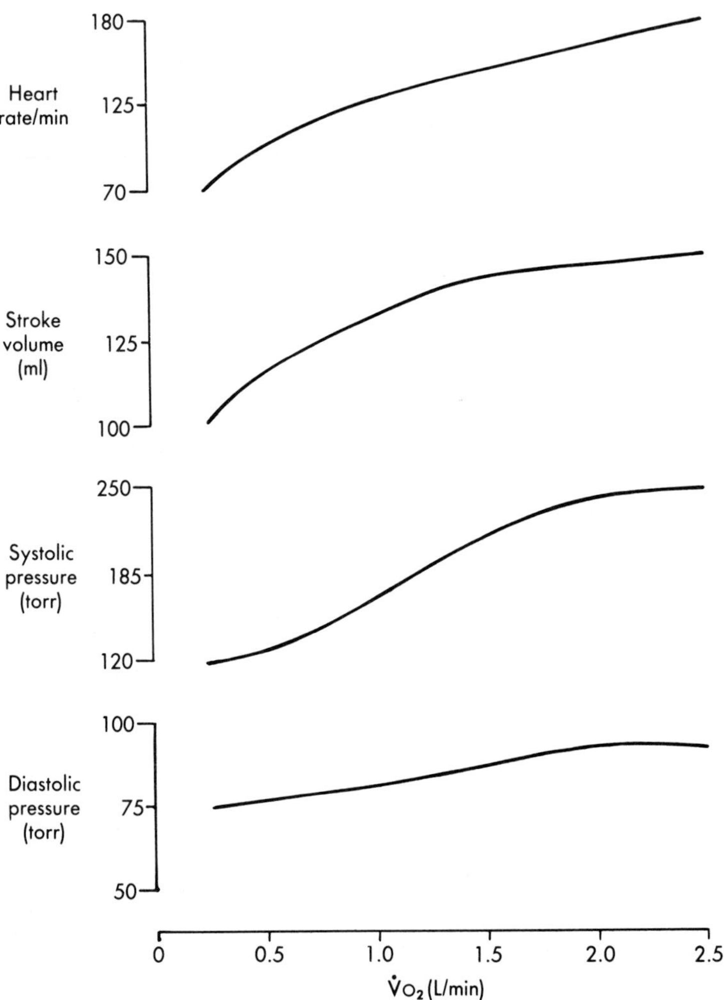

Fig. 7-8 Normal cardiovascular responses during exercise. Four cardiovascular parameters are plotted against $\dot{V}O_2$ as a measure of work rate, as they might appear in a normal healthy adult. HR increases linearly with work, with the maximum value attained declining with advancing age. SV increases initially at low to moderate work loads but then becomes fairly constant. Cardiac output, which equals HR $\times$ SV, is thus increased at low and moderate work loads by both HR and SV, but predominantly by HR at higher levels. Systolic BP increases by about 100 mm Hg (torr) in a linear fashion, while diastolic BP increases only slightly.

$$\dot{V}O_2 = \left(\left[\left(\frac{1 - FE_{O_2} - FE_{CO_2}}{1 - FI_{O_2}}\right) \times FI_{O_2}\right] - FE_{O_2}\right) \times \dot{V}E(STPD)$$

where

FE_{O_2} = Fraction of O_2 in the expired sample
FE_{CO_2} = Fraction of CO_2 in the expired sample
FI_{O_2} = Fraction of O_2 in inspired gas (room air = 0.2093)

$$\dot{V}E(STPD) = \dot{V}E(BTPS) \times \left(\frac{PB - 47}{760}\right) \times 0.881$$

$\left(\frac{1 - FE_{O_2} - FE_{CO_2}}{1 - FI_{O_2}}\right)$ = Factor to correct for the small difference between inspired and expired volumes

O_2 consumption at the highest level of work attainable by healthy individuals, called the $\dot{V}O_{2max}$, is characterized by a plateau of the O_2 uptake despite increasing external work loads. The $\dot{V}O_{2max}$ is useful for comparing endurance exercise ability between subjects, or for comparison to an age-related predicted $\dot{V}O_{2max}$ value. Equations for deriving predicted $\dot{V}O_{2max}$ are included in the Appendix. One measure of impairment is the percentage of expected $\dot{V}O_{2max}$ attained by the exercising subject. Because stature, gender, age, and fitness level all affect the "normal" maximal O_2 consumption, most prediction equations show a large variability (i.e., $\pm$ 20%). Subjects who have reductions in $\dot{V}O_{2max}$ of 20% to 40% may be considered to have mild to moderate exercise impairment, while those who have $\dot{V}O_{2max}$ values less than 60% of their predicted value may have severe exercise impairment.

Several studies have attempted to estimate $\dot{V}O_2$ based on the height and weight of the subject, along with the speed and slope of a treadmill, or length of time spent walking. O_2 uptake values estimated from treadmill walking vary so much that their value is limited. Power output from a well-calibrated cycle ergometer may be used to estimate $\dot{V}O_2$ more accurately than power output from treadmill exercise. The values obtained are typically less influenced by weight or stride, but the actual $\dot{V}O_2$ may differ significantly from the estimate.

$\dot{V}CO_2$ is a direct reflection of the state of metabolism and is expressed in liters, or milliliters, per minute, STPD. Pulmonary ventilation, consisting of alveolar ventilation ($\dot{V}A$) and dead space ventilation ($\dot{V}D$), may be related in terms of the $\dot{V}CO_2$. The fraction of alveolar carbon dioxide (FA_{CO_2}) is directly proportional to $\dot{V}CO_2$ and inversely proportional to the $\dot{V}A$; i.e., the concentration of CO_2 in the lung is determined by CO_2 production and the rate of removal from the lung by ventilation. This relationship may be expressed:

$$FA_{CO_2} = \frac{\dot{V}CO_2}{\dot{V}A}$$

The $\dot{V}CO_2$ in the healthy person at rest is about 0.20 L/min (STPD); in trained individuals, it may be more than 4.0 L/min, STPD during maximal exercise. The adequacy of $\dot{V}A$ in response to the increase in $\dot{V}CO_2$ is indicated by the maintenance of the Pa_{CO_2} in equilibrium with alveolar gas as determined by the FA_{CO_2} at low and moderate work loads, and the reduction of the Pa_{CO_2} at high work loads.

$\dot{V}CO_2$ may be calculated using this equation:

$$\dot{V}CO_2 = (FE_{CO_2} - 0.0003) \times \dot{V}E$$

where

FE_{CO_2} = Fraction of CO_2 in expired gas
0.0003 = Fraction of CO_2 in room air (may vary)
$\dot{V}E$(STPD) = Calculated as in the equation for $\dot{V}O_2$

RER, the repiratory exchange ratio, as defined by $\dot{V}O_2$ and $\dot{V}CO_2$ at the mouth, is calculated as the $\dot{V}CO_2$ divided by the $\dot{V}O_2$; it is expressed as a fraction. In some circumstances, RER is assumed to be 0.8, but for exercise evaluation or for metabolic studies, the actual value is reported. RER typically increases from a resting level of between 0.75 and 0.85 as work increases. When anaerobic metabolism begins to produce CO_2 from the buffering of lactate, the $\dot{V}CO_2$ approaches the $\dot{V}O_2$; as exercise continues, $\dot{V}CO_2$ exceeds $\dot{V}O_2$. The RER may be increased at submaximal work loads, or even at rest, if hyperventilation is present; RER represents the exchange ratio between CO_2 and O_2 in the lungs, but not necessarily at the cellular level. In exercise tests in which a steady state is allowed to develop (i.e., 4 to 6 minutes at a constant work load), RER approaches or equals the respiratory quotient (RQ), and reflects the ratio of $\dot{V}CO_2/\dot{V}O_2$ at the cellular level. Under steady-state conditions, the $\dot{V}CO_2$ reflects the CO_2 produced metabolically at the cellular level.

Sample calculations of $\dot{V}E$, $\dot{V}O_2$, $\dot{V}CO_2$, and RER, as used with one of the gas accumulation methods, are included in the Appendix.

VENTILATORY EQUIVALENTS FOR O_2 AND CO_2, AND O_2 PULSE IN EXERCISE

The minute ventilation during exercise may be related to the amount of work being performed (expressed as the $\dot{V}O_2$). This ratio is termed the ventilatory equivalent for O_2 ($\dot{V}E/\dot{V}O_2$), and is calculated by dividing the $\dot{V}E$ (BTPS) by the $\dot{V}O_2$ (STPD) and expressing the ratio in liters of ventilation per liter of O_2 consumed per minute. The $\dot{V}E/\dot{V}O_2$ is a measure of the efficiency of the ventilatory pump at various work loads.

Ventilation at low and moderate work loads increases linearly with increasing $\dot{V}O_2$ and $\dot{V}CO_2$; the absolute level of ventilation depends on the response to CO_2, the adequacy of VA, and the VD/VT ratio. At work loads in excess of about 60% to 75% of the maximum, $\dot{V}E$ is more closely related to $\dot{V}CO_2$. Because ventilation helps determine the volume of O_2 that can be transported per minute, it is often useful to evaluate the level of total ventilation required for a particular work load to assess the role of the lungs in exercise limitations. In healthy persons, the ratio remains in the range of 20 to 30 L/L of $\dot{V}_{O_2}$ until higher levels of work are reached. As ventilation increases to match the $\dot{V}CO_2$ above the anaerobic threshold, the ventilatory equivalent of O_2 also increases. In some pulmonary disease patterns, the $\dot{V}E/\dot{V}O_2$ may be close to normal at rest, but increases with exercise out of proportion to increases in either $\dot{V}O_2$ or $\dot{V}CO_2$. This usually occurs in individuals who have severe ventilation/perfusion abnormalities that worsen with increasing cardiac output during exercise. Similarly, some subjects who have pulmonary disease may have an elevated $\dot{V}E/\dot{V}O_2$ at rest (i.e., $VE/\dot{V}O_2 > 40$ L/L of $\dot{V}O_2$) that falls during exercise but does not return to the normal range. Many subjects hyperventilate during the resting phase at the beginning of an exercise evaluation and show an increased $\dot{V}E/\dot{V}O_2$ that usually returns to the normal range during exercise. This pretest hyperventilation is also usually denoted by an RER value greater than 1.0 that returns to a more normal level once the actual exercise begins.

The ventilatory equivalent for CO_2 ($\dot{V}E/\dot{V}CO_2$) is calculated similarly to the $\dot{V}E/\dot{V}O_2$, by dividing CO_2 production (STPD) by minute ventilation (BTPS). The normal level is in the range of 25 to 35 of L/L of $\dot{V}CO_2$. $\dot{V}E/\dot{V}CO_2$ may be useful for estimating the maximum tolerable work load of subjects who have moderate or severe ventilatory limitations. The ventilatory equivalents for O_2 and CO_2, measured by a breath-by-breath technique, may be useful in identifying the onset of the anaerobic threshold. Anaerobic metabolism is usually accompanied by a steady increase in the $\dot{V}E/\dot{V}O_2$ while the $\dot{V}E/\dot{V}CO_2$ remains constant or falls slightly. This same pattern may also be seen on a breath-by-breath display of end-tidal O_2 and CO_2 (see Fig. 7-7). Markedly elevated $\dot{V}E/\dot{V}CO_2$ (i.e., $\dot{V}E/\dot{V}CO_2 > 50$ L/L of $\dot{V}CO_2$) may also be observed in pulmonary hypertensive disease.

The efficiency of the circulatory pump may be related to the work load, expressed as the $\dot{V}O_2$, during exercise by the O_2 pulse. The O_2 pulse is defined as the volume of O_2 consumed per heartbeat and may be readily calculated from the electrocardiogram (ECG) recorded during the exercise evaluation. The heart rate (HR) may be read manually from a standard ECG tracing or from an accurate analog signal. The $\dot{V}O_2$ in milliliters, STPD, is divided by the HR, and the quotient is expressed as milliliters of $\dot{V}O_2$ per heart beat. In healthy individuals, the O_2 pulse varies between 2.5 and 4.0 ml O_2/beat at rest and increases to between 10 and 15 ml O_2/beat during strenuous exercise. In patients who have cardiac disease, the O_2 pulse may be normal or even low at rest, but does not rise to expected levels during exercise, consistent with an inappropriately high HR for a particular level of work. Because cardiac output, which normally increases linearly with exercise, is the product of HR and stroke volume (i.e., HR $\times$ SV), a low O_2 pulse is generally consistent with an inability to increase the stroke volume and may even fall in subjects who have poor left ventricular function. This pattern of low O_2 pulse with increasing work rate may be seen in subjects who have coronary artery disease or valvular insufficiency, but it is most pronounced in the cardiomyopathies. Tachycardia, or tachyarrythmias, tend to lower the O_2 pulse because of the abnormal elevation of HR. Conversely, beta-blocking agents, which tend to reduce HR, may falsely elevate the O_2 pulse. The O_2 pulse is often considered to be an index of fitness; at similar power outputs a fit subject will have a higher O_2 pulse than one who is deconditioned. This is evidenced by a lower HR, both at rest and at maximal work loads. Conditioning exercises (i.e., training) tend to increase stroke volume so that the heart beats less frequently to produce the same cardiac output. Trained subjects can thus achieve higher work rates before reaching their limiting cardiac frequency.

GAS EXCHANGE AND EXERCISE BLOOD GASES

Blood gas sampling during exercise testing, though invasive, is often indicated in subjects who have primary pulmonary disorders. An indwelling arterial catheter permits analysis of blood gas tensions (i.e., Pa_{O_2} and Pa_{CO_2}), saturation (Sa_{O_2}), O_2 content (Ca_{O_2}), pH, and lactate levels at various work loads. The indwelling catheter, in conjunction with a suitable pressure transducer (Fig. 7-9), allows continuous monitoring of systemic blood pressure as well. Arterial catheterization, at either the radial or brachial sites, has been demonstrated to be relatively safe, and is indicated if multiple blood specimens are required. An alternative technique is to obtain a specimen by a simple arterial puncture at peak exercise. Use of a cycle ergometer for testing allows better stabilization of the site. The sample should be obtained within 15 seconds of peak exercise because gas tensions, particularly Pa_{O_2}, may change rapidly.

Oxygen saturation during exercise may be monitored using an ear or finger pulse oximeter (see Chapter 9) and is sometimes referred to as the Sp_{O_2}. A distinct advantage of pulse oximetry is that it provides continuous measurements, unlike the conventional means of arterial sampling. Such "in vivo" measurements are extremely valuable in evaluating subjects who have pulmonary disease in whom rapid changes in Pa_{O_2} and Sa_{O_2} frequently occur during exercise. It should be noted that pulse oximetry may overestimate the true saturation if a significant concentration of COHb is present. A single arterial sample, preferably at peak exercise, may be used to correlate the Sp_{O_2} reading with true saturation if the specimen is analyzed with a multi-wavelength blood oximeter (see Chapter 9). Inadequate perfusion of the ear or finger may also confound oximetry during exercise testing. Motion artifact, light scattering within the tissue at the probe site, and dark skin pigmentation may all cause discrepancies between the Sp_{O_2} and the actual Sa_{O_2} (see Sa_{O_2}, Chapter 6).

In healthy persons, the Pa_{O_2} tends to remain constant even up to relatively high work loads. The alveolar P_{O_2}, calculated using the alveolar air equation (see Chapter 6), increases during maximal exercise because of the

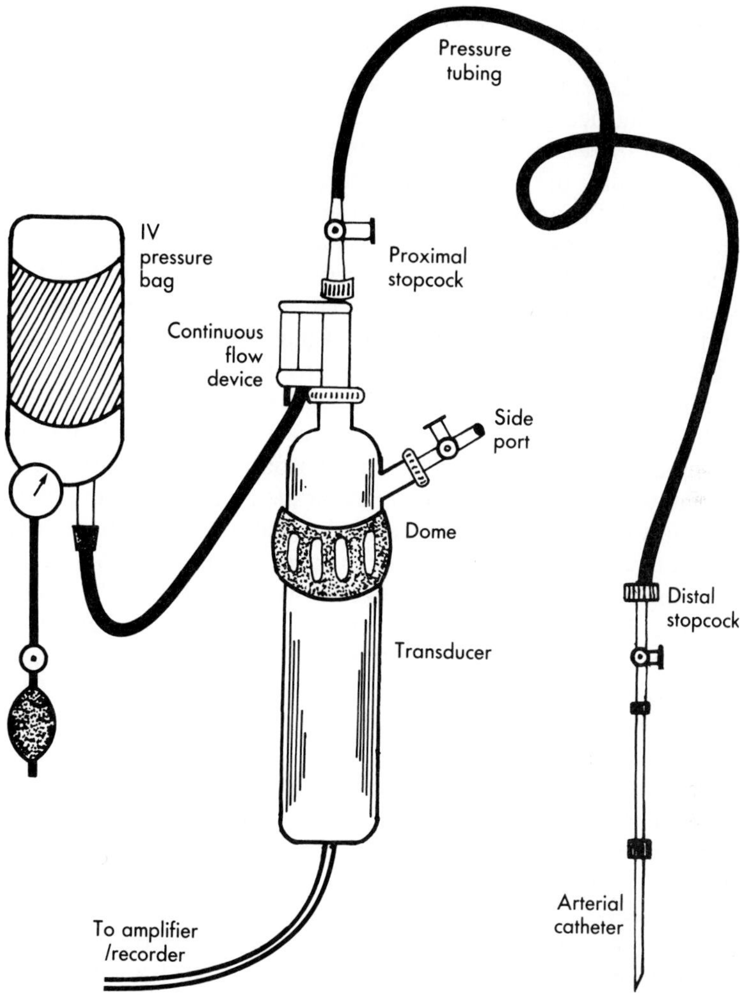

Fig. 7-9 Pressure transducer setup for continuous arterial monitoring—the components for continuous monitoring of systemic BP via an arterial catheter. The catheter is normally inserted into the radial or brachial artery. Pressure tubing connects the catheter to a continuous flow device that maintains a constant pressure and a small flow of solution against the arterial line to prevent back flow of blood into the system. The continuous flow device also allows flushing of the system. Connected in line with the tubing is the transducer assembly. Pressure changes in the system are transmitted via a thin membrane at the base of the dome to a pressure transducer. Blood samples may be drawn by inserting a heparinized syringe at the distal stopcock, closing the proximal stopcock to block the continuous flow device, and withdrawing (the BP signal is temporarily lost during sampling). A similar assembly can be used for connection to a Swan-Ganz catheter for pulmonary artery monitoring during exercise.

increased ventilation that accompanies the rise in $\dot{V}CO_2$. The alveolar-arterial (A-a) gradient, normally about 10 mm Hg, widens as a result of the increase in alveolar O_2 tension and because of a lower mixed venous O_2 content. The $P(A\text{-}a)_{O_2}$ may increase to 20 to 30 mm Hg in healthy individuals during heavy exercise because of these mechanisms. A fall in the Pa_{O_2} with increasing exercise can result from increased right-to-left shunting, inequality of $\dot{V}A$ in relation to pulmonary capillary perfusion, or a potential diffusion limitation at the alveolocapillary interface. Because exercise normally reduces the mixed venous O_2 tension ($P\bar{v}_{O_2}$), the presence of a shunt or $\dot{V}/\dot{Q}$ inequality may result in a decrease in the Pa_{O_2} or a widening of the $A\text{-}a_{O_2}$ gradient without an absolute change in the magnitude of the shunt. This is a direct result of the mixed venous blood with a lowered O_2 content (due to extraction by the exercising muscles) passing through abnormal lung units, then being mixed with normally arterialized blood. In some subjects who have decreased Pa_{O_2} and increased $P(A\text{-}a)_{O_2}$ at rest, increased cardiac output or redistribution of ventilation during exercise may actually cause an increase in the Pa_{O_2}. This improvement of the Pa_{O_2} may result from an increased PA_{O_2} caused by a reduction of PA_{CO_2} at moderate to high work rates, or because of improved $\dot{V}/\dot{Q}$ relationships resulting directly from the changes in ventilation and/or cardiac output. Because the Pa_{O_2} may either increase or decrease during exercise, depending on the pathologic mechanisms involved, measuring Pa_{O_2} during exercise may be particularly valuable in subjects who have known or suspected pulmonary disorders.

A Pa_{O_2} falling to less than 55 mm Hg or an Sa_{O_2} decreasing to less than 85% is sufficient reason for terminating the exercise evaluation. Subjects who have hypoxemia while at rest or at very low work rates should be tested with supplementary O_2 via a controlled delivery system (e.g. a nasal cannula) to determine an appropriate exercise prescription. Different levels of O_2 may be required for rest and various activities of daily living; correlation of Pa_{O_2} using supplementary O_2 at different exercise work loads allows relatively precise titration of therapy to the patient's needs.

In healthy individuals, the Pa_{CO_2} remains relatively constant at low and moderate work rates because $\dot{V}A$ increases to match the increase in $\dot{V}CO_2$. The end-tidal CO_2 increases at submaximal work loads, indicating that less ventilation is "wasted" (i.e., VD/VT decreases). At work loads higher than 50% to 60% of the $\dot{V}O_{2max}$, the metabolic acidosis resulting from anaerobic metabolism stimulates $\dot{V}E$ to increase in response to the augmented $\dot{V}_{CO_2}$. Ventilation thus increases more than required to keep the Pa_{CO_2} constant, causing a progressive decrease in Pa_{CO_2} and effecting a respiratory compensation for the acidosis associated with anaerobic metabolism (see Figs. 7-6 and 7-7). The PET_{CO_2} decreases along with the Pa_{CO_2} at high work rates. Some individuals who have airways obstruction may be able to increase their $\dot{V}A$ to maintain a normal Pa_{CO_2} at low work loads, but they may not be able to reduce the Pa_{CO_2} to compensate for the metabolic acidosis that occurs at very high exercise levels. In many subjects who have airway obstruction, the level of maximal exercise is limited by the lack of ventilatory reserve, such that these individuals typically do not reach the anaerobic threshold. In subjects who have severe air flow obstruction, $\dot{V}A$ may not be able to match the increase in $\dot{V}CO_2$, resulting in hypercapnia and respiratory acidosis. Increased work of breathing and reduced sensitivity to CO_2, combined with the increased $\dot{V}CO_2$ during exercise, allow the Pa_{CO_2} to rise.

The pH, like Pa_{CO_2}, is regulated by the $\dot{V}A$ at low work rates. The $\dot{V}A$ increases in proportion to the $\dot{V}CO_2$ up to the anaerobic threshold. At work rates above the anaerobic threshold, proportional increases in ventilation maintain the pH at normal levels with most of the buffering of lactic acid provided by HCO_3^- and a decrease in the Pa_{CO_2}. At the highest work rates, above 80% of the $\dot{V}O_{2_{max}}$, the pH decreases despite hyperventilation, as the compensation for lactic acidosis becomes incomplete. In the presence of airways obstruction, ventilatory limitations may prevent compensation above the anaerobic threshold, with the development of significant acidosis; however, subjects who have moderate or severe obstruction generally cannot exercise up to a level that elicits anaerobic metabolism, and acidosis occuring in these subjects is often caused directly by increased Pa_{CO_2}.

Arterial blood gases drawn during exercise allow several other parameters of gas exchange to be determined, namely physiologic dead space, $\dot{V}A$, and the VD/VT ratio.

VD, (see Chapter 2) comprised of anatomic and alveolar dead space, makes up that part of the $\dot{V}E$ that does not participate in gas exchange. The VD/VT ratio expresses the relationship between "wasted" and tidal ventilation for the average breath. The normal adult at rest has a $\dot{V}A$ of 4 to 7 L/min (BTPS) and a VD/VT ratio of approximately 0.25 to 0.35. The volume of dead space normally increases during exercise in conjunction with increased $\dot{V}E$. But, because of increases in VT and increased perfusion of well-ventilated lung units, such as the apices, the VD/VT ratio falls. This pattern is expected in healthy subjects (see Fig. 7-6). The VD/VT may fall in mild and moderate pulmonary disease; in severe airway obstruction or in pulmonary vascular disease, the VD/VT may remain fixed or even rise. An increase in the VD/VT indicates increased ventilation in relation to perfusion, and is most often associated with pulmonary hypertension. The $\dot{V}A$ during exercise normally increases proportionately more than the $\dot{V}E$ because the VD/VT falls. In subjects whose VD/VT ratio remains fixed or rises, the adequacy of $\dot{V}A$ must be assessed in terms of the Pa_{CO_2} and not simply by the magnitude of the $\dot{V}E$.

Calculation of VD, $\dot{V}A$, and VD/VT requires measurement of the Pa_{CO_2}. VD (BTPS) may be calculated using the following equation:

$$VD = \left(VT \times \left(1 - \frac{FE_{CO_2} \times (PB - 47)}{Pa_{CO_2}}\right)\right) - VD_{sys}$$

where

V_T = Tidal volume, in liters (BTPS)
FE_{CO_2} = Fraction of expired CO_2
$P_B - 47$ = Dry barometric pressure
Pa_{CO_2} = Arterial CO_2 tension
VD_{sys} = Dead space of the one-way breathing valve, in liters

Once the VD is determined, $\dot{V}_A$ (BTPS) can be calculated using this equation:

$$\dot{V}_A = \dot{V}_E - (f_b \times V_D)$$

where

$\dot{V}_E$ = Minute ventilation (BTPS)
f_b = Respiratory rate
V_D = Ventilatory dead space (BTPS)

The V_D/V_T ratio may be calculated as the quotient of the VD, as determined above, and the VT, averaged from the $\dot{V}_E$ and f_B, or derived simply from the difference between arterial and mixed expired CO_2 at each exercise level:

$$V_D/V_T = \frac{(Pa_{CO_2} - PE_{CO_2})}{Pa_{CO_2}}$$

where

PE_{CO_2} = partial pressure of CO_2 in expired gas

CARDIOVASCULAR MONITORS DURING EXERCISE

Continuous monitoring of heart rate (HR), and electrocardiogram (ECG), and intermittent or continuous monitoring of blood pressure (BP) during exercise are essential to safe performance of the test. Assessment of HR, ECG, and BP allows work limitations caused by cardiac or vascular disease to be identified and quantified. The level of fitness, or conditioning, can be gauged from the HR response in relation to the maximal work rate achieved during exercise.

Heart rate and electrocardiogram

HR and rhythm are monitored continuously using one or more modified chest leads. Standard precordial chest lead configurations (V_1-V_6) allow comparison with resting 12-lead tracings. Twelve-lead monitoring during exercise is practical with devices that incorporate adequate filters, digital or analog, to eliminate movement artifact, and may provide more sensitive ST segment monitoring. Limb leads normally must be moved to the torso for ergometer or treadmill testing, and resting ECGs should be performed to record differnces between the standard and modified leads. Single-lead monitoring allows only for gross arrhythmia detection and rate determination, and may not be adequate for testing subjects who have known or suspected cardiac disease. The ECG monitoring device should be able to provide tracings sufficiently free of motion artifact to allow assessment of intervals and segments up to the subject's maximal heart rate (HR_{max}). Computerized arrhythmia recording, or manual "freeze-frame" storage, may be of value for careful evaluation of conduction abnormalities, while allowing the testing protocol to be continued smoothly. Many digital ECG systems generate computerized "median" complexes averaged from a series of beats; these may be helpful in analyzing ST segment depression. The "raw" or nondigitized ECG should also be available. HR should ideally be analyzed by visual inspection of a tracing with manual measurement of the rate, rather than by an automatic sensor. Most HR meters average the R-R intervals over several beats. Inaccurate readings may occur because of variable rhythms, such as nodal or ventricular arrhythmias, or because of motion artifact. Tall T waves may be falsely identified as R waves and cause automatic calculation of HR to be incorrect. Accurate measurement of HR is necessary to determine the subject's maximal rate, as compared with his or her age-related predicted maximal. Significant ST segment changes should be easily identifiable from the tracing up to the predicted maximum HR. Because artifacts caused by movement are the most common cause of unacceptable recordings during exercise, it is useful to allow the subject to "practice" the exercise, whether ergometer or treadmill, not only to familarize the subject, but to check for adequacy of the ECG signal. Carefully applied electrodes, proper skin preparation, and secured lead wires greatly minimize movement artifact.

HR normally increases linearly with the work load, up to an age-related maximum. Although several formulas are available for predicting maximal HR, it should be noted that a variability of ± 10 to 15 beats/min exists in healthy adults. Two commonly-used equations for predicting maximal HR are:

1. $HR_{max} = 220 - Age_{years}$
2. $HR_{max} = 210 - (0.65 \times Age_{years})$

Equation 1 yields slightly higher predicted values in young adults, while equation 2 produces higher values in older adults. Other methods of predicting HR_{max} vary depending on the type of exercise protocol used in deriving the regression data. Specific criteria for terminating an exercise test should include factors based on symptom limitation as well as HR and BP changes (see Safety section).

HR increases almost linearly with increasing $\dot{V}O_2$, and is the main factor affecting the increase in cardiac output. Increases in stroke volume account for a smaller portion of the increase in cardiac output, primarily at low and moderate work loads. While the HR changes from around 70 beats/min to close to 200 beats/min, the stroke volume increases from 80 ml to approximately 110 ml in healthy upright subjects. Reduced HR response may occur in subjects who have ischemic heart disease or complete heart block, or who are treated with drugs that block the effects of the sympathetic nervous system (i.e., beta blockers). HR response may also be reduced if the autonomic nervous system is impaired, or if the heart is denervated, as in cardiac transplantation. Low HR contributes to low cardiac output and almos always results in a reduced $\dot{V}O_{2max}$. Reductions in stroke volume are usually related to the preload and afterload on the left ventricle. Increased HR response, in relation to the work load, implies that the stroke volume is compromised and that increased cardiac output is accomplished primarily by increased frequency. In subjects who have heart disease (i.e., coronary artery disease or cardiomyopathies), increased HR response is typically accompanied by ECG changes such as arrhythmias and/or ST segment depression. Deconditioned subjects who do not have heart disease show a high HR at lower than maximal work loads, but usually without ECG abnormalities. Depression of the ST segment greater than 1 mm for a duration of 0.08 seconds is usually considered evidence of ischemia. ST depression at low work loads that increases with HR and continues into the postexercise period is usually indicative of multivessel coronary artery disease. ST depression accompanied by exertional hypotension, or marked increase in diastolic pressure, is usually associated with significant coronary disease. The predictive value of ST segment changes during exercise must be related to the subject's clinical history and risk factors for heart disease.

The most common arrhythmia occurring during exercise testing is the ventricular premature contraction (VPC). VPCs are associated with an increased incidence of myocardial ischemia, and are considered dangerous because they may precede more serious lethal arrhythmias. Exercise-induced ventricular premature beats occurring at a rate of more than 10 per minute are often found in ischemic heart disease. Increased VPCs during exercise may also be seen in mitral valve prolapse. Coupled VPCs (couplets) often precede ventricular tachycardia or ventricular fibrillation; occurrence of couplets or frequent VPCs may be indications for terminating the exercise evaluation. Some subjects with VPCs at rest, or at low work loads, may have these ectopic beats suppressed as the exercise intensity increases. The most serious ventricular ectopic beats are sometimes seen in the immediate postexercise phase.

Blood pressure (BP)

Systemic BP may be monitored intermittently using the standard cuff method or continously by connection of a pressure transducer to an indwelling arterial catheter (see Fig. 7-8). An indwelling line allows continuous display and recording of systolic, diastolic, and mean arterial pressures. In addition, the catheter provides ready access for arterial blood sampling when multiple specimens are required. Arterial catheterization can normally be accomplished easily using either the radial or brachial site. The catheter must be adequately secured to prevent loss of patency during vigorous exercise. Automated BP monitors using a self-inflating cuff may also be used during exercise testing. These devices, as well as manual cuffs, may not be able to detect the usual BP sounds during vigorous exercise, particularly treadmill walking.

Systolic BP increases in healthy subjects during exercise from 120 mm Hg to approximately 200 to 250 mm Hg. Diastolic pressure normally rises only slighly (10 to 15 mm Hg), or not at all. The mean pressure rises from approximately 90 mm Hg to about 110 mm Hg, depending on the changes in systolic and diastolic pressures. The increase in systolic pressure is caused almost completely by the increase in the cardiac output, particularly the stroke volume. Even though the cardiac output may increase fivefold, (i.e., from 5 to 25 L/min), the systolic pressure only doubles, because of the tremendous decrease in peripheral vascular resistance. Most of this decrease in resistance results from vasodilatation in exercising muscles. Increases in the systolic pressure to greater than 250 to 300 mm Hg should be considered an indication for terminating the exercise evaluation. Similarly, if the systolic pressure fails to rise with an increasing work load, or if the diastolic pressure falls markedly, the cardiac output is not increasing appropriately. The exercise test should be terminated, and the subject's condition stabilized. Variations in BP during exercise are often caused by the subject's respiratory efforts. Differences of as much as 30 mm Hg between inspiration and expiration may be seen during continuous monitoring of arterial pressure. These wide pressure swings are common in patients who have pulmonary disease. In maximal tests, in which the subject is taken to HR_{max}, it may be impossible to obtain a reliable BP at peak exercise, even with an arterial catheter. In addition, the systolic pressure may transiently drop and the diastolic may fall to zero at the termination of exercise. To minimize the degree of hypotension resulting from the abrupt cessation of heavy exercise, the subject should "cool down," that is, continue working at a low work rate until BP and HR have stabilized at, or slightly above, baseline levels.

Safety

Safe and effective exercise testing for cardiopulmonary disorders requires careful pretest evaluation to identify contraindications to the test procedure. Such contraindications are included in the first box on p. 148. A preliminary workup should include a complete history and physical examination by either the referring physician or the physician performing the stress test. Preliminary laboratory tests should include a 12-lead ECG, a chest x-ray film, baseline pulmonary function studies with before and after bronchodilators, and routine laboratory examinations (i.e., complete blood count and serum electrolytes). Subjects receiving methylxanthines should have a recent theophylline level, particularly if the primary indication for

CONTRAINDICATIONS TO EXERCISE TESTING

Pa_{O_2} less than 40 mm Hg with subject breathing room air
Pa_{CO_2} greater than 70 mm Hg
$FEV_{1.0}$ less than 30% of the predicted value
Recent (within 4 weeks) myocardial infarction
Unstable angina pectoris
Second-degree or third-degree heart block
Rapid ventricular/atrial arrhythmias
Orthopedic impairment
Severe aortic stenosis
Congestive heart failure
Uncontrolled hypertension
Limiting neurologic disorders
Dissecting/ventricular aneurysms
Severe pulmonary hypertension
Thrombophlebitis or intracardiac thrombi
Recent systemic or pulmonary embolus
Acute pericarditis

INDICATIONS FOR TERMINATING EXERCISE TESTS

Monitoring system failure
2 mm horizontal or downsloping ST depression or elevation
T wave inversion or Q waves
Sustained supraventricular tachycardia
Ventricular tachycardia
Multifocal premature ventricular beats
Development of second-degree or third-degree heart block
Exercise-induced left or right bundle branch block
Progressive chest pain (angina)
Sweating and pallor
Systolic pressure greater than 250 mm Hg
Diastolic pressure greater than 120 mm Hg
Failure of systolic pressure to increase, or a drop of 10 mm Hg with increasing work load
Lightheadedness, mental confusion, or headache
Cyanosis
Nausea or vomiting
Muscle cramping

exercise testing is ventilatory limitation or exercise-induced bronchospasm.

The entire procedure, including the risks involved and benefits of the information obtained, should be explained or demonstrated to the subject and appropriate informed consent forms signed. A physician experienced in exercise testing should supervise the test. Submaximal tests on subjects less than 40 years of age with no known risk factors may be performed by qualified technologists or nurses, provided a physician is immediately available. Criteria for terminating the exercise evaluation before the specified endpoint or symptom limitation occurs are listed in the bottom box on p. 148.

Following termination of the exercise evaluation, regardless of the reason, the subject should be monitored until cardiac and vascular parameters return to pretest levels. Electrocardiographic monitoring should continue for at least 15 minutes, with tracings made at frequent intervals immediately postexercise.

Personnel conducting exercise tests should be trained in handling cardiovascular emergencies and should be certified in cardiopulmonary resuscitation. The laboratory should have available resuscitation equipment, including:

1. Standard intravenous (IV) medications (i.e., epinehrine, atropine, lidocaine, isoproterenol, propranolol, procainamide, sodium bicarbonate, and calcium gluconate)
2. Syringes, needles, and IV infusion apparatus
3. Portable O_2 and suction equipment
4. Airway equipment, endotracheal tubes, and laryngoscope
5. Direct current (DC) defibrillator and appropriate monitor

CARDIAC OUTPUT (FICK METHOD)

Cardiac output is commonly measured by thermal or dye dilution, or by the direct or indirect Fick method. The Fick methods require exhaled gas analysis and are often used in conjunction with exercise testing.

The direct Fick method is as follows:

$$\dot{Q}_T = \frac{\dot{V}O_2}{C(a\text{-}\bar{v})_{O_2}} \times 100$$

where:

$\dot{Q}_T$ = Cardiac output, in liters per minute

$\dot{V}O_2$ = Oxygen consumption, in liters per minute

$C(a\text{-}\bar{v})_{O_2}$ = Arterial-mixed venous O_2 content difference

100 = Factor to correct $C(a\text{-}\bar{v})_{O_2}$ to liters (content differnces are normally reported in vol% or milliliters per deciliter)

The $\dot{V}O_2$ is measured as described previously; the $C(a\text{-}\bar{v})_{O_2}$ is obtained by measuring or calculating (see Chapter 6) the O_2 content in both the arterial and mixed venous samples.

The indirect Fick method, also termed the CO_2 rebreathing technique is as follows:

$$\dot{Q}_T = \frac{\dot{V}_{CO_2}}{C(a\text{-}\bar{v})_{CO_2}} \times 100$$

where:

$\dot{Q}_T$ = Cardiac output, in liters per minute
$\dot{V}_{CO_2}$ = CO_2 production, in liters per minute
$C(a\text{-}\bar{v})_{CO_2}$ = Arterial-mixed venous CO_2 content difference
100 = Factor to correct $C(a\text{-}\bar{v})_{CO_2}$ to liters (content differences are normally reported in vol% or milliliters per deciliter

The $\dot{V}_{CO_2}$ is measured as described previously. The content difference for CO_2 can be obtained completely noninvasively or in conjunction with arterial blood gas analysis. To calculate the mixed venous CO_2 content, the $P\bar{v}_{CO_2}$ must be measured using a rebreathing technique. This measurement is accomplished while the subject is connected to the typical circuit used for exhaled gas analysis during exercise. The subject, either at rest or during exercise, is switched to a rebreathing bag containing a mixture of CO_2 in air that is slightly higher than the $P_{A_{CO_2}}$ and has a volume of 1 to 2 times the V_T. In general, fractional concentration of CO_2 in the bag must be adjusted between 7% and 15%, and the volume must be between 1 and 3 L. The bag CO_2 is usually estimated from the subject's end-tidal CO_2, so that a rapid equilibrium between the bag and mixed venous blood can be achieved. The subject rebreathes rapidly from the bag until an equilibrium between the CO_2 in the bag and in the alveoli occurs (Fig. 7-10). If equilibrium is not accomplished, because of either too much or too little CO_2 in the bag, a different concentration is prepared and the maneuver repeated. Because no CO_2 is removed during the rebreathing, because of the slightly higher CO_2 concentration in the bag, the fractional concentration at equilibrium closely resembles that in the pulmonary capillaries. From the fractional concentration, the partial pressure, and hence the content, can be determined. A similar method of rebreathing does not require a special mixture of CO_2, but simply monitors the rise in the concentration of CO_2 in the bag during rebreathing. An equilibrium value can be estimated from the exponential increase in CO_2. The most accurate application of the exponential method requires computerized curve fitting. Once the mixed venous tension of CO_2 is known, the CO_2 content may be calculated or read from a standard nomogram. (The reader is referred to the excellent text by Jones, et al, listed in the Selected Bibliography at the end of this chapter.) The CO_2 content of arterial blood can be estimated similarly using either a measured Pa_{CO_2} or an estimated value derived from the end-tidal and mixed-expired CO_2 values, the V_T, and the respiratory rate:

$$Pa_{CO_2} = P_{ET_{CO_2}} + 4.4 - 0.0023V_T + 0.03f_b - 0.09P_{E_{CO_2}}$$

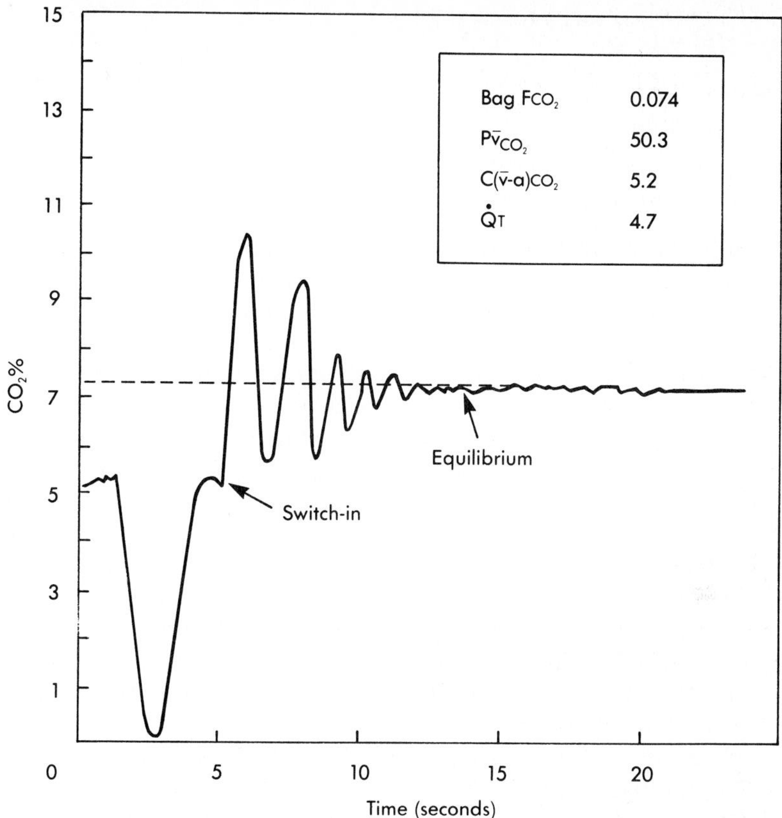

Fig. 7-10 Cardiac output determination by CO_2 rebreathing. Expired CO_2, sampled at the mouth with a breath-by-breath system, is plotted against time as the subject is switched from breathing room air to rebreathing from a bag containing 7% to 15% CO_2. After switch-in, the subject takes several fast deep breaths until an equilibrium is established, as identified by a flat CO_2 tracing. For the maneuver to work correctly, the CO_2 concentration in the bag must be slightly higher than the subject's alveolar CO_2. The fractional concentration of CO_2 in the bag (bag F_{CO_2}) is then used to estimate the mixed venous CO_2. A modified form of the Fick equation, using CO_2 content in arterial and mixed venous blood instead of O_2 content), is then used along with the V_{CO_2} to determine the cardiac output.

where:

$P_{ET_{CO_2}}$ = Partial pressure of end-tidal CO_2
V_T = Tidal volume
f_b = Frequency of breathing (respiratory rate)
$P_{E_{CO_2}}$ = Partial pressure of mixed-expired CO_2

Or, Pa_{CO_2} can be estimated:

$$Pa_{CO_2} = P_{E_{CO_2}} \div \left(1 - \frac{V_D + V_{D_{sys}}}{V_T}\right)$$

where:

$P_{E_{CO_2}}$ = Partial pressure of mixed-expired CO_2
V_D = Subject's ventilatory dead space (estimated)
$V_{D_{sys}}$ = Dead space of the breathing circuit

Both of these methods of estimating Pa_{CO_2} presume normal lung function; completely noninvasive cardiac output may not be practical if the subject has lung disease by static measures of pulmonary function.

After the CO_2 contents of mixed venous and arterial blood are calculated, the difference is divided into the $\dot{V}_{CO_2}$, measured immediately before the rebreathing maneuver. These calculations may be performed manually or, because of their complexity, by computer. Corrections to the calculated CO_2 contents must be made if the subject's Hb is less than 15 gm%, or if the Sa_{O_2} is much less than 95%, because of the effects of Hb and O_2 saturation on the CO_2 dissociation curve. A correction for slight differences between the alveolar and arterial CO_2, which occurs primarily during exercise, may be necessary so that the bag P_{CO_2} accurately reflects $P\bar{v}_{CO_2}$.

Because equilibrium must be achieved quickly, before recirculation occurs, a rapid-responding CO_2 analyzer is necessary; thus the CO_2 rebreathing method lends itself well to breath-by-breath analysis. Attainment of a true equilibrium can also be complicated by having a CO_2 concentration in the rebreathing bag that is either too high or too low, as well as by an inadequate volume to match the subject's tidal breathing. To rapidly adjust the gas concentrations and bag volume during exercise, a computerized gas mixing system may be helpful.

The cardiac output is approximately 4 to 6 L/min at rest, and rises during exercise to 25 to 35 L/min in healthy subjects. Cardiac output is the product of HR and stroke volume:

$$\dot{Q}_T = HR \times SV$$

where:

HR = Heart rate in beats per minute
SV = Stroke volume in liters or milliliters

SV is approximately 70 to 100 ml at rest and increases to 100 to 140 ml with low or moderate exercise. The HR increases almost linearly with increasing work rate as described above, so that at low work loads the increase in cardiac output is caused by a combination of HR and SV. At moderate and high work loads, further increases in $\dot{Q}_T$ are caused mainly by increases in the HR. The SV increases very little during exercise in the supine position, but is slightly higher at rest than in the upright subject. Derivation of the SV from $\dot{Q}_T$ and HR is useful in quantifying poor cardiac performance in subjects who have coronary artery disease, cardiomyopathy, or other diseases that affect myocardial contractility.

Subjects who reach their predicted $\dot{V}O_{2max}$ and their predicted HR_{max} typically have a normal cardiac output and SV. A subject who has a reduced $\dot{V}O_{2max}$, but achieves a maximal predicted HR, often has a low cardiac output due to a low SV. This limited cardiac output in the face of increasing exercise loads is often accompanied by an early onset of anaerobic metabolism. Reduced cardiac output is typical in both atrial and ventricular arrhythmias, valvular insufficiency, and cardiomyopathies.

In subjects who are fit, the SV may be increased both at rest and during exercise. Endurance (aerobic) training normally results in increased SV; other benefits include reductions in systolic BP and ventilation. Fit subjects typically have lower resting heart rates than their sedentary counterparts, and are able to reach a higher $\dot{V}O_2$. Depending on the frequency, intensity, and duration of training, fit indidivuals are able to maintain a higher level of work for longer periods because of improved cardiac performance.

The main disadvantage of the direct Fick method is that placement of a pulmonary artery catheter is required to obtain a mixed venous sample. The indirect Fick method, CO_2 rebreathing, is somewhat complicated, and requires careful attention to the correct CO_2 concentration in the rebreathing bag. Additionally, if arterial PCO_2 is estimated rather than measured, the content differences may be in error. In subjects who have obstructive pulmonary disease, this may be a serious limitation, although the CO_2 rebreathing technique appears to work well despite uneven distribution of ventilation.

SELF-ASSESSMENT QUESTIONS

1. Which of the following exercise protocols would allow measurement of heart rate and ventilation under steady-state conditions:
   a. Constant speed treadmill, grade increase of 5% each minute
   b. 10% grade treadmill, speed increase of 2.5 MPH every minute
   c. Cycle ergometer ramp test, 16 watts/minute
   d. Cycle ergometer, increasing resistance 50 watts every 6 minutes

2. Which of the following are true concerning the use of a cycle ergometer for exercise evaluation:
   I. Power output can be calculated from resistance and pedaling rate
   II. $\dot{V}O_{2max}$ is slightly higher than on a treadmill
   III. Ventilation and blood lactate are higher than on a treadmill
   IV. Work load is independent of the subject's weight
   a. I, II, III, IV
   b. I, III, IV
   c. I, II, III
   d. II, IV

3. A patient who weighs 50 Kg has her $\dot{V}O_{2max}$ measured during an incremental treadmill exercise test; the reported value is 1.75 L/min, STPD. This represents a maximum exercise capacity of ________ METS.

a. 87.5
b. 35.0
c. 17.5
d. 10.0

4. Measurements of $\dot{V}O_2$ and $\dot{V}CO_2$ during exercise are commonly performed using which of the following:
a. Breath-by-breath integration of flow and fractional gas concentrations
b. Mixed expired gas analysis from a mixing chamber
c. Mixed expired gas analysis from a bag or balloon
d. All of the above

5. An incremental exercise test produces the following results (values in parentheses are percents of predicted values):

$\dot{V}O_{2max}$ L/min, STPD	1.77	(51%)
$\dot{V}E_{max}$ L/min, BTPS	31.0	(49%)
HR_{max} beats/min	177	(101%)

Which statement best describes these results:
a. Moderate exercise impairment
b. Severe exercise impairment, with cardiovascular limitation
c. Severe exercise impairment, with ventilatory limitation
d. Severe exercise impairment, with cardiovascular and ventilatory limitations

6. Which of the following are required for breath-by-breath analysis of $\dot{V}O_2$ and $\dot{V}CO_2$:
I. Integration of flow and fractional gas concentrations
II. Rapid response gas analyzers
III. Measurement of "phase delay" of the gas analyzers
IV. 5 liter (or larger) mixing chamber
a. I, II, III, IV
b. I, III, IV
c. I, II, III
d. II, IV

7. Which of the following exercise variables is a measure of the work performed:
a. $\dot{V}O_2$
b. Heart rate
c. Treadmill speed/slope
d. $\dot{V}E$

8. A subject at rest has a $\dot{V}E/\dot{V}O_2$ of 24 L/L of O_2; after 5 minutes of exercise the ventilatory equivalent for O_2 is still 24 L/L of O_2. This response is:
a. Consistent with normal lung function
b. Indicative of airway obstruction
c. Consistent with pulmonary hypertension
d. Both b and c

9. A subject performs an exercise test in which he reaches 100% of his predicted maximum heart rate at 50% of his predicted $\dot{V}O_{2max}$; if there are no ECG abnormalities, the best description of this response would be:
   a. Cardiomyopathy
   b. Ventilatory limitation to exercise
   c. Deconditioning
   d. Abnormally large stroke volume

10. Which of the following may result during an exercise test when ischemic heart disease is present:
    I. Ventricular premature contractions
    II. $\dot{V}O_{2max}$ less than predicted
    III. ST segment depression
    IV. A reduced O_2 pulse
    a. I, II, III, IV
    b. I, II, IV
    c. II, III, IV
    d. III only

11. Which of the following are indications for terminating an exercise evaluation:
    I. Sweating and pallor
    II. Systolic blood pressure greater than 190 mm Hg
    III. Diastolic blood pressure greater than 140 mm Hg
    IV. Nausea and vomiting
    a. I, II, III, IV
    b. I, II, IV
    c. I, III, IV
    d. II, III only

12. At low and moderate work loads, increased cardiac output is accomplished by:
    a. Increased systemic vascular resistance
    b. Increased heart rate
    c. Increased stroke volume
    d. All of the above
    e. b and c only

SELECTED BIBLIOGRAPHY

General references

American College of Sports Medicine: Guidelines for graded exercise testing and exercise prescription, ed 3, 1986, Lea & Febiger.

Astrand PO and Rodahl K: Textbook of work physiology, New York, 1970, McGraw-Hill Inc.

Hansen JE: Exercise instruments, schemes, and protocols for evaluating the dyspneic patient, Am Rev Respir Dis (suppl) 129:S25, 1984.

Hansen JE, Sue DY, and Wasserman K: Predicted values for clinical exercise testing, Am Rev Respir Dis (suppl) 129:S49, 1984.

Hellerstein HK, Brock LL, and Bruce RA: Exercise testing and training of apparently healthy individuals: a handbook for physicians, New York, 1972, Committee on Exercise, American Heart Association.

Jones NL: Clinical exercise testing, ed 3, Philadelphia 1988, WB Saunders Co.

Lange-Anderson K, et al: Fundamentals of exercise testing, Geneva, 1971, World Health Organization.

Spiro SG: Exercise testing in clinical medicine, Br J Dis Chest 71:145, 1977.

Ventilation, gas exchange, and blood gases

Jones NL: Exercise testing in pulmonary evaluation: rationale, methods and the normal respiratory response to exercise, Parts I and II, New Engl J Med 293:541, 1975.

Jones NL: Normal values for pulmonary gas exchange during exercise, Am Rev Respir Dis (suppl) 129:S44, 1984.

Neuberg GW et al: Cardiopulmonary exercise testing: the clinical value of gas exchange data, Arch Intern Med 148:2221, 1988.

Sue DY et al: Measurement and analysis of gas exchange during exercise using a programmable calculator, J Appl Physiol 49:456, 1980.

Wasserman K and Whipp BJ: Exercise physiology in health and disease, Am Rev Respir Dis 112:219, 1975.

Weber KT et al: Concepts and applications of cardiopulmonary exercise testing, Chest 93:843, 1988.

Whipp BJ, Ward SA, and Wasserman K: Ventilatory responses to exercise and their control in man, Am Rev Respir Dis (suppl) 129:S17, 1984.

Cardiovascular monitoring during exercise

Bruce RA: Value and limitations of the electrocardiogram in progressive exercise testing, Am Rev Respir Dis (suppl) 129:S28, 1984.

Ellestad MH et al: Maximal treadmill stress testing for cardiovascular evaluation, Circulation 39:517, 1969.

Pollack ML et al: A comparative analysis of four protocols for maximal stress testing, Am Heart J 92:39, 1976.

Stone HL and Liang IYS: Cardiovascular response and control during exercise, Am Rev Respir Dis (suppl) 129:S13, 1984.

8

Specialized Test Regimens

The diagnosis of specific pulmonary disorders requires that an appropriate battery of tests be performed. It may not be necessary to perform all of the various tests available; in many instances, simple spirometry and/or blood gas analysis provide sufficient information to delineate a disease process or recommend a course of therapy. The addition of lung volume determination and diffusing capacity may be necessary to quantitate changes to the pulmonary parenchyma or to assess the overall gas exchange. Specialized test regimens, such as those described in this chapter, consist of one or more standard tests performed under specific conditions. The $FEV_{1.0}$, for example, may be analyzed before and after bronchodilator, inhalation challenge, or exercise to quantify airway reactivity. The subject's pulmonary history and clinical condition at the time of testing often aid in the selection of appropriate tests and assist in the interpretation of the results.

PULMONARY HISTORY AND RESULTS REPORTING

Accurate interpretation of pulmonary function studies—from simple screening spirometry to the complete cardiopulmonary evaluation—requires clinical information pertinent to possible pulmonary disorders. An ordered array of questions that can be easily answered by the subject provides the most useful type of history. Often, the interpreter of pulmonary function studies may have little clinical information concerning the subject, other than that obtained at the time of testing. An appropriate history should be taken as a routine part of pulmonary function testing, including the following:

1. Age, sex, standing height, weight, race, current diagnosis
2. Family history—Did anyone in your immediate family (mother, father, brother, or sister) ever have:

   Tuberculosis
   Emphysema
   Chronic bronchitis
   Asthma
   Hay fever or allergies
   Cancer
   Other lung disorders

3. Personal history—Have you ever had, or been told that you had:

Tuberculosis
Emphysema
Chronic bronchitis
Asthma
Recurrent lung infections
Colds
Pneumonia or pleurisy
Allergies or hay fever
Chest injury
Chest surgery

4. Occupation—Have you ever worked:

In a mine, quarry, or foundry
Near gases or fumes (if so, what kind?)
In a dusty place (if so, what kind?)

5. Smoking habits—Have you ever smoked:

Cigarettes (________/day)
Cigars (________/day)
Pipe (________/day)
How long? (________years)
Do you still smoke?
Do you live with a smoker?

6. Cough—Do you ever cough:

In the morning
At night
At a particular time of the year
Blood (when _____________)
Phlegm (when _____________)
(color _____________)
(volume _____________)

7. Dyspnea—Do you get short of breath:

At rest
On exertion (when ________)
At night

8. Subject disposition at time of test

Dyspneic
Wheezing
Coughing
Cyanotic
Apprehensive
Cooperative/uncooperative

9. Current medications

____________________ (Last Taken: ________)
____________________ (Last Taken: ________)

Most of these types of questions can be answered yes, no, or circling an appropriate response. In addition, space may be provided for comments either by the subject or history taker. An outline history of this type provides a basis for evaluation of the various tests. When the physician performs the test, such a history may be redundant if a medical history is available.

Standardized reporting helps simplify test interpretation; a common method of recording test results follows a format such as that outlined in Fig. 8-1. Test results are usually reported in conjunction with the appropriate predicted normal values and a corresponding percent of normal value. Because many studies providing predicted normal values are available for the more common pulmonary function tests, the normal values chosen for a particular laboratory should represent the methodology employed, as well as the patient population being tested. For example, a laboratory using a water-sealed spirometer at or near sea level might select predicted values obtained using similar equipment. Because trying to match methodologies may not always be practical, predicted normal values that represent a large and diverse population are usually most appropriate. (See the Appendix for a more detailed discussion of selecting normal values). In addition to the predicted value itself, the standard deviation (SD) or standard error of estimate (SEE) for any predicted normal value should be considered in the final evaluation of lung dysfunction. The SD or SEE are measures of the *variability* that exists in the sample population tested to generate the predicted values. Using a statistical approach (i.e., SD or SEE) to define the difference between the subject's measured value and the predicted value is usually more sound than using simple percentages.

Perhaps the best method to estimate the extent of abnormality is to calculate the *confidence interval* (CI) for each predicted value. The CI is defined as:

$$CI = 1.65 \times SD$$

where:

SD = the standard deviation for a particular parameter

1.65 = the number of SDs *below* the mean that includes 95% of the normal population

This method accounts for the variability associated with each individual pulmonary function parameter. For tests in which the subject could be considered abnormal if the derived value is either higher or lower than the predicted value, such as RV, the CI is calculated using 1.96 SDs. One drawback of reporting the relation between measured and predicted values in this way is that some parameters (for example, $FEF_{25\%\text{-}75\%}$) are so variable in the normal population that one CI may include extremely low or even negative values. Considering how variable a specific parameter is in the normal population is important when using that parameter to diagnose

NAME ______________________________ SEX ______________

AGE ____________ HEIGHT ____________________ WEIGHT ____________

Test	Subject	Predicted	% Normal
Lung Volumes			
VC i-e e-i			
FRC			
RV			
TLC			
RV/TLC x 100%			
Ventilation			
V_T			
$\dot{V}_E$			
f			
Pulmonary Mechanics			
FVC			
FEV 0.5			
FEV 1.0			
FEV 1.0%			
FEF 25-75%			
MVV			
Arterial Blood Gases			
Pa_{O_2}			
% Sat.			
Pa_{CO_2}			
pH			
Distribution			
SBN_2			
7 Minute N_2			
Miscellaneous			

INTERPRETATION:

DIAGNOSIS:

Interpreted by ______________________

Performed by ______________________

Fig. 8-1 Typical data record sheet.

pulmonary abnormalities (see the Appendix, "Selecting and Using Predicted Values").

In addition to comparison with predicted normal values, the reported pulmonary function results should be referenced to any previous studies of the subject. Comments on serial tests should include whether or not there has been a significant change in function in relation to previous tests, and, if so, to what extent. Some pulmonary function software allows calculation of percent change for serial tests in a manner similar to that used for before and after bronchodilator studies (see next section). Reporting of serial test results is important in longitudinal studies designed to assess the rate of decline of a specific pulmonary function parameter (i.e., $FEV_{1.0}$, FVC).

Reporting of results should include any other information that is pertinent to the interpretation of the test. Some laboratories "adjust" predicted values for certain ethnic groups to more accurately reflect the expected values. If predicted values are race-corrected or standardized in some other way, that fact should be included in the final report. If multiple predicted sets are used to accommodate subjects of different ethnic origins or to provide a complete set of normal values, the source of the reference equations should be reported. When a computer-assisted interpretation is generated, it should be clearly marked as such. Some test parameters are corrected before reporting; for example, the $D_{L_{CO}}$ may be corrected for HB, COHb, or altitude. If corrections to the measured value are made, both the uncorrected and corrected data should be available so that the interpreter can evaluate the effect of the correction on the measurement. Questionable test results should not be reported, but often it is impossible to differentiate between an abnormal finding and an erroneous one. In such an instance, the questionable value should be noted as such. Following predefined criteria for acceptability for each test may be helpful in elucidating the causes of questionable results (see Chapter 11, for "Criteria for Acceptability").

BEFORE AND AFTER BRONCHODILATOR STUDIES

One of the most practical applications of pulmonary function testing is the determination of a course of therapy in the management of airway obstructive disease. Pulmonary function tests, particularly spirometry, can be performed before and after bronchodilator administration to determine the reversibility of airways obstruction. An $FEV_{1\%}$ of less than 70% is a good indication for performing bronchodilator studies; except in older adults, low $FEV_{1.0}$/FVC ratios are associated with obstruction. Some subjects whose $FEV_{1.0}$ and FVC are within normal limits may display a low $FEV_{1\%}$ if the FVC is greater than 100% of the predicted value while the $FEV_{1.0}$ is slightly reduced. Bronchodilator studies may be indicated anytime there is clinical evidence of altered airway reactivity. Although any pulmonary function parameter may be measured before and after bronchodilator therapy, tests of pulmonary mechanics are usually evaluated. The subject is typically given a normal array of tests, including spirometry, lung volumes, and diffusing capacity. FRC determinations done by He dilution or the open-circuit N_2 method should be performed before bronchodilator administration to provide an accurate baseline on which to judge any changes in the lung volume compartments that occur as a result of the dilator. Even though indices of flow such as the $FEV_{1.0}$ and $FEF_{25\%-75\%}$ usually show the greatest change, lung volumes and DL_{CO} may also respond to bronchodilator therapy.

Subjects referred for bronchodilator testing should withhold routine bronchodilator therapy before the procedure, beta-agonists for 8 hours, sustained-action beta-adrenergics and methylxanthines for 12 hours, and cromolyn sodium for 24 hours. Prednisone and other corticosteroids may be continued before testing at a stable dosage.

The bronchodilator, usually a beta-adrenergic agent, can be administered by an aerosol generator, intermittent positive pressure breathing (IPPB), or a metered-dosage device. A metered-dose inhaler (MDI) typically provides a more reproducible, and thus more quantifiable, administration of bronchodilator. For subjects who are unable to coordinate the activation of the metered-dose device with a slow deep inspiration, the use of an aerosol reservoir, or spacer, may provide a more consistent delivery of medication. Depending on the type of bronchodilator used and the means of administration, the therapy should last long enough to achieve the maximum effects. With MDIs, two or more "puffs" spaced over several minutes may result in greater bronchodilation. Most aerosolized bronchodilators begin taking effect upon inhalation and continue for an indefinite period, usually at least an hour. Some beta-adrenergic preparations have a slower onset, and peak response may not occur for 10 to 15 minutes following inhalation of the drug. Evaluation of atropine-like drugs may require a delay of 45 to 60 minutes or longer following inhalation.

Reversibility of airway obstruction and improvement in flow rates are considered significant for increases of greater than 15% to 20%. The percent of change may be calculated:

$$\% \text{ Change} = \frac{\text{Postdrug} - \text{Predrug}}{\text{Predrug}} \times 100$$

where:

Postdrug = The test parameter value after administration
Predrug = The test parameter value before administration

Any pulmonary function parameter that worsens following bronchodilator will produce a negative value using this equation. In addition, parameters that have small absolute values (for example, an $FEF_{25\%-75\%}$ less than 0.5 L/sec) may show large percent changes even though the actual improvement in flow is minimal. The $FEV_{1.0}$ is the most commonly assessed parameter for quantifying bronchodilator effects, but the $FEF_{25/75\%}$, $\dot{V}_{max50\%}$, and SGaw are also useful. If the FVC increases more than the $FEV_{1.0}$ following bronchodilator, the $FEV_{1\%}$ may actually decrease; changes in the $FEV_{1\%}$ following bronchodilator should be interpreted carefully. Increases in the FVC also usually indicate that the flow rates determined at a specific fraction of the vital capacity (i.e., $\dot{V}_{max50\%}$) should be reported using the isovolume technique (see Chapter 3). Spirometry software that allows superimposition of flow-volume loops at TLC provides graphic analysis of the extent of improvement in flows at all lung volumes.

Disease patterns involving the bronchial and bronchiolar musculature show the most pronounced change from "before" to "after." Improvements of greater than 50% in parameters such as the $FEV_{1.0}$ and $FEF_{25\%-75\%}$ may occur in uncomplicated asthma. Moderate or severe chronic obstructive diseases may fail to show any improvement, and may sometimes yield poorer results for the "after" tests because of the exertion of performing the forced expiratory tests several times. A common cause of little or no bronchodilator response is inadequate deposition of the inhaled drug because of a poor inspiratory maneuver. Because bronchodilators effect the greatest change in flows, repetition of the lung volume tests and DL_{CO} are usually unnecessary. An increase in VC is normally at the expense of the previously increased RV. However, if symptomatic improvement occurs with bronchodilator in the absence of increased flows, it may be a result of changes in the lung volume compartments, changes in DL_{CO}, or changes in the matching of ventilation to perfusion. A common change is one in which the VC increases only slightly, but the $FEF_{25\%-75\%}$ or $FEV_{1.0}$ shows significant increase. This may be caused by the opening of previously obstructed airways without notable increase in the actual volume of air moved by a forced expiratory maneuver.

Failure of the $FEV_{1.0}$ to increase by more than 15% to 20% does not preclude the use of bronchodilator therapy, particularly if symptomatic improvement or increased exercise tolerance is demonstrated. Many subjects who have obstructive lung disease may show minimal response to inhaled bronchodilator on initial testing, but significant improvement on subsequent tests. Repeat testing may be indicated in subjects with clinical signs of obstruction who would benefit from bronchodilator therapy.

A paradoxical fall in Pa_{O_2} may occur in some subjects following administration of inhaled bronchodilator. This hypoxemia is thought to result from alterations in the matching of ventilation and blood flow in the lungs, which occurs when a beta-adrenergic drug enters the circulatory system via the lungs and then is distributed to poorly ventilated lung regions during recirculation. An increased blood flow to poorly ventilated lung units results in an increased venous admixture, with a fall in Pa_{O_2}. Blood gas analysis before and after bronchodilators may be required to document the paradoxical hypoxemia, particularly if flows improve but symptoms of hypoxemia worsen. Other complications of inhaled beta-adrenergic drugs usually center on aggravation of cardiac arrhythmias or hypertension. Careful monitoring of heart rate and blood pressure in susceptible subjects before and after bronchodilator administration should be part of the testing regimen. If a subject develops tachycardia, sweating, or other signs of adverse cardiovascular response, testing should be terminated and the subject should be evaluated immediately by a physician.

QUANTITATIVE METHACHOLINE CHALLENGE TEST

Bronchial provocation testing is useful in determining the extent of airway reactivity, particularly in subjects with symptoms of bronchospasm who have normal pulmonary function studies or uncertain results of bronchodilator studies. The objective of the test is to determine if airway hyperreactivity is present. A positive test results when inhalation of methacholine precipitates a 20% decrease in the $FEV_{1.0}$. The metacholine concentration at which this decrease occurs is referred to as the provocative dose, or $PD_{20\%}$. Methacholine increases parasympathetic tone in bronchial smooth muscle, resulting in bronchoconstriction. In the doses usually employed (see Table 8-1), healthy persons do not display decreases greater than 20% in the $FEV_{1.0}$; thus, the methacholine challenge test is highly specific for airway hyperreactivity. Because bronchospasm may be induced in asthmatic subjects by physical, chemical, or allergic stimuli, the degree of response to methacholine may vary.

Subjects to be tested should be asymptomatic and should have a baseline $FEV_{1.0}$ equivalent to at least 80% of their highest previously observed value. If the subject is taking bronchodilators, the following steps are recommended:

1. Beta-adrenergic agents should be withheld for 8 hours.
2. Sustained-action beta-adrenergic and methylxanthines should be withheld for 12 hours.

Table 8-1 Units for methacholine challenge*

Methacholine concentration (mg/ml)	Cumulative # of breaths	Cumulative units/five breaths	Cumulative # of minutes
0.075	5	0.375	3
0.15	10	1.125	6
0.31	15	2.68	9
0.62	20	5.78	12
1.25	25	12.00	15
2.50	30	24.50	18
5.00	35	49.50	21
10.00	40	99.50	24
25.00	45	225.00	27

*One metacholine unit is arbitrarily defined as one inhalation of 1 mg/ml of methacholine in diluent. The quantity of drug required to provoke a 20% decrease in $FEV_{1.0}$ is expressed in x units/x min; for example, 12 methacholine units/15 min.

3. Cromolyn sodium should be withheld for 24 hours.
4. Antihistamines should be withheld for 48 hours.
5. Subjects receiving corticosteroids should be challenged while taking a stable dosage.

Baseline spirometry is performed to establish that the subject's $FEV_{1.0}$ is above 80% of the previously observed best values and that overt obstruction is not present. Subjects who demonstrate obstruction based on reduced $FEV_{1\%}$ or other flows do not require challenge testing to document airway obstruction, but may be tested to establish the degree of hyperreactivity. A simple gas-powered nebulizer may be used to generate the methacholine aerosol, but a dosimeter provides a true "quantitative" challenge test. The dosimeter or nebulizer should be activated during inspiration, either automatically by a flow sensor or manually by the subject. Ideally, the dosimeter or nebulizer should have an output sufficiently high so that 1 ml of solution can be aerosolized during the course of the inhalations at each level.

The subject begins by inhaling five breaths of nebulized diluent, usually normal saline. The breaths should be slow and deep, usually to TLC, with a short (i.e., 1 to 2 seconds) breathhold at TLC to maximize aerosol deposition. After 3 minutes, spirometry is performed. The $FEV_{1.0}$ following inhalation of the diluent value then becomes the "control," and if the $FEV_{1.0}$ is not reduced 10% from the baseline, the quantitative challenge is performed. Some subjects, usually those with highly reactive airways, will have a positive response to the diluent alone. The following methacholine dilutions may be used:

0.075	mg/ml
0.15	mg/ml
0.31	mg/ml
0.60	mg/ml
1.25	mg/ml
2.50	mg/ml
5.00	mg/ml
10.00	mg/ml
25.00	mg/ml

Each of these dilutions may be prepared from a 25 mg/ml stock. Methacholine is fairly stable after mixing and may usually be kept for 2 weeks under refrigeration. The lowest dosages (i.e., 0.075 mg/ml or less) are the least stable and may need to be prepared immediately before testing. One milliliter volumes are suitable for five inhalations in commonly used nebulization devices. Other dilutions may be used but should be arranged in such a way that the dosages range from approximately 0.1 mg/ml up to 25 mg/ml. An adequate number of intermediate concentrations should be used, usually five, so that a 20% decrease in $FEV_{1.0}$ can be detected without inducing a more severe response.

The subject inhales five breaths, as described for the diluent above, from the nebulizer beginning with the most dilute solution (i.e., 0.075 mg/ml). Spirometry is repeated at 3 minutes, with the "best" test selected from duplicate or triplicate efforts. The percent of decrease is calculated as follows:

$$\% \text{ Decrease} = \frac{x - y}{x} \times 100$$

where:

x = Control (following diluent) $FEV_{1.0}$
y = Current $FEV_{1.0}$ following methacholine inhalation

A 20% or greater decrease in the $FEV_{1.0}$ is considered a positive test. The decrease should be sustained; additional spirometry efforts may be necessary to distinguish an actual decrease from variability in the maneuvers. If the test is negative, then five breaths of the next higher dilution are administered and the measurements are repeated. If the test is borderline positive, less than five inhalations of the next dilution may be given.

At each dilution, the subject should be observed and questioned for the perception of symptoms such as chest tightness and wheezing. Auscultation may be helpful in detecting the beginning of bronchospasm. As soon as a 20% fall in the $FEV_{1.0}$ is observed, administration of the methacholine is terminated. The bronchospasm may be reversed by means of an appropriate bronchodilator, usually by inhalation. Spirometry should be performed following reversal to document the efficacy of the bronchodilator in reversing the effects of the methacholine.

Several methods of quantifying the results of the procedure are commonly used. The dilution that produced the 20% decrease in $FEV_{1.0}$ is most often reported as the $PD_{20\%}$. A more precise method totals the amount of methacholine inhaled to produce the requisite decrease by multiplying the number of breaths times the dilution. This method requires a dosimeter or metered-dosage type of nebulizer, so that a known quantity of drug is given with each inhalation. Table 8-1 lists the cumulative amounts of methacholine delivered using the five-breath routine and the dosage schedule listed above.

Methacholine challenge testing presents some risk to the subject; therefore, a physician familiar with the procedure should be immediately available. Technologists administering bronchial challenge tests should be thoroughly familiar with the procedure and with the signs and symptoms of bronchospasm. Medications for reversal of the bronchospasm, as well as for resuscitation, should be immediately available in the event of an untoward reaction.

The spirometer used should meet the minimal standards set by the American Thoracic Society (see Chapter 11) and should provide spirometric tracings or flow-volume loops for later evaluation.

Similar protocols may be employed for antigen and histamine challenge testing, both for testing and for expressing results. Antigen inhalation challenge requires intradermal (cutaneous) testing to establish a safe initial dosage for inhalation challenge.

TESTING FOR EXERCISE-INDUCED ASTHMA (EIA)

Exercise-induced asthma is typified by bronchospasm during or immediately following vigorous exercise. It is thought to be related to heat loss from the upper airway that accompanies increased ventilation during exercise. Evaluation of exercise-induced bronchospasm is helpful in quantifying the extent of reversible airway obstruction in the following instances:

1. In subjects who have shortness of breath on exertion, but who exhibit normal resting pulmonary functions
2. In symptomatic subjects in whom bronchial provocation tests (methacholine) produce negative or ambiguous results
3. In subjects with known EIA in whom therapy is being evaluated
4. In screening subjects for an activity that may present some risk to asthmatics, such as athletics

Subjects being tested by exercise challenge should be evaluated by means of an appropriate history, physical examination, and laboratory studies, including ECG, to ascertain potential contraindications to exercise testing (see Chapter 7). Methylxanthine and beta-adrenergic bronchodilators should be withheld for 8 to 12 hours before testing, depending on the preparation. Some sustained-release theophylline preparations may need to be withdrawn 24 to 48 hours before testing. Cromolyn sodium should be excluded for 24 hours, but corticosteroids may be maintained in subjects receiving stable dosages. Before exercise, the subject's pulmonary functions should be greater than 80% of the previously determined "best" values and the $FEV_{1.0}$ should be not less than 65% of the predicted value. Subjects with overt obstruction typically do not require an exercise challenge to demonstrate airway hyperreactivity.

Either a treadmill or cycle ergometer may be used, depending on the type of physiologic measurements being made. The exercise should be vigorous enough to elicit work rates between 60% and 85% of the subject's predicted maximal O_2 consumption for 6 to 8 minutes. The subject's response to an increasing work load should be monitored via continuous ECG and blood pressure. Ventilatory parameters, such as $\dot{V}_E$ and V_T, may be helpful in assessing the pattern of pulmonary response to exercise. A spirometer that meets the American Thoracic Society requirements (see Chapter 11) is necessary. The device should be simple enough for repeated measurements following the exercise and should allow for multiple recordings of either volume-time tracings or flow-volume curves, or both. Some automated systems provide software specifically for challenge testing, either by inhalation or exercise, with capability for superimposing MEFV curves, etc. Resuscitation equipment, as described in Chapter 7, must be available.

One to two minutes of low-intensity exercise allow evaluation of ventilatory and cardiovascular responses to work. As soon as a normal cardiovascular response is obtained, the work load should be increased to a level that will allow the subject to attain 85% of the predicted maximum HR or predicted maximum $\dot{V}O_2$. Usually, a short period of moderately heavy work is all that is required to trigger exercise-induced bronchospasm. Normally, bronchospasm occurs immediately following the exercise, not during it, unless the test is extended over a longer interval. Repeated testing within 2 hours may result in a "refractory period" during which the severity of the bronchoconstriction lessens, presumably due to the build-up of catecholamines. An extended warm-up period before the actual exercise may also protect the airways and lessen the subsequent bronchoconstriction.

Pulmonary function baseline values are established before testing and are compared to the subject's usual values. Following exercise, measurements should be taken at 1 to 2 minutes and then every 5 minutes as the selected parameter (usually $FEV_{1.0}$ or SGaw) decreases to a minimum and continued until the parameter returns to baseline. Maximal decreases are typically seen in the first 5 to 10 minutes following cessation of exercise, and spontaneous recovery occurs within 20 to 40 minutes. The best value of duplicate measurements is recorded. Ambient temperature, relative humidity, and PB should be recorded because of their influence on airway muscle tone. Several common methods of reporting the response to exercise are:

1. Maximum percent of decrease of baseline function:

$$\frac{x - y}{x} \times 100$$

where

x = Baseline value (FEV_1)
y = Lowest after-exercise value

2. Maximum decrease as a percentage of the predicted value:

$$\frac{x - y}{P} \times 100$$

where

x = Baseline value (FEV_1)
y = Lowest after-exercise value
P = Subject's predicted value

3. Lowest value as a percent of predicted value:

$$\frac{y}{P} \times 100$$

where

y = Lowest after-exercise value
P = Subject's predicted value

The advantage of the first method is that the baseline parameter is included in both the numerator and denominator and provides a unit that is independent of the absolute values, making it useful for comparisons between subjects. The second method can be used similarly. Baseline values should always be reported, particularly if the third method is used.

Exercise-induced asthma (i.e., bronchospasm) has been demonstrated to be related to respiratory heat and/or water loss in the upper airway as a result of increased minute ventilation. Some individuals with EIA are protected from bronchospasm during exercise if warm moist air is inhaled. The stimulus to bronchospasm during exercise testing is likely to be the level of ventilation achieved, as well as the ambient temperature and humidity. Recently, cold air inhalation has been suggested as a means of evaluating airway responsiveness. The difficulties associated with control of temperature and humidity in the testing context may limit the usefulness of this type of challenge. The exercise-induced asthma test, particularly if used to evaluate prophylactic therapy, is a quite practical means of quantifying airway reactivity.

PREOPERATIVE PULMONARY FUNCTION TESTING

Preoperative pulmonary function testing is one of several means available to clinicians to evaluate surgical candidates who are at risk of developing respiratory complications. Preoperative testing, in conjunction with history and physical examination, ECG, and chest X-ray, is indicated for one or more of the following reasons:

1. To determine the level of risk involved in the surgical procedure (i.e., morbidity and mortality)
2. To plan perioperative care, including preoperative preparation, type, and duration of anesthetic during surgery; and postoperative care to minimize complications
3. To estimate postoperative lung function in candidates for pneumonectomy or lobectomy

The surgical candidate who needs preoperative pulmonary function testing is determined by the type of surgical procedure and the individual's risk factors. Many investigations, both prospective and restrospective, have identified that the risk of postoperative pulmonary complications are highest in *thoracic procedures,* followed by *upper abdominal* and *lower abdominal* procedures. Increased incidence of complications appears in both healthy subjects and those who have pulmonary disorders, with the latter being at higher risk in proportion to the degree of pulmonary impairment.

Preoperative pulmonary function testing is *definitely* indicated in:

1. Subjects with a history of smoking
2. Subjects with symptoms of pulmonary disease (i.e., cough, sputum

production, shortness of breath)

3. Subjects with abnormal physical examination findings, particularly of the chest (i.e., abnormal breath sounds, ventilatory pattern, respiratory rate)
4. Subjects with abnormal chest x-ray

Preoperative testing may also be indicated in:

1. Subjects with morbid obesity (i.e., greater than 30% above ideal body weight)
2. Subjects advanced in age, usually greater than 70 years
3. Subjects with current or recent respiratory infections, or a history of respiratory infections
4. Subjects with marked debilitation or malnutrition

In each of these subjects, the primary purpose of pulmonary function testing is to uncover preexisting pulmonary disease. Decreases in the VC of more than 50% of the preoperative value place individuals with compromised function at high risk of developing atelectasis and pneumonia. Decreases in the FRC and increases in closing volume (CV) may lead to $\dot{V}/\dot{Q}$ abnormalities and hypoxemia. Abnormal ventilatory function, both in terms of the central control of respiration and the status of the ventilatory muscles, may also play a role in postoperative complications.

Certain tests of pulmonary function appear to be better predictors of postoperative complications, and hence should be used for both risk evaluation and to assist in planning the perioperative care of the individual.

1. *Spirometry.* FVC, $FEV_{1.0}$, $FEF_{25\%-75\%}$, and MVV. Because obstructive disease can easily be identified with simple spirometry, a significant percentage of subjects who might develop postoperative problems can be detected with minimal screening. Subjects whose FVC is reduced, with or without airways obstruction, typically have impaired ability to cough effectively when the VC decreases further during the immediate postoperative period. The MVV, although dependent on subject effort, appears to be uniquely suited to detecting postoperative risk. This may be due in part to the fact that the MVV tests lung parenchyma, airway function, ventilatory muscle function, and subject cooperation. The measured MVV correlates better with the incidence of postoperative problems than the estimated MVV (i.e., $FEV_{1.0} \times 35$ or 40); this may be attributable to measurement of both inspiratory and expiratory flow during the MVV, whereas the $FEV_{1.0}$ assesses just expiration. Because the ventilatory muscles may be involved in the development of postoperative complications, a test such as the MVV may be a more sensitive predictor than expiratory flow tests.
2. *Bronchodilator studies.* Operative candidates with obstruction, either known or demonstrated via spirometry, should also be tested with bronchodilators. Postbronchodilator values for FVC, $FEV_{1.0}$, $FEF_{25\%-75\%}$, and MVV may be used in estimating the surgical risk

and may make a significant difference in the degree of risk if there is substantial reversibility. Bronchodilator studies are similarly helpful in planning perioperative care; bronchodilator therapy may improve the subject's bronchial hygiene preoperatively as well as postoperatively.

3. *Blood gas analysis.* Arterial blood gases are helpful in subjects with documented lung disease to assess their overall response to the pulmonary changes known to occur postoperatively. The Pa_{O_2} itself is not a good prognosticator of postoperative problems, but individuals with hypoxemia at rest usually also have abnormal spirometry, and hence are at risk. The Pa_{O_2} may actually improve postoperatively in subjects undergoing thoracotomy for lung resection, if the resected portion was contributing to $\dot{V}/\dot{Q}$ abnormalities. The Pa_{CO_2} appears to be the most useful blood gas indicator of surgical risk. If the Pa_{CO_2} is above 45 mm Hg, there is a marked increase in postoperative morbidity and mortality. Elevated Pa_{CO_2} values are most commonly encountered in subjects who have significant airways obstruction.
4. *Lung volumes.* Lung volumes, even though they may be reduced dramatically in the immediate postsurgical phase, do not correlate well preoperatively with postoperative complications, and do not enhance the estimate of complications.
5. *DL_{CO}.* Diffusion studies, like lung volume determinations, do not appear to improve the prediction of postoperative complications.
6. *Exercise testing.* Exercise studies can accurately predict subjects at risk in that those who fail to tolerate moderate work loads typically have airways obstruction or similar ventilatory limitations. Subjects who can attain an O_2 uptake of less than 20 ml/min/Kg typically have a low incidence of cardiopulmonary complications, while those unable to attain 15 ml/min/Kg almost always have complications.

In addition to these tests for predicting postoperative problems, several other tests are employed specifically in predicting postoperative lung function in candidates for pneumonectomy or lobectomy. These procedures are normally used in conjunction with spirometry and blood gas analysis.

1. *Perfusion* and *$\dot{V}/\dot{Q}$ scans.* Lung scans (see Chapter 4) are particularly useful in estimating the remaining lung function in patients who are likely to require removal of all or part of a lung. Split-function scans are performed; these allow partitioning of lungs into right and left halves or into multiple lung regions. Although $\dot{V}/\dot{Q}$ scans give the best estimate of overall function, simple perfusion scans yield quite similar information. Lung scan data, in the form of regional function percentages, are used in combination with simple spirometric indices to calculate the patient's postoperative capacity. For example:

Table 8-2 Preoperative pulmonary function

Test	Increased postop risk	High postop risk	Candidate for pneumonectomy*
FVC	Less than 50% of predicted	Less than 1.5 L	—
$FEV_{1.0}$	Less than 2.0 L or 50% of predicted	Less than 1.0 L	Greater than 2.0 L
$FEF_{25\%-75\%}$	Less than 50% of predicted	—	—
MVV	—	Less than 50 L/min or 50% of predicted	Greater than 50 L/min or 50% of predicted
Pa_{CO_2}	—	Greater than 45 mm Hg	—
Predicted Postop $FEV_{1.0}$	—	—	Greater than 0.8 L
Pulmonary Artery Occlusion	—	—	Less than 35 mm Hg

*Values in this column determine if the subject is to be considered a candidate for lung resection.

$$\text{Postop } FEV_{1.0} = \text{Preop } FEV_{1.0} \times \text{\%Perfusion to unaffected portions}$$

Subjects whose postoperative $FEV_{1.0}$ is calculated to be less than 800 ml are typically not considered surgical candidates.

2. *Pulmonary artery occlusion pressure.* In some candidates for pneumonectomy, the development of postoperative pulmonary hypertension may be a limiting factor. To estimate the effect of redirecting the entire right ventricular output to the remaining lung, a catheter is inserted into the pulmonary artery of the affected lung and blood flow is occluded by means of a balloon. The resulting pressure increase in the remaining lung is then measured. A pressure increasing to less than 35 mm Hg is usually considered consistent with acceptable postoperative pressures. The effect of redirected blood flow on oxygenation may also be a consideration, and this can also be examined during occlusion to estimate postoperative Pa_{O_2}.

These tests to predict the effects of resection on the remaining lung are normally used in series, with spirometry done first, followed by split function lung scans if the spirometry is acceptable, and then pulmonary artery occlusion pressure, if the development of cor pulmonale is a concern. Table 8-2 summarizes some general ranges of values used for preoperative pulmonary function testing.

PULMONARY FUNCTION TESTING FOR DISABILITY

Pulmonary function tests are one of several means of determining a subject's inability to perform certain tasks. Respiratory impairment and disability, however, are not synonymous. Respiratory impairment relates to the failure of one or more of the functions of the lungs, which is what most pulmonary function studies measure. Disability is the inability to perform tasks that are required either for employment or everyday activities. Those pulmonary function tests used to determine impairment leading to disability should characterize the type, extent, and cause of the impairment. Pulmonary function testing may not completely describe all of the factors involved in the disabling impairment; other factors involved may be the age, educational background, and motivation of the subject, and the energy requirements of the task in question.

Determination of the level of impairment usually consists of the following:

1. *Physical examination,* which does not allow quantification of disabling symptoms but is useful in grading shortness of breath. Shortness of breath is the most prominent feature of respiratory impairment, but, like pain, is subjective. Tachypnea, cyanosis, and abnormal respiratory patterns are not indicative of the extent of impairment, but may be helfpul in elucidating the findings from pulmonary function studies.
2. *Chest X-ray,* which does not correlate well with shortness of breath or pulmonary function studies, except in advanced cases of pneumoconioses. Absence of usual findings in the pneumoconioses may be helpful in excluding occupational exposure as part of the impairment.
3. *Pulmonary function studies,* which should be objective and reproducible, and most importantly, specific to the disorder being investigated.
   a. *FVC and $FEV_{1.0}$.* Spirometry is the most useful index for the assessment of impairment caused by airway obstruction. A permanent record of the tracings should be kept. The volume-time tracing should have the time sensitivity marked on the horizontal axis and the volume sensitivity marked on the vertical axis. The paper speed should be at least 20 mm/sec and the volume excursion at least 10 mm/L. The three largest FVC and FEV_1 values should be within 5%, and each maneuver should be continued for at least 10 seconds. The largest FVC and $FEV_{1.0}$ value from three acceptable maneuvers is reported. $FEV_{1.0}$ calculated from a flow-volume curve is not acceptable. Spirometry is normally repeated following bronchodilator therapy.
   b. *MVV.* The MVV has some drawbacks in that it is influenced by subject effort, which may be in question in disability determinations. The test may also be affected by muscular coordination, cardiac disease, neurologic function, and chest wall compliance. One satisfactory MVV maneuver is required (see Chapter 11), but it should not be calculated from the $FEV_{1.0}$. The tracing

should show both inspiratory and expiratory excursions, rather than just accumulated volume; the recording should be continued for 10 to 15 seconds.

c. *Lung volumes.* Lung volume determination correlates poorly with shortness of breath and disability, but may be necessary to assess the extent of restriction present. The VC may be required for disability determination, but other lung volumes are not.

d. DL_{CO}. The diffusion capacity is useful in determining impairment in restrictive disorders such as fibrosis. Either single-breath or steady-state methods may be used; the predicted normal value for the method should also be reported.

e. *Arterial blood gas analysis.* Although blood gas results are objective, they are largely nonspecific in determining impairment. The A-aO_2 gradient is not reliable because it may be affected by hyperventilation. Blood gas analysis may be required in diffuse pulmonary fibrosis, and should include both the Pa_{O_2} and the Pa_{CO_2}. Blood gases and A-aO_2 gradient are helpful if measured during exercise. The requirement for supplementary O_2 may also be quantified by exercise blood gas analysis.

f. *Exercise testing.* Exercise testing may be indicated if the results of simple spirometry, diffusing capacity, or blood gases are uncertain with regard to the extent of respiratory impairment. The $\dot{V}E_{max}$, compared to the MVV, helps to determine the ventilatory reserve, if any, that remains. Similarly, the HR_{max}, if much less than predicted for the work load, indicates a ventilatory rather than cardiovascular limitation. Ventilatory equivalents for O_2 and CO_2 ($\dot{V}E/\dot{V}O_2$ and $\dot{V}E/\dot{V}CO_2$) are most useful if measured during sustained exercise. They may be used to estimate functional limits that can be compared to the job requirements of the individual. The dyspnea index (see Chapter 7) is considered normal if it is less than 12% of the MVV, values between 35% and 50% are equivocal, and values greater than 50% are almost always considered abnormal.

Limits for determining disability on the basis of respiratory impairment have been set for the United States by the Social Security Administration. Criteria are set according to the disease category (see box on p. 175):

In reporting impairment for disability purposes, the remaining functional capacity is as important in determining the subject's ability to carry out a certain task as the percentage of lost function. Some statement of the subject's ability to understand and cooperate with the pulmonary function measurements should accompany the tabular and graphic data.

PULMONARY FUNCTION TESTING IN CHILDREN

Pulmonary function testing of children employs many of the same basic tests as testing of adults. Differences between adult and pediatric testing

DISEASE CATEGORY CRITERIA

COPD

$FEV_{1.0}$ less than 1.0 to 1.4 L (for heights of 57″ to 73″, respectively)
MVV less than 32 to 48 L/min (for heights of 57″ to 73″, respectively).

Asthma

(Same as for COPD)
OR
Episodes of severe attacks despite treatment every 2 months
OR
six times per year with wheezing between attacks.

Diffuse pulmonary fibrosis

VC less than 1.2 to 2.0 L (for heights of 57″ to 73″, respectively)
OR
$DL_{CO}SS$ less than 6 ml CO/min/mm Hg
$DL_{CO}SB$ less than 9 ml CO/min/mm Hg
OR
Pa_{O_2} less than 65 mm Hg (at a Pa_{CO_2} of 30 mm Hg)
Pa_{O_2} less than 55 mm Hg (at a Pa_{CO_2} of 40 mm Hg)

Other restrictive ventilatory disorders (kyphoscoliosis, thoracoplasty, lung resection)

VC less than 1.0 to 1.4 L (for heights of 59″ to 70″, respectively)

Pneumoconioses (demonstrated by chest x-ray)

Nodular focal fibrosis evaluated as for COPD
OR
Interstitial disseminated fibrosis evaluated as for pulmonary fibrosis

exist not only in the absolute dimensions of the developing pulmonary system but in two main areas concerned with the testing regimens themselves:

1. Newborns, infants, and very young children cannot strictly perform those tests that require and depend on subject cooperation.
2. Young children and adolescents may perform variably on those tests that are effort dependent or that require considerable cooperation.

Testing infants and young children

Tests of lung function in infants and very young children can be used to assess lung volumes, flows, and mechanical factors, including compliance and resistance. Inability to perform maximal efforts eliminates such parameters as FVC, $FEV_{1.0}$, or maximal expiratory flow-volume curves. A number of new techniques have recently emerged that are particularly applicable to young children.

Partial expiratory flow-volume (PEFV) curves. The partial expiratory flow-volume (PEFV) curve is a record of the maximal flow developed over a portion of the VC. In infants, the forced exhalation is obtained by applying either a positive pressure to the thorax and abdomen or a negative pressure to the airway. Infants who are intubated, and usually deeply sedated, can have their lungs inflated to TLC and then connected to a source of negative pressure, with expiratory flow plotted against volume to derive the usual flow-volume curve. This technique is usually reserved for the measurement of flows in infants in the critical care setting, and is not performed routinely in the infant laboratory. In infants who are not intubated, the pressure necessary to drive exhalation is generated by an inflatable bag that encircles the infant's chest and abdomen. The PEFV curve is obtained by rapidly applying a pressure around the thorax and abdomen at end-inspiration, increasing the pleural pressure and generating the forced expiratory maneuver. The pressure bag must fill rapidly, requiring approximately 100 ms to reach 95% peak pressure, and must be connected to a reservoir that has a volume ten times that of the bag to ensure a relatively constant pressure. Flow is usually measured using an infant face mask sealed with lubricant and attached to a low dead space pneumotachometer. The infant is evaluated after falling asleep spontaneously or after mild sedation with chloral hydrate. Chloral hydrate should be used with caution if the child has clinical signs of wheezing. The flow-volume curve may either be displayed on a storage oscilloscope or digitized for computerized storage.

In young children (i.e., ages 3 to 6) cooperation is essential to obtain reliable PEFV curves; some children in this age group who have a good attention span and coordination may even be capable of performing full MEFV curves. The child must be relaxed and able to follow instructions. The technologist's ability to elicit cooperation and to motivate the child are crucial. Several attempts may be necessary to generate an adequate, reproducible effort. The young child is tested breathing through a mouthpiece with a nose clip in place. Flow is measured by a penumotachometer and volume determined by analog or digital integration of the flow signal, with the tracing display on a storage oscilloscope or computer screen. Tidal breathing is recorded to obtain a consistent end-expiratory point (i.e., FRC) on the volume axis. The child is then instructed to exhale forcefully from end-inspiration and to continue exhaling past the end-expiratory level to produce the PEFV curve.

The PEFV curve is quantitated by measuring flow at FRC (Fig. 8-2). The highest flow obtained is reported as the $\dot{V}_{max}$FRC. In infants, the reservoir pressure that supplies the inflatable cuff is gradually increased until a maximal flow is reached. Theoretically, the pressure in the bag is increased until no further increases in flow result, indicating that flow limitation has been reached. It is not clear, however, whether the applied pressure can be directly related to the pleural pressure under dynamic conditions; hence, flow limitation may not be achieved in a reproducible fashion. PEFV curves in young children very likely do represent maximal flows (i.e., flow limitation) if two or more reproducible curves can be obtained. Infants with obstructive disease (i.e., severe air flow limitation) have intrathoracic obstruction that suggests that true flow limitation is reached during external compression. In healthy infants, inspiratory efforts or upper airway resistance (i.e., glottic closure) may impede forced expiratory flow, causing the flow at FRC to appear less than it would be if true flow limitation occurred. Flow limitation occurs, but not in an effort-independent manner.

To standardize measurements, the $\dot{V}_{max}$FRC may be divided by the absolute FRC determined either by He dilution, by N_2 washout, or ple-

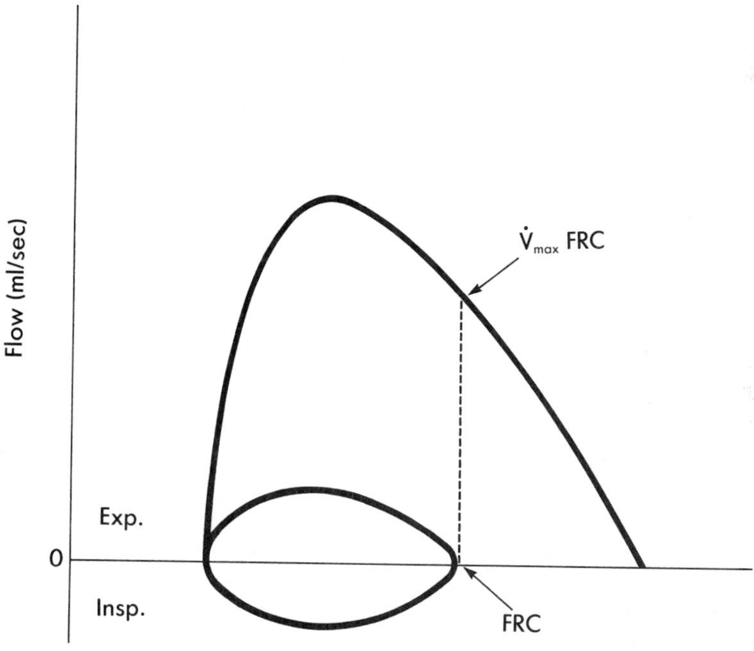

Fig. 8-2 Partial expiratory flow-volume (PEFV) curve—A flow-volume curve typical of that which might be obtained in a normal infant or child. The term "partial" refers to the fact that flow is plotted only over a portion of the VC, rather than over the entire VC, as is normally done. This maneuver can be performed in young children who may not be able to inspire to TLC or expire completely to RV by having them exhale forcefully after a normal inspiration. In infants, PEFV curves may be obtained by applying positive pressure to the thorax and abdomen using a pressure jacket. The primary flow measurement is the $\dot{V}_{max}$ FRC, which is determined by recording tidal breathing (small loop) to identify the end-expiratory point, then reading the flow at that volume. Abnormal PEFV curves show a concave appearance much like those in adults with airway obstruction (see Chapter 3).

thysmograph (VTG). The maximal flow at FRC is expressed as FRC/sec. The $\dot{V}_{max}$FRC displays a variability similar to flow measures at low lung volumes (i.e., $\dot{V}_{max\ 50}$, $\dot{V}_{max\ 25}$) in older children or adults. The variability among subjects (approximately 30%) makes the $\dot{V}_{max}$FRC less sensitive than the $FEV_{1.0}$ for detecting differences between healthy children and those with asthma.

PEFV curves in infants and young children have been used to assess normal lung growth and development. Persons who have asthma, cystic fibrosis, or bronchopulmonary dysplasia all show reduced $\dot{V}_{max}$FRC values. Inhalation challenge studies using metacholine, histamine, or cold air as the stimulus and $\dot{V}_{max}$FRC as the dependent variable have shown that a significant number of infants and young children have nonspecific airway hyperreactivity. Because young children and infants typically cannot perform a forced expiratory maneuver to determine $FEV_{1.0}$ the $\dot{V}_{max}$FRC may be helfpul in tracking the effectiveness of bronchodilators or related therapies. The $FEV_{1.0}$ is still the parameter of choice for detecting airway reactivity in older children and adolescents.

Lung volumes. Lung volume determinations, specifically the FRC, in infants and young children are usually accomplished using the closed-circuit He dilution, open-circuit N_2 washout, or body plethysmograph techniques. Special procedures are typically required to adapt the general methods for each of these techniques to the pediatric patient. In the commonly-used He dilution technique, a small-volume spirometer is used for infants, with special attention to reduction of system volume and dead space components to accommodate the small FRC volumes commonly encountered. Infant plethysmography is accomplished using a small constant-volume chamber in which the infant reclines; the infant's nose and mouth rest against a cuffed opening in the plethysmograph. Flows can be measured using a close-fitting face mask, as for PEFV curves, with airway occlusion at end-expiration for determination of VTG and airways resistance. Plethysmographic lung volumes may be measured in young children by allowing a parent to hold the child on their lap while sitting in the plethysmograph. The adult is instructed to hold his or her breath while the child breathes through a pneumotachometer, and the mouth shutter is closed at end-expiration. Nonpanting VTG maneuvers are normally obtained, but some children can be coached to perform the closed-shutter panting acceptably. Corrections for the gas displacement of both the child and parent, based on their combined weights, are used in the calculation of the VTG.

Since VC may not be obtained in infants or young children, FRC is often the only lung volume that can be reproducibly discerned. The FRC in infants is a function not only of the recoil forces of the lung and chest wall, but it is dynamically maintained by the laryngeal "braking" (of flow) and by shortening of the expiratory time. Because of these mechanisms, FRC may change rapidly from breath to breath, confounding measurements by the foreign gas techniques. The variability of the FRC may lead to errors in measurements based on lung volumes such as $\dot{V}_{max}$FRC or compliance, and variation of FRC values may occur with changes in lung function in young children as well as in infants. Despite the mechanisms by which the FRC can change dynamically, the FRC has been shown to be reproducible in sedated children.

Pulmonary mechanics. Measurements of lung compliance and resistance are of greatest importance in infants who have abnormal pulmonary physiology. The compliance of the respiratory system (CRS) can be determined noninvasively by one of several methods. The infant may breathe spontaneously into a small-volume (i.e., approximately 1 L) water-filled spirometer, while two or more weights are added to the bell. The weights produce pressure changes in the circuit, which are measured and related to the change in end-expiratory lung volume on the breathing tracing. CRS is then calculated as the slope between the pressure-volume changes. CRS may also be derived by occlusion of the airway at end-inspiration and recording of the pressure plateau that occurs as the respiratory muscles relax. By recording the difference between the relaxed volume of expiration and the volume at end-inspiration, a pressure-volume slope (i.e., compliance) can be determined. This technique may be modified to allow multiple occluded breaths and determining the slope of the pressure-volume points at the end of each breath. Dynamic compliance and resistance measurements require the measurement of flow, volume, and esophageal pressure: such testing is usually reserved for infants that require ventilatory support. Two problems that interfere with these groups of measurements are long time constants and the effects of changes in the upper airway. Measurement of a stable pressure during airway occlusion may be impossible in infants who have marked differences in the compliance/resistance characteristics in different lung units; this occurs if equilibration of pressures within the lung is incomplete when a subsequent breath begins. Because the infant chest wall is extremely compliant, distortion of pleural pressure within the thorax may occur during inspiration and may affect measurements of esophageal pressure. Similarly, the upper airway (i.e., the larynx) may influence the time constants because of its contribution to the total resistance.

Testing in older children and adolescents

Pulmonary function testing in older children and adolescents is often directed toward diagnosis and evaluation of the most common disease states in this group of pediatric subjects. These are asthma, cystic fibrosis, and chest deformities. In each of these diseases basically the same tests are used as in adults who have either obstructive or restrictive disorders.

The presence and severity of *asthma* in children is evaluated using a method similar to that used for testing the extent of reversible obstructive lung disease in adults.

1. *Lung volume measurements* (VC, TLC, RV, FRC, RV/TLC) provide information concerning air trapping and/or hyperinflation, particularly in acute asthmatic episodes.
2. *Flow measurements* (FEF_X, FEV_T, $FEV_{T\%}$, MEFV curves, and PEFR) help to quantify the degree of obstruction and determine the effectiveness of bronchodilators. The PEFR may be particularly useful, because it can be measured conveniently at the bedside with a portable peak flow meter, providing serial measurements for planning and evaluating therapy. PEFR should be correlated with the $FEV_{1.0}$ or other flow measurements to detect changes that may be caused by obstruction and not just effort.
3. *Blood gas analysis* may be indicated in acute asthmatic episodes to detect hypoxemia and hypercapnia. Impending respiratory failure may be signaled by worsening hypoxemia accompanied by hypocapnia turning to hypercapnia.
4. *Exercise testing* may be used to determine the presence of exercise-induced bronchospasm and to evaluate the effectiveness of particular therapeutic regimens.

The alterations in lung function in children who have *cystic fibrosis* may be followed using the same group of tests as is used in adults who have COPD.

1. *Lung volumes* (VC, FRC, RV, TLC, RV/TLC) are most useful in detecting increases in FRC and RV associated with air trapping typical of advanced obstruction.
2. *Flow measurements* (FEF_X, FEV_T, $FEV_{T\%}$, MEFV curves, and PEFR) assess the extent of obstruction caused by mucus plugging, bronchospasm, and edema. The efficacy of bronchodilators, aerosol therapy, chest physical therapy, and other modalities aimed at management of secretions is determined largely by the changes in $FEV_{1.0}$ and FVC before and after treatment.
3. *Arterial blood gas studies* may provide information concerning the degree of respiratory insufficiency, particularly the effects of $\dot{V}/\dot{Q}$ mismatching on oxygenation.

Chest deformities that are commonly evaluated by pulmonary function studies include kyphoscoliosis and pectus excavatum. Measurements include those parameters that are useful in assessing restrictive ventilatory patterns, such as lung volumes and DL_{CO}. Flow studies such as $FEV_{1.0}$ and MEFV curves may provide additional information if the chest deformity contributes to abnormalities of large airways. Spirometry, lung volumes, and blood gas analysis may all be used to follow postoperative changes if surgical intervention is employed. Calculation of predicted values based on height should be performed using the "wing-tip" method (i.e., arm span distance) instead of standing height.

Normal values of lung function for children in all cases depend on height (length in infants), sex, and age. Lung function predicted values in children vary mainly with height, and some parameters change dramatically at the onset of puberty. For spirometric variables (i.e., FVC, $FEV_{1.0}$) lung function increases up to about age 18 in boys and about age 16 in girls. After these ages, volumes and flows plateau, then begin to decline. Because of this "peaking" of lung function in the late teens, separate regression equations are often used for young children, adolescents, and adults. Problems can arise if gaps occur in the ranges over which the predicted normal values are valid. For example, regressions from a study of children might include ages 6 to 17 and regressions from a study of adults from 20 to 80 years; it may not be valid to extrapolate either set of equations to determine expected values in 18- or 19-year-olds. Rather, reference equations should be selected that eliminate these gaps. Nomograms and regression equations for common lung volumes and flows are included in the Appendix.

CRITICAL CARE MONITORING

Measurement of selected pulmonary function parameters is often indicated in subjects who are critically ill, particularly those who require mechanically supported ventilation. Some of these parameters, such as the vital capacity, closely resemble tests used in day-to-day pulmonary function evaluation, while others, such as capnography and reflective spectrophotometry, are highly specific for patients in an intensive care setting. Monitoring of the respiratory system includes the broad areas of pulmonary mechanics and gas exchange.

Pulmonary mechanics

Ventilation ($\dot{V}_E$,V_T,f) Assessment of minute ventilation and its components, tidal volume (V_T) and respiratory rate (f), is usually accomplished by means of a flow-sensing spirometer attached to the patient's airway. While the range of flows measured in spontaneously breathing subjects is usually much narrower than maximal flows (i.e., 0 to 12 L/sec), some bedside spirometers may not accurately measure very low or very high flows. In spontaneously breathing subjects, a mouthpiece and nose clip, or a close-fitting face mask, may be used. A low-resistance, unidirectional valve is normally employed so that only expired gas is collected. In subjects who are intubated, the valve and spirometer combination is attached directly to the artificial airway. The patient then breathes normally while the $\dot{V}_E$, respiratory rate, and time are recorded. The interval for measuring $\dot{V}_E$ may be dictated by the patient's condition and ability to cooperate. If the respiratory pattern is stable, a 1-minute interval usually provides an acceptable estimate of the resting ventilation. V_T is derived by dividing the $\dot{V}_E$ by the rate (see Chapter 2). Most subjects change their breathing pattern when a mouthpiece/nose clip or mask are applied, so measurements of resting ventilation should be continued long enough to ensure a stable pattern. The dead space of the valve system (i.e., the valve plus mouthpiece or mask) may also influence the resting ventilation. Subjects with very small VT (i.e., VT less than 200 ml) may not tolerate the addition of a valve system with a dead space in excess of 100 ml; the addition of a significant dead space volume may also result in a pattern of ventilation that differs markedly from the subject's true resting level. Low dead space systems typically also offer higher resistance because they have smaller aperture valves, which may be a consideration in subjects who have high resting respiratory rates. Measurements of resting ventilation can also be accomplished indirectly by means of inductive plethysmography (see Chapter 9). The respiratory inductive plethysmograph records the motion of the rib cage and abdomen, and with appropriate calibration, can derive the volume and timing of individual breaths. The advantage of this approach is that no connection to the airway is required; the disadvantage is that calibration must be done carefully and checked often.

Patients receiving supplementary O_2 or being mechanically supported offer special problems for measurements of ventilation. Many mechanical ventilators incorporate volume-displacement or flow-sensing spirometers as an integral part of their monitoring/alarm systems. When practical, these built-in spirometers should be used to assess ventilation. The patient may be left connected to the ventilator support system if it allows spontaneous breathing through the ventilator circuit. Some systems that allow spontaneous ventilation (i.e., intermittent mandatory ventilation, or IMV) may have inappropriately high resistance and/or dead space, resulting in patient discomfort or inability to reach a stable ventilatory level. In such a case, ventilation measurements may require a separate spirometer and removal of the patient from the support system for the test. Subjects receiving supplementary O_2 should have an appropriate F_{IO_2} maintained while ventilatory parameters are measured. This may require addition of O_2 to the inspiratory side of the one-way valve; care should be taken that the flow of supplementary O_2 does not directly enter the spirometer to avoid falsely elevated $\dot{V}E$.

Minute ventilation is usually assessed in relation to the patient's Pa_{CO_2}. A normal or elevated Pa_{CO_2} with a markedly elevated $\dot{V}E$ usually indicates increased physiologic dead space. A less common cause of increased Pa_{CO_2} is increased $\dot{V}CO_2$. Patients who have limited ventilatory reserves may not be able to compensate for increased CO_2 production. Adjustment of the source of caloric intake from high carbohydrates to high fat (see Metabolic Studies, this chapter) may be necessary to reduce the CO_2 load to a level that can be accommodated by the patient. An elevated $PaCO_2$ with a low minute ventilation suggests decreased respiratory drive or neuromuscular dysfunction. Inability to wean from mechanical ventilation often accompanies low VT values (i.e., VT 300 ml) and high respiratory rates (i.e., 22 to 30 breaths per minute). Subjects who are disconnected from mechanical support for the purpose of measurement of ventilation or other spontaneous parameters may show markedly different patterns as the time off the ventilator increases. Respiratory muscle fatigue, worsening hypoxemia or hypercapnia, and anxiety may cause deterioration of the pattern of breathing and make interpretation of rate, V_T, and minute ventilation difficult.

VC *flows, and MVV.* The VC is routinely measured in the management of patients who require ventilatory support or in impending ventilatory failure. The VC is usually measured using a portable spirometer, often employing a pneumotachometer or rotameter-type device. The spirometer should meet the American Thoracic Society's recommendation for volume accuracy (i.e., ± 3% or 100 ml, whichever is greater); accuracy for flow measurements may be unnecessary if the device is used only for VC determinations. Patients who are alert and cooperative can often perform reproducible VC maneuvers, usually by inspiring to TLC and expiring slowly to RV. Measurement of the MVV also requires patient cooperation and effort; in addition, the spirometer must be accurate over the range of flows developed. Although healthy persons may generate flows in excess of 200 L/min during the MVV maneuver, patients who are critically ill seldom achieve such high levels. The measuring device should have a low resistance, particularly over the flow range of 0 to 50 L/min.

The VC may be reduced in critically ill patients because of either obstruction, restriction, or neuromuscular disease. Poor effort or inability to perform the VC maneuver may also result in low values. Healthy adults have VC values in excess of 50 ml/Kg; the ability to move a VC breath of 10 to 12 ml/Kg is usually required to maintain unsupported ventilation. Values less than 10 ml/Kg are typically indicative of patients who are difficult to wean from mechanical support of ventilation. The maximal voluntary ventilation maneuver (MVV) helps in estimating the ventilatory reserve available to the patient. If the resting $\dot{V}_E$ exceeds approximately 50% of the MVV, the subject probably will not be able to ventilate spontaneously for an extended interval.

Measurements of FVC and flow rates in the critical care setting provide a quantitative basis for therapy in obstructive airway processes, particularly asthma. Portable spirometers allow serial measurements, on a daily or even hourly basis, to assess the effectiveness of bronchodilators, aerosol therapy, or chest physical therapy. If the FVC and $FEV_{1.0}$ are to be measured in the intensive care setting, the spirometer should meet the minimum American Thoracic Society requirements (see Chapter 11) for volume as well as for flows. PEFR, although commonly used, may not quantify the reversibility of obstruction, because normal peak flows may be developed early in a forced expiration despite decreased $FEV_{1.0}$ or FEF_X values. Ideally, PEFR should be correlated with the $FEV_{1.0}$. Peak flows, as measured with a small portable device, may be beneficial in evaluating the control of asthma in subjects who use the device routinely and for whom conventional spirometric measurements are well documented. Serial measurements, daily or more often, can serve as an index for evaluation of therapeutic maneuvers to control bronchospasm.

Respiratory pressures. Respiratory muscle strength is assessed by measuring the maximal pressure that can be generated at the airway. Negative inspiratory force (NIF) is similar to the maximal inspiratory pressure (MIP, see Chapter 3) and is measured by connecting a pressure manometer to an occluded airway and noting the maximum negative pressure that can be developed. While the MIP is normally measured by having the subject inspire from RV, the NIF is measured at or near FRC. The NIF, also referred to as the maximum inspiratory force, is used in obtunded individuals in whom a VC cannot be obtained. Occlusion of the airway produces maximal values within 10 to 20 seconds, but may not be tolerated well by subjects whose cardiovascular status is unstable. A VC of 15 ml/Kg requires development of approximately -20 cm H_2O, and this value is considered the minimum below which a subject usually will not be able to maintain adequate spontaneous ventilation over an extended period. Values greater than -80 cm H_2O) are observed in healthy individuals, but negative pressures greater than -20 cm H_2O are not predictive of a specific VC.

Gas exchange

Capnography. Continuous analysis of expired CO_2 (see Chapter 6) may be used as a respiratory monitor in patients who are intubated, as well as those who are not. CO_2 is analyzed either by means of an infrared analyzer or mass spectrometer. Most infrared analyzers withdraw a small continuous flow of gas from the patient and direct it into a sample cell. Accurate analysis depends on a constant flow and adequate removal or compensation for water vapor; the CO_2 analyzer is usually zeroed by sampling room air and spanned by sampling a 5% CO_2 mixture. Some analyzers, specially designed for use with mechanical ventilators, feature a heated infrared chamber that is placed directly in the gas flow, usually near the artificial airway; the infrared light passes through the gas in the breathing circuit without the necessity of a sample pump. Response time of in-line analyzers is very rapid, and there are no changes in sample flow rate to alter calibration. As described in Chapter 6, capnography is used to monitor end-tidal CO_2, to calculate the $Pa\text{-}P_{ET_{CO_2}}$ gradient, and to estimate dead space. Exhaled CO_2 analysis can detect acute reductions in cardiac output, because dead space usually increases as cardiac output falls. Simple trend monitoring serves to ascertain changes in respiratory rate, such as disconnection from the mechanical ventilator.

Pulse oximetry. Noninvasive oximetry to measure Sa_{O_2} is widely used to monitor patients on mechanical ventilation or being supported by supplementary O_2. The measurement of Sa_{O_2} by means of two wavelength pulse oximetry is described in Chapter 6. In the critical care setting, pulse oximetry is used for continuous monitoring, employing probes located on either the ear or finger. Most of the pulse oximeters currently available use a microprocessor to analyze arterial pulsations in a capillary bed; computerization allows the oximeter to adjust light output to accommodate different tissues and conditions to obtain an optimal signal. In addition, the microprocessor permits alarms to be triggered when saturation or pulse rate exceed preset limits. Many instruments provide digital and/or analog outputs for connection to recorders or computerized monitoring systems.

Oxygen saturation by pulse oximetry (Sp_{O_2}) is particularly well-suited to detecting changes in saturation across the physiologic range often encountered in critically ill patients, namely 75% to 95%. Clinical decisions regarding changes in mechanical ventilator settings or O_2 therapy are often made when the saturation falls below 90%. Conversely, pulse oximetry is relatively insensitive to changes in O_2 content when the Pa_{O_2} is greater than 100 mm Hg, because of the relatively flat upper portion of the O_2Hb dissociation curve. Although the accuracy of many oximeters differ, confidence limits of $\pm$ 4% are realistic for most instruments; at low saturations (i.e., <75%) almost all pulse oximeters tend to become less accurate (see Chapter 9). Despite this large variability, detection of acute changes in Sa_{O_2} can be made if the pulse oximeter is correlated with blood oximetry and careful attention is paid to those factors that can affect the pulse oximeter's accuracy. COHb, MetHb, jaundice, cardiac output dyes, high-intensity light, skin pigmentation, and hypoperfusion are all interfering substances that are not uncommon in the critical care setting. Motion artifact, particularly shivering, interferes with the detection of the pulse waveform that is necessary to distinguish arterial absorption from venous and tissue absorption. Decreased local perfusion, caused by hypothermia or vasopressor drugs, is known to result in an Sp_{O_2} that is less than the Sa_{O_2}. Response times of some oximeters may also present problems, particularly if saturation falls rapidly, as sometimes occurs with bradycardia.

Transcutaneous blood gases. Transcutaneous electrodes for measuring Po_2 ($tcPo_2$) and Pco_2 ($tcPco_2$) are used in some intensive care units. Transcutaneous gas monitoring, specifically measuring the $tcPo_2$, is widely used in neonatal units, because the gradients between arterial blood and the skin tend to be smaller. Transcutaneous Po_2 monitors use a Clark electrode (see Chapter 9); the attachment site is heated by the electrode itself to produce local hyperemia. The hyperemia helps to "arterialize" the capillary flow in the skin, but also necessitates periodic repositioning of the electrode to prevent burns. Transcutaneous Po_2 electrodes have also been designed that can be attached to the conjunctiva of the eye and to the mucous membranes of the oropharynx, but they are not widely used. The $tcPco_2$ is monitored by a modified Severinghaus electrode, attached in a manner similar to the $tcPo_2$ electrode. The $tcPco_2$ electrode has a slower response time than the $tcPo_2$ electrode, and it is somewhat more tedious to calibrate. A combination $tcPo_2$ and $tcPco_2$ electrode is available.

$tcPo_2$ correlates well with Pa_{O_2} in patients who have a stable cardiovascular status. Decreases in cardiac output normally result in a reduction in cutaneous blood flow and localized hypoxia. In adults, because of the thickness of the keratin layer of the skin, the $tcPo_2$ tends to be about 20% less than the Pa_{O_2} when the subject is at rest. This gradient widens in the face of reduced blood flow, either systemically or locally. The $tcPo_2$ is useful for detecting large swings in Po_2 such as sometimes occur when lung function changes while supplementary O_2 is being administered. $tcPo_2$ may be particulary valuable in distinguishing abrupt increases in Po_2 in susceptible patients such as neonates. The $tcPco_2$, like Po_2, depends largely on the local perfusion and metabolism. The $tcPco_2$ usually exceeds the Pa_{CO_2} because of the increased CO_2 production caused by the heated electrode.

Mixed venous oxygen saturation ($S\bar{v}_{O_2}$). The use of a fiberoptic pulmonary artery catheter employing reflective spectrophotometry (see Chapter 9) allows continuous measurement of mixed venous saturation. This catheter uses a fiberoptic bundle to transmit light, at either two or three wavelengths, to blood flowing in the pulmonary artery; the reflected light returns via a second fiberoptic pathway to a photodetector. A microprocessor then calculates the $S\bar{v}_{O_2}$ based on the absorption of light by O_2Hb and reduced Hb and displays the value continuously. In addition, all of the other data normally obtained from a pulmonary artery catheter (i.e., mixed venous blood samples, PA pressure, wedge pressure) are available.

$S\bar{v}_{O_2}$ is useful in monitoring cardiac status and O_2 delivery. The $S\bar{v}_{O_2}$ is the average of the venous blood returning from all parts of the body; it may be affected by O_2 consumption, cardiac output, and the content of the arterial blood. Normal subjects have an $S\bar{v}_{O_2}$ of 75% to 85%. The $S\bar{v}_{O_2}$ may fall if the cardiac output decreases and the tissues continue consuming the same amount of O_2. $S\bar{v}_{O_2}$ in the range of 60% to 70% represents a slightly reduced cardiac output, and values less than 60% are usually associated with a significant reduction in cardiac output. However, a low $S\bar{v}_{O_2}$ may also be caused by increased O_2 extraction by the tissues, such as occurs during exercise, while the cardiac output is actually increasing. Redistribution of the cardiac output to organs that have a high O_2 consumption may also reduce the $S\bar{v}_{O_2}$ without an actual decrease in cardiac output. Conversely, the $S\bar{v}_{O_2}$ may increase if the tissue O_2 consumption decreases, as sometimes occurs with sepsis. Arterial content, as determined by the Sa_{O_2} and Hb, may also influence the $S\bar{v}_{O_2}$. If arterial content falls, because of pulmonary disease or anemia, while cardiac output and O_2 consumption remain constant, $S\bar{v}_{O_2}$ will decrease. Interpretation of changes in $S\bar{v}_{O_2}$ should always be considered in the context of the multiple factors that influence it.

METABOLIC MEASUREMENTS (INDIRECT CALORIMETRY)

Description

Measurements of $\dot{V}o_2$ and $\dot{V}co_2$ and their ratio, the RER may be used to determine the caloric energy expenditure and to partition the calories among the various substrates (i.e., fat, carbohydrate, protein). In combination with measurements of caloric intake and other laboratory values, such as urinary nitrogen, indirect calorimetry allows nutritional assessment and management.

Technique

Indirect calorimetry is performed using either an open-circuit or closed-circuit system to measure O_2 consumption, CO_2 production, and RER.

Open-circuit calorimetry. Exchange of O_2 and CO_2 may be measured by recording $\dot{V}_E$ and the fractional differences of O_2 and CO_2 between inspired and expired gas. These measurements are accomplished using either a mixing chamber or breath-by-breath system similar to those used for expired gas analysis during exercise (see Chapter 7). $\dot{V}O_2$ and $\dot{V}CO_2$ are measured as described for exercise testing; $\dot{V}_E$, V_T, and respiratory rate (f) are also measured. Connection to the subject may be made by a standard unidirectional valve, a ventilated hood or canopy (Fig. 8-3), or by connection to a mechanical ventilator circuit. A hood or canopy allows long-term measurements without direct connection to the patient's airway. The hood is ventilated by drawing a flow of gas that exceeds the patient's peak inspiratory demand through it; 40 L/min is usually adequate. By measuring the change in flow into and out of the hood during breathing (i.e., "bias" flow), ventilation can be calculated. Connection to a ventilator requires a means of measuring exhaled volume, along with both the inspired and expired fractional gas concentrations. Breath-by-breath measurements usually sample gas at the patient/ventilator connection.

Closed-circuit calorimetry. The simplest type of closed-circuit calorimeter is that which measures $\dot{V}O_2$ volumetrically. The subject rebreathes gas from a closed system that contains a spirometer that has been filled with O_2. CO_2 is scrubbed from the circuit and a recording of the decrease in system (spirometer) volume equals the rate of O_2 removal or $\dot{V}O_2$. A similar approach uses a closed spirometer system that allows measured amounts of O_2 to be added as the subject rebreathes and removes O_2. $\dot{V}O_2$ is then equal to the volume of O_2 added per minute. CO_2 production cannot be measured using a closed-circuit system unless a CO_2 analyzer is added to the device. $\dot{V}_E$, V_T, and respiratory rate may all be determined from volume excursions of the spirometer. Closed-circuit systems may be used with spontaneously-breathing patients by means of a simple breathing valve and mouthpiece. Use of a closed-circuit calorimeter with a mechanical ventilator requires that the spirometer system be connected betwen the patient and ventilator. The ventilator then "ventilates" the spirometer, which in turn ventilates the patient. This technique usually requires a bellows-type spirometer in a fixed container so that the bellows can be compressed by the positive pressure generated by the ventilator. The volume delivered by the ventilator (the V_T) must be increased to compensate for the volume of gas compressed in the closed-circuit spirometer during positive pressure breaths.

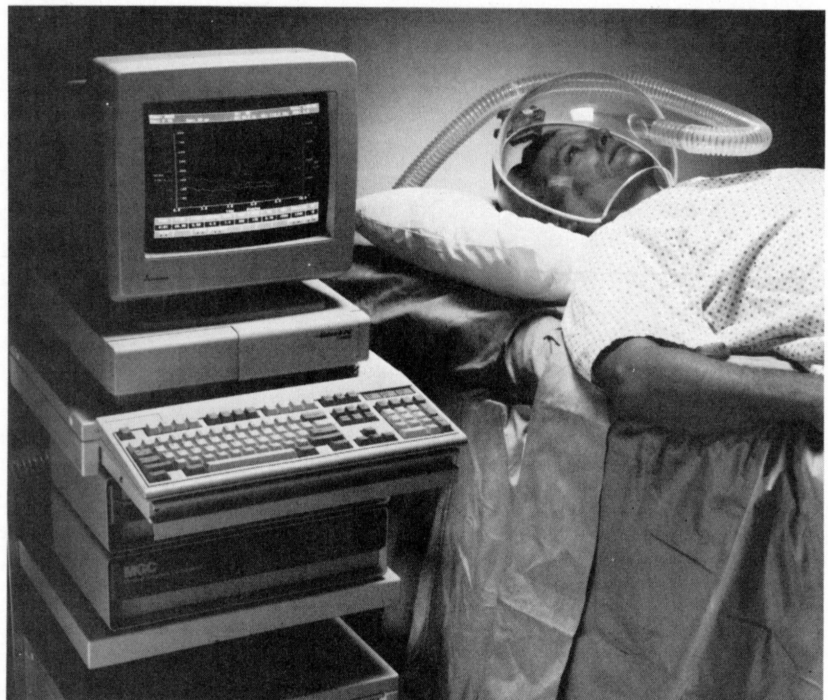

Fig. 8-3 Canopy for metabolic measurements. REE may be measured by assessing the changes in gas flow and fractional concentrations of expired air drawn from a hood or canopy. A continuous or "bias" flow of gas is drawn from the device and changes in flow are measured to determine ventilation; fractional gas concentrations are determined either breath-by-breath or after passing the gas through a mixing chamber. The canopy offers the advantage of not requiring direct connection to the subject's airway, which may affect ventilation and the measurement of REE. Although useful for spontaneously breathing subjects, the hood cannot be used with patients requiring mechanical support of ventilation. (Courtesy Medical Graphics Corporation, St. Paul, Minn.)

Because the purpose of indirect calorimetry is primarily to estimate resting energy expenditure (REE) over an extended period (i.e., 24 hours), the subject's condition during the measurement is critical. The following guidelines help ensure that measurements are made under steady-state conditions:

1. The subject should be recumbent or supine for 20 to 30 minutes before beginning measurements and should stay quiet during the test. The testing apparatus should not cause discomfort or exertion on the part of the subject.
2. The subject should be fasting for 2 to 4 hours before the test starts. If the subject is receiving feedings, either enteral or parenteral, they

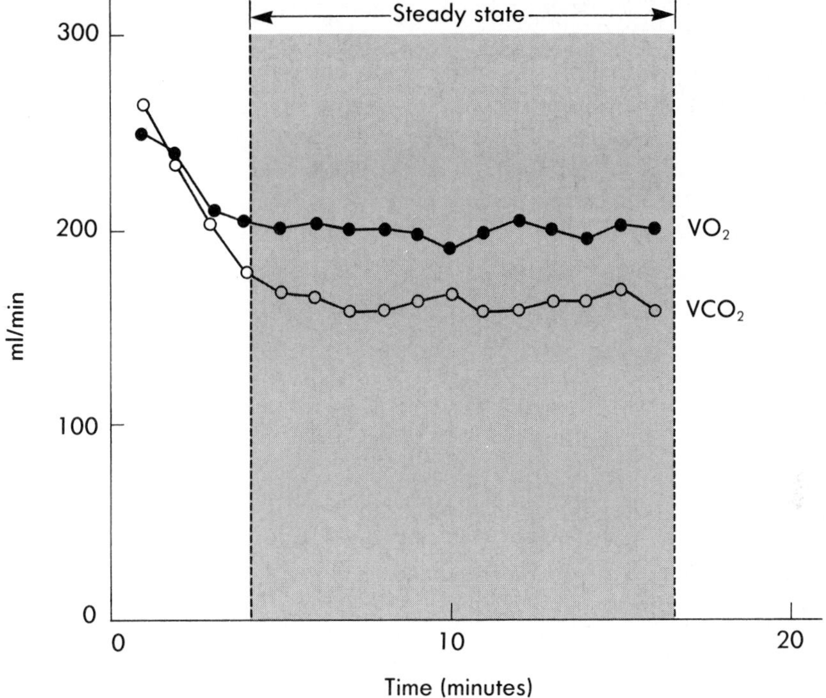

Fig. 8-4 Indirect calorimetry—Typical tracing of continuous measurement of $\dot{V}O_2$ and $\dot{V}CO_2$ as performed during open-circuit indirect calorimetry. The subject's expired gas is analyzed to determine O_2 consumption, CO_2 production, and RQ during a resting state; the measurements are continued for a long enough interval so that values representative of REE can be determined. From these measurements, the daily caloric requirements can be estimated, and the percentages of energy derived from fats, carbohydrates, and proteins can be calculated.

should be continuous, not in bolus form.

3. The subject should be in a neutral thermal environment. Special corrections may be required for subjects who are febrile or hypothermic.
4. Drugs or substances that alter metabolism should be avoided. Substances related to caffeine (methylxanthines) and nictoine are particularly common stimulants.
5. Data collection should continue long enough so that a stable baseline is established and steady-state conditions can be verified (Fig. 8-4). Common indicators of steady-state conditions are the parameters assessed as part of the metabolic study itself; $\dot{V}O_2$, $\dot{V}CO_2$, $\dot{V}E$, and heart rate should not change by more than $\pm 5\%$ over the testing interval. If the subject does not demonstrate steady-state conditions, longer test intervals may be required to average represen-

tative periods of metabolic activity.

6. Patients on ventilators should be in a stable condition; no ventilator adjustments should be made for 1 to 2 hours preceding the test period. Modifications in minute ventilation or F_{IO_2} settings can cause gross changes in the patterns of gas exchange, particularly in subjects who have pulmonary disease.

Metabolic calculations.

1. *Harris-Benedict equations* for estimating REE:

   Males

$$\text{REE (in kcal/24 hrs)} = 66.47 + 13.75W + 5.00H - 6.76A$$

   Females

$$\text{REE (in kcal/24 hrs)} = 655.10 + 9.56W + 1.85H - 4.68A$$

   where

   W = Weight in kilograms
   H = Height in centimeters
   A = Age in years

   The REE determined by these formulas was originally described as the basal metabolic rate (BMR). These equations may be used to estimate the caloric expenditure in normal subjects under conditions of no activity; the BMR in these circumstances is related to lean body mass. To determine the optimum level of calorie intake, the BMR must be adjusted upward, because trauma, surgery, infections, and burns all cause the REE to increase.

2. *Weir equation* for calculating REE from respiratory gas exchange and urinary N_2,:

$$\text{REE (in kcal/24 hrs)} = 1.44(3.941\dot{V}O_2 + 1.106\dot{V}CO_2) - 2.17(\text{UN})$$

   where

   $\dot{V}O_2$ is expressed in ml/min
   $\dot{V}CO_2$ is expressed in ml/min
   UN = Urinary N_2 (in gm/24 hrs)
   1.44 = Correction from ml/min to L/24 hrs

   Indirect calorimetry by the open-circuit method provides measures of both O_2 consumption and CO_2 production. The RER is the ratio of $\dot{V}CO_2/\dot{V}O_2$; under steady-state conditions the RER approximates the mean respiratory quotient (RQ) at the cell level. RQ normally varies from 0.71 to 1.00 depending on the substrate; carbohydrate oxidation produces an RQ near 1.0, fat oxidation produces an RQ near 0.71, and protein oxidation produces an RQ of 0.82. The RQ attributable to carbohydrates and fats may be determined by subtracting the $\dot{V}CO_2$ and $\dot{V}O_2$ derived from protein. This form of the

RQ is termed the nonprotein RQ or RQ_{NP} and is calculated:

$$RQ_{NP} = \frac{(\dot{V}CO_2 \text{ (in L/24 hrs)} - 4.8UN)}{(\dot{V}O_2 \text{ (in L/24 hrs)} - 5.9UN)}$$

where

$$\dot{V}CO_2 \text{ (in L/24 hrs)} = 1.44\ \dot{V}CO_2 \text{ (in ml/min)}$$
$$\dot{V}O_2 \text{ (in L/24 hrs)} = 1.44\ \dot{V}O_2 \text{ (in ml/min)}$$

Because CO_2 production varies with O_2 uptake, deviations of the RQ from the average value of 0.85 result in differences of less than 5% in the calculation of REE if the $\dot{V}O_2$ and RQ are used. Indirect calorimetry by the closed-circuit (volumetric) method takes advantage of this small difference by assuming a fixed RQ, usually 0.85, and measuring only $\dot{V}O_2$. Urinary N_2 is obtained from a 24-hour collection. Since protein metabolism accounts for only a small proportion of the total calories per day (about 12%), omission of the UN in the Weir equation changes the calculated REE by only 2%.

3. *Consolazio equations* for determination of energy expenditure from gas exchange ($\dot{V}O_2$, $\dot{V}CO_2$), urinary N_2 (UN), and the caloric equivalents of carbohydrates, fats, and proteins:

$$\text{Carbohydrates (in gm)} = (4.12\dot{V}O_2) - (2.91\dot{V}CO_2) - (1.94UN)$$
$$\text{Fat (in gm)} = (1.69\dot{V}O_2) - (1.69\dot{V}CO_2) - (2.54UN)$$
$$\text{Protein (in gm)} = (6.25UN)$$

From the grams used by each substrate, the kilocalories (kcal) derived from that source can be computed:

$$\text{Carbohydrates (in kcal)} = 4.18 \text{ Carbohydrates (in gm)}$$
$$\text{Fat (in kcal)} = 9.46 \text{ Fat (in gm)}$$
$$\text{Protein (in kcal)} = 4.32 \text{ Protein (in gm)}$$
$$\text{Total (in kcal)} = \text{Carbohydrate} + \text{Fat} + \text{Protein (in kcal)}$$

The percentage of calories attributable to each of the substrates may also be calculated by dividing the kilocalories derived from the substrate by the total kilocalories. Since the Consolazio equations are intended for analysis of normal substrate partitioning, RQ values outside of the range of 0.71 to 1.00 will result in negative values for either carbohydrates or lipids. These negative values are artifactual if the RER does not equal the RQ (i.e., the patient is not in a metabolic steady state).

Significance

Indirect calorimetry is most often used to assess nutritional status of patients whose daily energy expenditure is altered by disease, injury, or therapeutic interventions. The REE accounts for approximately two thirds of the daily energy requirements in healthy subjects. The Harris-Benedict equations (see above) or similar predictive equations are commonly used to estimate the REE, with the addition of various "factors" to account for the extra requirements imposed by the patient's clinical status. Because of the variability in metabolic requirements of patients who are critically ill, indirect calorimetry can be used to detect undernourishment, overnourishment, or the use of inappropriate substrates.

Undernourishment or starvation can occur during illness; it is detected by caloric expenditure in excess of caloric intake (i.e., negative energy balance). Both fat stores and protein, from muscle breakdown, may contribute to metabolism during periods of undernourishment. Indirect calorimetry, along with measurement of body weight, triceps skin fold measurements, and other approximations of energy reserves allow planning of nutritional therapy to replete diminished reserves. Overnourishment occurs when any substrate is supplied in excess of the energy requirements, and is most deleterious when the patient's nutritional status is already adequate. Excess lipid or carbohydrate calories are stored as fat, which may place stress on one or more organ systems.

Patients who have pulmonary disease present a special dilemma in that excessive carbohydrate intake results in increased CO_2 production; the RQ of carbohydrates is 1.00. In patients with respiratory failure, this excess production of CO_2 places an increased ventilatory load on the respiratory muscles. Adjustments in substrate use can be made after the nonprotein RQ is determined by indirect calorimetry. Lipids are typically substituted for glucose so that the RQ can be reduced while the caloric intake is maintained. Patients with respiratory failure may also experience atrophy of ventilatory muscle. Substrate analysis can also be used to assess N_2 balance, which is related to the breakdown of muscle protein, and to determine the nutritional requirements necessary to maintain N_2 balance.

Technical considerations involved in indirect calorimetry include accurate gas analysis and accurate measurement of $\dot{V}E$ during the test interval. The most common problem related to gas analysis during metabolic measurements is attainment of a true "steady state," in which the measured metabolic rate is representative of the caloric expenditure over 24 hours. Hyperventilation caused by connection to a mask or mouthpiece or by ventilator manipulation is a frequent occurrence; head hoods or continuous flow canopies can eliminate much of the stimulation associated with connection to the metabolic measurement system (see Fig. 8-3), but cannot be used for patients on mechanical ventilators. An RER greater than 1.00 should always be evaluated in relation to the $\dot{V}E$ and end-tidal CO_2; abnormally high $\dot{V}E$ and low end-tidal CO_2 values may indicate hyperventilation. RER values in excess of 1.00 that cannot be explained as hyperventilation may be due to the storage of excess calories as fat (i.e., lipogenesis). RER values below 0.70 may occur in ketosis occurring during extreme fasting or diabetic ketoacidosis. More commonly, however, low RER values signal improper calibration of the gas analyzers or hypoventilation. Inaccurate calibration or improper performance of either the CO_2 or O_2 analyzer can result in RER values outside of the usual metabolic range of 0.7 to 1.00.

Special problems may be encountered in performing metabolic measurements on patients requiring mechanical ventilatory support. The most common difficulty relates to measurements of O_2 consumption when the patient is receiving supplmentary O_2. Measurement of $\dot{V}_{O_2}$ by respiratory gas exchange requires analysis of the difference between inspired and expired O_2 and the minute ventilation. In subjects breathing room air, the inspired $F_{I_{O_2}}$ is constant; many O_2 blending systems, such as those used on ventilators, may not provide a constant fraction of inspired O_2. Large differences in the calculated $\dot{V}O_2$ can result from small fluctuations in the $F_{I_{O_2}}$ even if the $F_{E_{O_2}}$ remains relatively constant. Small differences in the inspired and expired volumes, caused by the RER, are corrected by adjusting the inspired fraction of oxygen according to the equation:

$$\frac{(1 - F_{E_{O_2}} - F_{E_{CO_2}})}{(1 - F_{I_{O_2}})} \times F_{I_{O_2}}$$

This correction of inspired $F_{I_{O_2}}$ for gas balance in the lung (i.e., the Haldane transformation; see $\dot{V}O_2$, Chapter 7) limits the accuracy of the open-circuit method of determining $\dot{V}O_2$. As the $F_{I_{O_2}}$ is increased, the value in the denominator of the equation becomes smaller. Even with very accurate gas analysis, measurement of differences between the $F_{I_{O_2}}$ and $F_{E_{O_2}}$ when the $F_{I_{O_2}}$ is above 0.50 is quite variable. Indirect calorimetry by the volumetric method (i.e., closed system) avoids this problem by measuring the actual volume of O_2 removed during rebreathing. Measurement of $\dot{V}O_2$ and $\dot{V}CO_2$ in spontaneously breathing patients who require supplementary O_2 can usually be accommodated by allowing the subject to breath from a high flow Venturi device or from a reservoir bag containing an increased $F_{I_{O_2}}$.

Other considerations involved in metabolic measurements on ventilated patients include the effects of positive pressure on gas analysis and on volume determination. Analysis of O_2 and CO_2 in the ventilator circuit must take into account the effect of positive pressure breaths on the gas analyzers. Depending on the sampling method employed, positive pressure swings during each breath may generate falsely high partial pressure readings. Closed-circuit calorimetry places a volumetric device in the breathing circuit between the ventilator and the patient. The volume delivered by the ventilator must be increased to accommodate the higher compressible gas volume in the circuit, approximately 1 ml/cm H_2O for each liter of added volume.

SELF-ASSESSMENT QUESTIONS

1. A pulmonary history for use in conjunction with pulmonary function testing should include:
   a. A smoking history

b. An occupational history
c. A description of cough and sputum production
d. A description of shortness of breath
e. All of the above

2. A subject is given a before and after bronchodilator study (spirometry) and these values are recorded:

		Predrug	**Postdrug**	**Predicted**
FVC	(L)	2.30	2.80	3.40
$FEV_{1.0}$	(L)	1.38	1.73	2.72
$FEV_{1\%}$		60	62	–

The percent improvement following bronchodilator is:
a. 25%
b. 22%
c. 14%
d. 2%

3. A subject is given a methacholine challenge test and the following results are recorded:

Dosage (mg/ml)	$\mathbf{FEV_{1.0}}$
Baseline	3.90
Control (saline)	3.71
0.075	3.11
0.150	2.92
0.310	2.50

These findings are consistent with:
a. Positive methacholine challenge after normal saline control
b. Positive methacholine challenge; PD_{20} = 0.075 mg/ml
c. Positive methacholine challenge; PD_{20} = 0.150 mg/ml
d. Positive methacholine challenge; PD_{20} = 0.310 mg/ml

4. Before an exercise-induced asthma (EIA) test, the patient should be instructed to:
I. Withhold beta-adrenergic bronchodilators for 8 to 12 hours
II. Withhold sustained action theophylline preparations for four hours
III. Continue steroids if so ordered
IV. Continue cromolyn sodium if prescribed
a. I, II, III, IV
b. I, III, IV
c. II, IV
d. I, III

5. The point for standardization of flow measured from the PEFV curve in infants and small children is:

a. TLC
b. FRC
c. End-inspiration
d. RV

6. The measurement of respiratory system compliance (CRS) in infants may be accomplished by:
   a. Use of a weighted spirometer
   b. Airway occlusion at end-inspiration
   c. Whole body plethysmography
   d. a and b

7. Which of the following pulmonary function measurements are found in patients who require mechanical support of ventilation:
   I. VT less than 50 ml/kg
   II. VC less than 10 ml/kg
   III. $\dot{V}$E greater than 50% of the MVV
   IV. Negative inspiratory force less than 50 cm H_2O
   a. I, II, III, IV
   b. II, III
   c. I, IV
   d. II, IV

8. Which of the following are known to interfere with Sa_{O_2} measured by pulse oximetry:
   I. Motion, such as shivering
   II. COHb and MetHB
   III. Sinus tachycardia
   IV. Hypoperfusion of the sensor site
   a. I, II, III, IV
   b. II, III, IV
   c. I, II, IV
   d. I, III

9. A patient scheduled for thoracic surgery is referred for pulmonary function evaluation of postoperative risk; which of the following would best predict pulmonary complications:
   a. $DL_{CO}SB$
   b. Indirect calorimetry
   c. End-tidal PCO_2
   d. Spirometry (FVC, $FEV_{1.0}$, etc.)

10. A patient scheduled for lung resection has an $FEV_{1.0}$ of 1.1 L; postoperative $FEV_{1.0}$ could be estimated by:

a. Measuring $\dot{V}E$ at maximal exercise
b. Multiplying the preop $FEV_{1.0}$ by the percent of perfusion to the unaffected lung
c. Multiplying the preop FVC by the physiologic shunt fraction
d. Multiplying the sum of the FVC and $FEV_{1.0}$ by 0.5

11. For spirometric tracings to be acceptable for determining respiratory impairment for disability, which of the following must be met:
I. The $FEV_{1.0}$ must be indicated on the F-V loop
II. The recorder must have a volume excursion of at least 10 mm/L
III. The $FEV_{1.0}$ must be recorded at a paper speed of 20 mm/second
IV. The $FEV_{1.0}$ should be the largest value from three acceptable maneuvers
a. I, II, III, IV
b. I, III, IV
c. II, III, IV
d. III, IV only

12. Which of the following conditions must be met for indirect calorimetry to accurately measure the resting energy expenditure (REE):
I. The patient should be supine or semirecumbent for 20 to 30 minutes
II. The patient should be fasting for 12 hours
III. No caffeine-like stimulants should be administered before testing
IV. The measurements should be completed within 5 minutes or less
a. I, II, III, IV
b. I, II, IV
c. I, III
d. II, IV

13. A patient has an RQ of 0.71 measured by indirect calorimetry; if the patient is in a steady state, which substrate is most likely being used for energy production:
a. Lipids (fat)
b. Carbohydrates (glucose)
c. Proteins
d. A combination of protein and carbohydrate

14. Which of the following conditions might result in inaccurate measurement of $\dot{V}O_2$ by indirect calorimetry on a mechanically ventilated patient:
I. An FI_{O_2} greater than 0.60
II. A tidal volume greater than 1000 ml
III. A unsteady FI_{O_2}
IV. An RER greater than 0.95
a. I, II, III, IV
b. I, III
c. II, IV
d. III, IV

SELECTED BIBLIOGRAPHY

Testing regimens

Becklake MR and Permutt S: Evaluation of tests of lung function for screening for early detection of chronic obstructive lung disease. In Macklem P et al, editors: The lung in transition between health and disease, New York, 1979, Marcel Dekker, Inc.

Cotes JE: Lung function throughout life; determinants and reference values. In Cotes JE, editor: Lung function: assessment and application in medicine, ed 4, Oxford, 1979, Blackwell Scientific Publications Ltd.

Before and after bronchodilator studies

Girard WM and Light RW: Should the FVC be considered in evaluating response to bronchodilator, Chest 84:87, 1983.

Light RW, Conrad SA, and George RB: The one best test for evaluating the effects of bronchodilator therapy, Chest 72:512, 1977.

Sourk RL and Nugent KM: Bronchodilator testing: confidence intervals derived from placebo inhalations, Am Rev Respir Dis 128:153, 1983.

Bronchial challenge and exercise-induced asthma

Bhagat RG and Grunstein MM: Comparison of responsiveness to methacholine, histamine, and exercise in subgroups of asthmatic children, Am Rev Respir Dis 129:221, 1984.

Chai H et al: Standardization of bronchial inhalation challenge procedures, J Allergy Clin Immunol 56:323, 1975.

Cockroft DW and Berscheid BA: Standardization of inhalational provocation test: dose vs concentration of histamine, Chest 82:572, 1982.

Cockroft DW et al: Bronchial reactivity to inhaled histamine: a method and clinical survey, Clin Allergy 7:235-43, 1977.

Cropp GJA et al: Guidelines for bronchial inhalation challenges with pharmacologic and antigenic agents, ATS News, Spring: 11-19, 1980.

Eggleston PA and Rosenthal RR: Guidelines for the methodology of exercise challenge testing of asthmatics, J Allergy Clin Immunol 64:642, 1979.

Fish JE and Kelly JF: Measurements of responsiveness in bronchoprovocation testing, J Allergy Clin Immunol 64:592-6, 1979.

McLaughlin FJ and Dozor AJ: Cold air inhalation challenge in the diagnosis of asthma in children, Pediatrics 72:503, 1983.

Michoud MC, Ghezzo H, and Amyot R: A comparison of pulmonary function tests used for bronchial challenges, Bull Eur Physiopathol Respir 18:609-21, 1982.

Pepys G and Hutchcroft BJ: Bronchial provocation tests in etiologic diagnosis and analysis of asthma, Am Rev Respir Dis 112:829, 1975.

Preoperative Pulmonary Function Testing

Boysen PG: Preoperative pulmonary function tests and complications after coronary artery by-pass, Anesthesiology 57:A499, 1982.

Cain HD, Stevens PM, and Adaniya R: Preoperative pulmonary function and complications after cardiovascular surgery, Chest 76:130, 1979.

Olsen GN et al: Pulmonary function evaluation of the lung resection candidate: a prospective study, Am Rev Respir Dis 111:379, 1975.

Reichel J: Assessment of operative risk of pneumonectomy, Chest 62:570, 1972.

Tisi GM: Preoperative evaluation of pulmonary function: validity, indications, and benefits, Am Rev Respir Dis, 119:293, 1979.

Respiratory impairment for disability

Gaensler EM and Wright GW: Evaluation of respiratory impairment, Arch Environ Health 12:146, 1966.

Harber P et al: Statistical 'biases' in respiratory disability determinations, Am Rev Respir Dis 128:413, 1983.

Morgan WKC: Pulmonary disability and impairment: can't work? won't work?, Basics of RD, American Thoracic Society 10:No. 5, 1982.

US Dept of Health and Human Services: Social Security Regulations: rule for determining disability and blindness, SSA Pub No 64-014, Washington, DC, 1981, US Government Printing Office.

Pulmonary function testing in children

England SJ: Current techniques for assessing pulmonary function in the newborn and infant: advantages and limitations, Pediatr Pulmonol 4:48, 1988.

Falliers CF: Why test function in children routinely?, J Respir Dis 3(1):37, 1982.

Kanner RE et al: Spirometry in children: methodology for obtaining optimal results for clinical and epidemiologic studies, Am Rev Respir Dis 127:720, 1983.

LeSoeuf PN, Hughes DM, and Landau LI: Effect of compression pressure on forced expiratory flow in infants, J Appl Physiol 61:1639, 1986.

Morgan WJ et al: Partial expiratory flow-volume curves in infants and young children. Pediatr Pulmonol 5:232, 1988.

Polgar G and Promadhat V: Pulmonary function testing in children: techniques and standards, Philadelphia, 1971, WB Saunders Co.

Stocks J et al: Improved accuracy of the occlusion technique for measuring total respiratory compliance in infants, Pediatr Pulmonol 3:71, 1987.

Taussig LM: Standardization of lung function testing in children, J Pediatr 97:668, 1980.

Tepper RS, Pagtakhan RD, and Taussig LM: Noninvasive determination of total respiratory compliance in infants by the weighted spirometer method, Am Rev Respir Dis 130:461, 1984.

Wall MA, Misley MC, and Dickerson D: Partial expiratory flow-volume curves in young children, Am Rev Respir Dis 129:557, 1984.

Critical care monitoring

Fahey PJ, Harris K, and Vanderwarf C: Clinical experience with continuous monitoring of mixed venous oxygen saturation in respiratory failure, Chest 86:748, 1984.

Marini JJ: Monitoring during mechanical ventilation, Clin Chest Med 9:73, 1988.

Maunder RJ and Hudson LD: Respiratory monitoring in the intensive care unit. In Shoemaker WC and Abraham E, editors: Diagnostic methods in critical care, New York, 1987, Marcel Dekker, Inc.

Rebuck AS and Chapman KR: Measurement and monitoring of exhaled carbon dioxide. In Nochomovitz ML and Cherniack NS, editors: Non-invasive respiratory monitoring, New York, 1986, Churchill Livingstone Inc.

Taylor MB and Whitman JG: The current status of pulse oximetry: clinical value of continuous noninvasive oxygen saturation monitoring, Anaesthesia 41:943, 1986.

Tobin MJ: Respiratory monitoring in the intensive care unit, Am Rev Respir Dis 138:1625, 1988.

Tobin MJ et al: The pattern of breathing during successful and unsuccessful trials of weaning from mechanical ventilation, Am Rev Respir Dis 134:1111, 1986.

Tremper KK and Waxman KS: Transcutaneous monitoring of respiratory gases. In Nochomovitz ML and Cherniack NS, editors: Non-invasive respiratory monitoring, New York 1986, Churchill Livingstone Inc.

Yamanaka MK and Sue DY: Comparison of arterial-end-tidal P_{CO_2} difference and dead space/tidal volume ratio in respiratory failure, Chest 92:832, 1987.

Metabolic measurements (indirect calorimetry)

Askanazi J et al: Nutrition for the patient with respiratory failure: glucose vs fat, Anesthesiology 54:373, 1981.

Consolazio CF, Johnson RE, and Pecora LJ: Physiological measurements of metabolic functions in man, New York, 1963, McGraw-Hill Inc.

Feurer I and Mullen JL: Bedside measurement of resting energy expenditure and respiratory quotient via indirect calorimetry, Nutrition in Clinical Practice 1:43, 1986.

Harris JA and Benedict FG: Biometric studies of basal metabolism in man, Pub No 279, 1919, Carnegie Institute of Washington.

Weir JB: New methods for calculating metabolic rate with special reference to protein metabolism, J Physiol 109:1, 1949.

Weissman C et al: Evaluation of a non-invasive method for the measurement of metabolic rate in humans, Clin Sci 69:135, 1985.

Weissman C et al: The energy expenditure of the mechanically ventilated critically ill patient—an analysis, Chest 89:2, 254, 1986.

9

Pulmonary Function Testing Equipment

The forerunner of the modern spirometer was introduced by Hutchinson in the midnineteenth century, and some vestiges of the original device are still evident in today's spirometers. Analysis of respiratory gases by volumetric methods was pioneered by Haldane in the early part of the twentieth century; modern gas analyzers use indirect means of assessing the partial pressures of gases. Many of the instruments in the pulmonary function laboratory today combine physical transducers, analog signal generators, and digitized representations of those signals. Some devices, such as the pulse oximeter, are based almost entirely on electronic components, for which the technology is less than 10 years old. The use of small computers (see Chapter 10) has eliminated many tedious calculations and has made sophisticated data processing available, even at the bedside.

This chapter enumerates and attempts to explain the principles of the most common pulmonary function test equipment in terms of specific testing applications. Included are volume-displacement and flow-sensing spirometers, gas analyzers, blood gas electrodes and oximeters, body plethysmographs, the respiratory inductive plethysmograph, breathing valves, and recording devices.

VOLUME-DISPLACEMENT SPIROMETERS

Water-sealed spirometers

For many years, the basic tool in the determination of lung volumes and flow rates has been the water-sealed spirometer. The water-sealed spirometer consists of a large (7 to 10 L) bell suspended in a container of water, with the open end of the bell below the surface of the water (Fig. 9-1). A system of breathing tubes into and out of the interior of the bell allows for the accurate measurement of gas volumes. The subject breathes into the spirometer, which causes the bell to move a proportional distance. The movement of the bell can be used to move a pen across a rotating drum or kymograph, or to activate one of several types of potentiometers to produce an analog DC voltage signal. For simple spirometry, a single large-bore hose carries both inspiratory and expiratory gases. For rebreathing studies, the breathing circuit necessarily includes a CO_2 absorber (soda lime), and separates inspiratory and expiratory circuits by means of one-way valves to eliminate dead space. Water-sealed spirometers are typically used for spirometry, flow-volume curves, lung volumes by helium dilution, and resting ventilation (i.e., $\dot{V}$E, tidal volume, and rate). In combination with an appropriate reservoir for the test gas, water-sealed spirometers can be used to perform diffusing capacity tests (both single-breath and rebreathing). A water-sealed spirometer can itself be used as a reservoir for special gas mixtures such as those used for diffusing capacity tests or for helium-air flow volume curves.

Two types of water-sealed spirometers (the Collins and the Stead-Wells) have been widely used, but only the latter is in common use today. Although it is no longer commonly used, the Collins spirometer was the basic tool of pulmonary function testing for many years (Fig. 9-1). This water-sealed spirometer was available in a variety of sizes. Older models featured a 9- or 13.5-L bell, and the later modular units were available with interchangeable 7- and 14-L bells. The spirometer employed a metal bell counterweighted by means of a pulley and chain assembly, which served to move two recording pens and a variable-speed kymograph, or paper drum. One pen recorded respiratory excursions during inspiration as well as expiration, the other during inspiration only, thus tracing accumulated volumes (i.e. $\dot{V}$E, MVV). The pen of the Collins spirometer moved in the

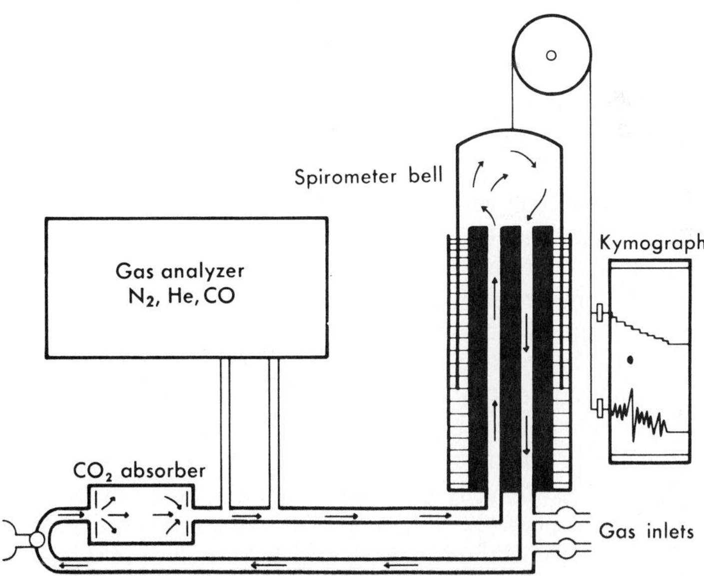

Fig. 9-1 Water-seal type spirometer. Typical water-seal spirometer apparatus, including a one-way breathing circuit with free breathing valve, CO_2 absorber, inlets for addition of gases, outlets for sampling by gas analyzers, and recording kymograph. (From Clinical spirometry, Braintree, Mass., Warren E. Collins, Inc.)

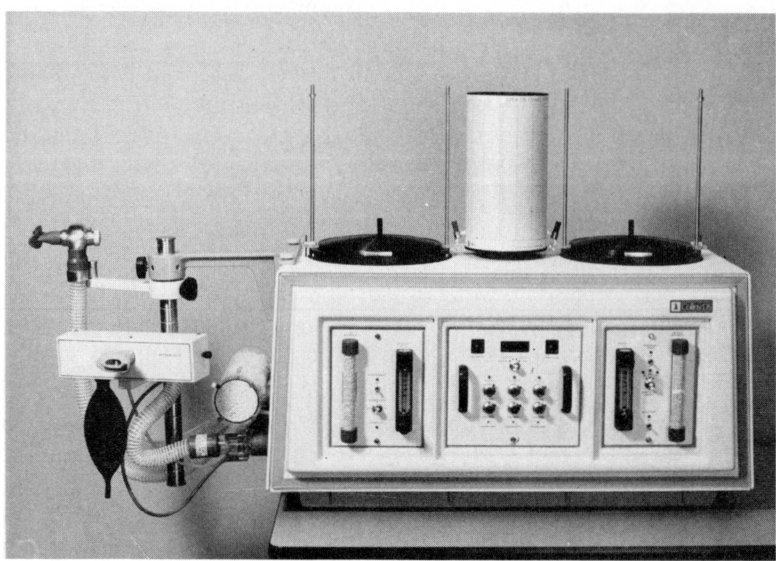

Fig. 9-2 Automated Stead-Wells water-seal spirometer. The Stead-Wells spirometer uses a lightweight plastic bell that is not counterweighted, shown here completely empty. The spirometer bell carries a pen that traces directly on a rotating kymograph. The bell also moves a linear potentiometer to generate analog signals for computerized measurements. With appropriate circuitry and gas analyzers, He dilution FRC determinations and $D_{L_{CO}}$ measurements are easily performed. (Courtesy Warren E. Collins, Inc., Braintree, Mass.)

opposite direction from the bell itself; when the bell rose, during expiration, the pen moved downward. Many spirograms are still depicted with expired volume causing a downward deflection on volume-time tracings. The kymograph had rotational speeds of 32, 160, and 1920 mm/min, so that timed capacities (i.e., $FEV_{1.0}$, MVV) could be conveniently recorded. The Collins-type water-sealed spirometer was also fitted with a rotary potentiometer on the pulley that supported the chain assembly to provide analog output signals for volume and flow.

The Stead-Wells type of water-sealed spirometer (Fig. 9-2) operates on principles quite similar to those outlined above, except that it employs a lightweight plastic bell that is not counterweighted or supported by pulleys. The plastic bell "floats" in the water well, and rises and falls during breathing. The Stead-Wells spirometer carries a recording pen mounted against a variable-speed (32, 160, and 1920 mm/min) kymograph, but, unlike the Collins spirometer, respiratory excursions deflect the pen in the same direction as the bell. Expiration is traced upward on the volume-time graph (see Fig. 3-1). The Stead-Wells spirometer bell can also be directly attached to a linear potentiometer to provide analog signals proportional to volume and flow, allowing either analog recording or analog-digital conversion of the signals.

The primary advantages of the water-sealed spirometer are its simplicity and its accuracy. Because the spirometer bell can be used to directly drive a pen against the chart drum, "manual" tracings can be obtained for comparison to those derived by computer from the analog outputs. Measurements of volumes and flows can be taken from the kymographic tracings if the bell factor and paper speed are known. The bell factor is simply the volume displacement per unit of vertical movement, usually expressed in ml/mm. Although most laboratories use computer-derived measurements, the capability to perform tests manually may be useful for quality assurance or for calibration.

The Collins water-sealed spirometer is no longer widely used for measuring forced vital capacity or flow parameters derived from that maneuver. The inertia of the counterweighted bell limits its ability to faithfully record the change in flows occurring during forced expiration, particularly in normal subjects. The Stead-Wells design, however, is capable of meeting the minimum requirements for flow and volume accuracy as outlined by the American Thoracic Society (see Chapter 11). For manual measurements from kymograph tracings, corrections from ATPS to BTPS are necessary. The problems encountered with water-sealed spirometers usually arise from leaks in the bell or in the breathing circuit; gravity causes volume loss in the presence of such leaks. Improper positioning of the spirometer (i.e., either too high or too low) can cause the bell to rise out of the water or to empty completely, resulting in water being drawn into the breathing circuit. Inadequate water in the device may also lead to erroneous readings that are sometimes difficult to detect. The size of the water-sealed spirometer and the weight when it is filled with water make it somewhat difficult to transport.

Maintenance of water-sealed spirometers include routine draining of the water well and checking for cracks or leaks in the bell itself. Chemical absorbers for water vapor must be routinely checked; they are rapidly exhausted because the gas in the spirometer is almost completely saturated with water vapor. Cleaning of water-sealed spirometers typically involves replacing breathing hoses and mouthpieces after each subject. Although the subject's expired gas comes into direct contact with the water in the spirometer, cross contamination is not common. Some systems allow the use of low-resistance bacteria filters to protect those parts of the breathing circuit that are not changed after each patient use from contamination. Such filters should be used only for maneuvers that are not flow dependent; the volume of these filters may need to be taken into account when calculating system volume or system dead space.

Dry rolling-seal spirometers

A recent innovation in volume-displacement spirometers is the dry rolling-seal spirometer. A typical unit consists of a piston mounted horizontally in a cylinder and supported by a rod that rests on bearings (Fig. 9-3). The

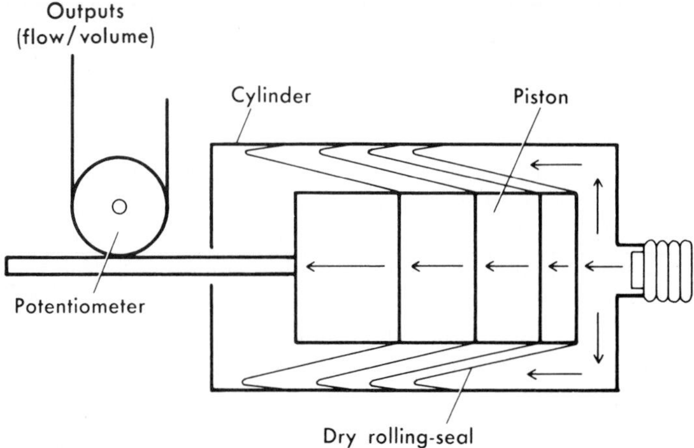

Fig. 9-3 Cutaway view of the main components of a dry rolling-seal spirometer. The figure gives an exaggerated view of the rolling-seal, which actually fits closely between the piston and the cylinder wall. The piston has a large surface area, so that its horizontal movement is minimized. This allows recording of normal breaths and maximal respiratory excursions with only a small amount of mechanical movement and hence, little resistance. The piston is supported by a rod that activates a rotary potentiometer. The rotational movement of the potentiometer is translated into analog signals for both flow and volume. Alternately, the rod may carry the recording pen across moving graph paper for direct tracing of volume-time curves. (From Form 370, Ohio Medical Products, Madison, Wis.)

piston is coupled to the cylinder wall by a flexible plastic seal that rolls on itself rather than sliding as the piston moves. A similar type of rolling-seal is also used with a vertically mounted, lightweight piston that rises and falls with breathing. The maximum volume of the cylinder with the piston fully displaced is usually 10 to 12 L; a large-diameter piston is employed so that excursions of just a few inches are all that is necessary to record large volume changes. The piston is normally constructed of lightweight aluminum to reduce inertia. Mechanical resistance is kept to a minimum by the bearings supporting the piston rod and by the rolling-seal itself.

Some dry rolling-seal spirometers employ a mechanically-driven graphing device in which the piston rod has a pen attached. The pen moves across graph paper or a strip chart recorder as the subject inspires and expires. Most dry rolling-seal spirometers use a potentiometer, either linear or rotating, that responds to the movement of the piston to provide a DC voltage output for volume and flow. A typical system might employ a 10-V potentiometer attached to a 10-L spirometer with an output of 1 V/L. The analog outputs for both volume and flow are most often directed to an analog-to-digital convertor (see Chapter 10) so that the data can be

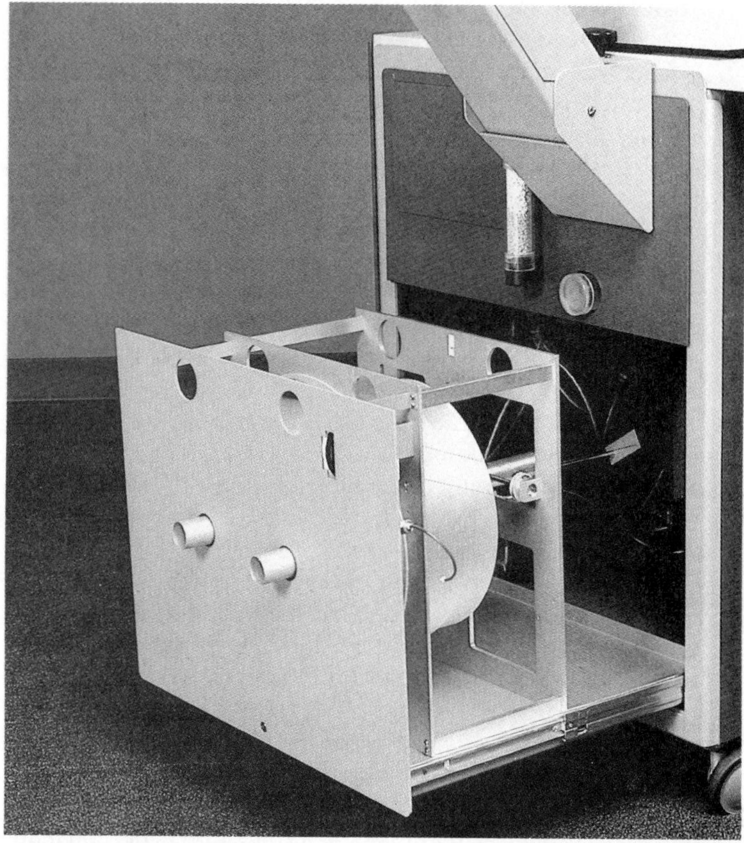

Fig. 9-4 Dry rolling-seal spirometer. A typical dry-seal spirometer consisting of a large aluminum piston mounted in a cylinder, with two ports to accommodate simple spirometry and rebreathing maneuvers, with a CO_2 absorber (see Fig. 9-3). (Courtesy Gould Medical Instruments, Inc., Dayton, Ohio.)

stored by computer. The piston of the standard dry rolling-seal spirometer (Fig. 9-4) travels horizontally, eliminating the need for counterbalancing. The vertically mounted spirometer depends on the lightweight piston and the rolling-seal to reduce resistance to breathing. Temperature corrections are made either by adjusting the analog signal or by modifying the digital value stored in the computer. One-way circuits and CO_2 scrubbers can be added to the inlets of the device so that dry rolling-seal spirometers can be used for rebreathing tests in the same way as water-sealed spirometers. To perform studies in which gas volumes larger than the spirometer itself are measured, such as the open-circuit N_2 washout, a "dumping" mechanism is attached to the spirometer. The dumping device empties the spirometer after each breath or after a predetermined volume is reached. Addition of an automated valve and sampling device allows the dry rolling-seal spirometer to be used for single-breath diffusion studies.

As with most volume-displacement-type spirometers, the dry rolling-seal spirometer can be used for manual or computerized testing. Manual testing, using a mechanical recorder, may be used for bedside or screening tests. Despite their large size, most dry rolling-seal spirometers can be transported rather easily. However, the addition of a computer, gas analyzers, or recorder may make the system too bulky for bedside testing. Common problems encountered with dry rolling-seal spirometers are sticking of the rolling-seal and increased mechanical resistance in the piston-cylinder assembly. These difficulties can usually be avoided by adequate maintenance of the spirometer. Cleaning of the dry rolling-seal involves disassembling the piston-cylinder assembly. The interior of the cylinder and the face of the piston are usually wiped with a mild antibacterial solution. The rolling-seal itself is also wiped with disinfectant; alcohol or similar drying agents may cause deterioration of the seal and should not be used. The seal may be lubricated with cornstarch to prevent sticking, but care must be taken to avoid excessive powder being left in the spirometer. The seal should be routinely checked for leaks or tears. After reassembly, the piston should be positioned at the maximum volume position. When the rolling-seal is completely extended, the material of the seal is less likely to develop creases that can result in uneven movement of the piston.

Bellows-type spirometers

A third general type of volume-displacement spirometer is the bellows or wedge bellows, both of which consist of collapsible bellows that fold or unfold in response to breathing excursions. The conventional bellows design is a flexible accordion-type container that has one end fixed while the other end is displaced in proportion to the volume injected during expiration. The wedge bellows operates similarly, except that it expands and contracts like a fan (Fig. 9-5). One side of the bellows remains stationary, while the other side moves with a pivotal motion around an axis through the fixed side. This displacement of the bellows by a volume of gas is translated either to movement of a mechanical recording device or to a potentiometer. For mechanical recording, chart paper moves at a fixed speed under the pen while a spirogram is traced. For computerized testing, displacement of the bellows is transformed into a DC voltage by a linear or rotating potentiometer.

The conventional bellows and wedge bellows may be mounted either horizontally or vertically. Horizontal bellows, either conventional or wedge, with a large surface offer little mechanical resistance and are normally used in conjunction with a potentiometer to produce analog volume and flow signals. Several types of small (approximately 7-L) vertically mounted bellows are currently available and are used widely for portable spirometry and bedside testing. Most of these offer simple mechanical

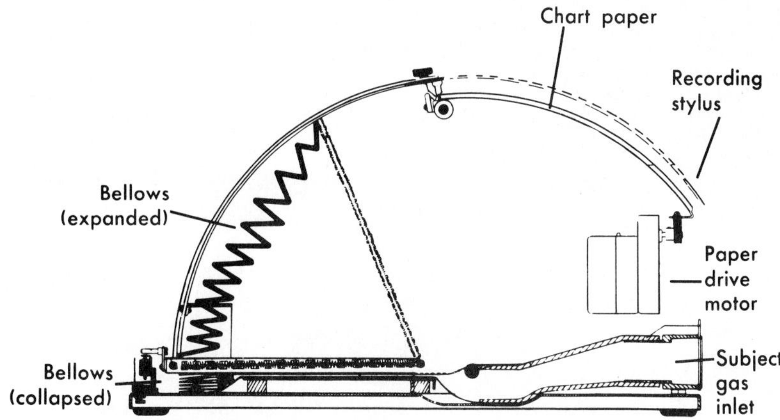

Fig. 9-5 Cross-sectional diagram of a wedge bellows type of spirometer. The fan-like movements of the wedge bellows produce mechanical movement, which is usually translated directly to a recording device. Some manufacturers suspend the bellows so that the primary movement is in a horizontal rather than vertical direction; large wedge bellows offer little mechanical resistance and are comparable to dry-seal or water-seal spirometers in accuracy and linearity. (Modified from Vitalograph Medical Instrumentation: Product brochure, Lenexa, Kan.)

recording and/or digital data reduction by means of a small dedicated microprocessor.

Both types of bellows (Fig. 9-6, *A* and *B*) are suitable for measurement of the vital capacity and its subdivisions, as well as the FVC, $FEV_{1.0}$, expiratory flow rates, and the MVV. Some bellows-type spirometers, especially those that are mounted vertically, are designed specifically for measurement of expiratory flows, because they empty spontaneously under their own weight. Horizontally mounted bellows can usually be set in a mid-range so as to record both inspiratory and expiratory maneuvers such as the flow-volume loop. In conjunction with the appropriate gas analyzers and breathing circuitry, bellows systems may be used for lung volume determinations and DL_{CO} measurements.

A common problem with the bellows spirometers is inaccuracy resulting either from sticking of the folds of the bellows caused by dirt or moisture or from aging of the bellows material. Leaks may also develop in the bellows material or at the point where the bellows is mounted. Leaks can usually be detected by filling the bellows with air, plugging the breathing port, and attaching a weight or spring to pressurize the gas inside. Cleaning bellows-type spirometers depends on the method of construction. In some instruments, the bellows can be entirely removed, while in others, the interior of the bellows must be wiped clean. Many bellows are made from rubberized or plastic-based material that can be cleaned with a mild detergent and dried thoroughly before reassembly.

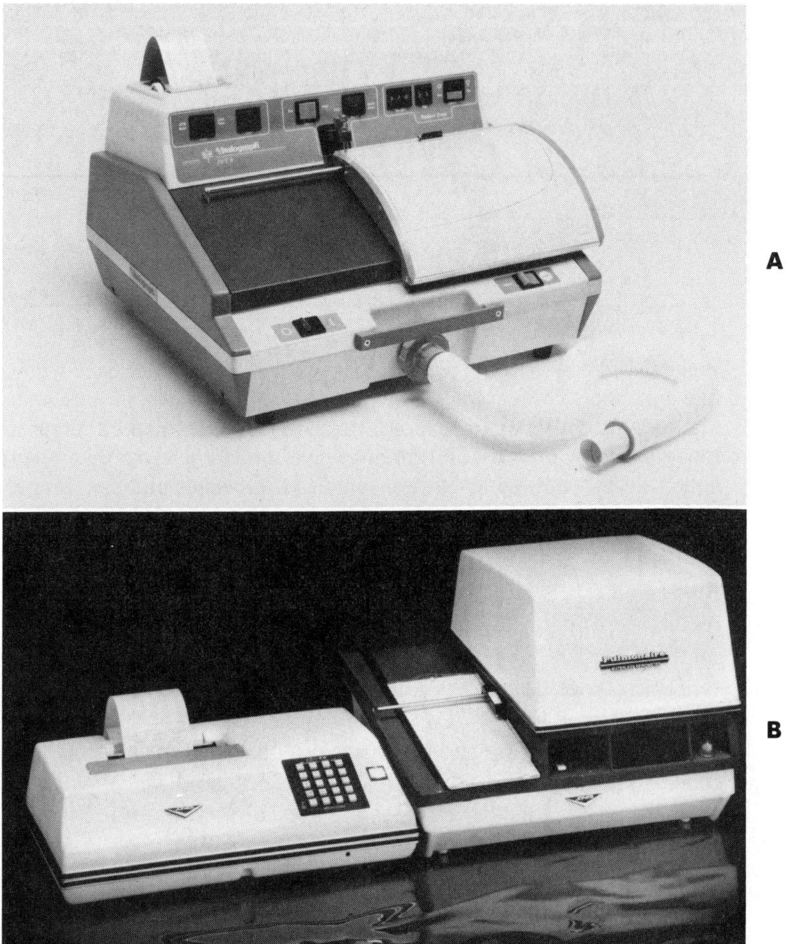

Fig. 9-6 Two types of bellows spirometers. **A**, Wedge bellows spirometer with direct-writing recorder, digital displays, and built-in printer for automated data reduction. (Courtesy Vitalograph Medical Instrumentation, Lenexa, Kan.) **B**, Conventional bellows-type spirometer with the bellows mounted horizontally and driving a pen across moving graph paper. A potentiometer allows analog output to a dedicated microprocessor with a built-in printer for automatic data reduction. (Courtesy Jones Medical Instrument Co., Oakbrook, Ill.)

Flow-sensing spirometers

In contrast to the volume-displacement spirometers described above is the flow-sensing spirometer, or pneumotachometer. The term pneumotachometer describes a device that measures flow. Flow-sensing spirometers use various physical principles to produce a flow signal that can be integrated to allow measurement of volumes as well as the flows. Integration is a process in which flow (i.e., volume per unit of time) is divided into a large number of small intervals (time) and the volume from each interval summed. Integration can be performed quite easily by an electronic circuit. Accurate determination of volumes by integration of flow requires accurate flow signals, accurate timing, and sensitive detection of low flows. One type of device that responds to bulk flow of gas is the turbine or impeller; integration is unnecessary because the turbine flow device directly measures gas volumes. The remaining types of flow-sensing spirometers all use tubes through which laminar air flow is possible (see Appendix, Some Useful Equations). Although a wide variety of flow-sensing spirometers is presently available, four basic designs are commonly used: turbines, pressure differential, heated wire, and ultrasonic flow sensors.

Turbines. The simplest type of flow-sensing device is the turbine or respirometer, which consists of a vane connected to a series of precision gears. Gas molecules flowing through the body of the instrument rotate the vane, which registers a volume (Fig. 9-7). The respirometer is suitable not only for measurement of lung volumes such as vital capacity but it can also be used for ventilation tests such as V_T and $\dot{V}_E$. One typical device, the Wright respirometer, can be used to measure volumes at flows between 3 and 300 L/min. At flows above 300 L/min, the vane is subject to distortion; therefore, it should not be used to measure FVC when the subject is capable of flows greater than 300 L/min. At low flows, less than 3 L/min, the inertia of the vane–gear system may cause erroneous measurements. The special advantage of the respirometer is its compact size and practicality in the bedside setting. Most respirometers register a wide range of volumes, from 0.1 up to 1 L on one scale and up to 100 L on another scale. Turbine devices are also widely used for bulk measurements in various dry gas meters.

An adaptation of the turbine flow device includes a photocell and light source that is interrupted by the movement of a vane or impeller. A pulsing of the light beam is caused by the interruption of the rotating vane, with each of the pulses equivalent to a fixed gas volume. The pulse count is summed and is proportional to the volume of gas flowing through the tube. The signal thus produced may not be linear at high or low flows, because of inertia or distortion of the rotating vane.

Pressure-differential flow sensors. A second type of flow-sensing device consists of a tube containing a resistive element that allows gas to flow through it but causes a pressure drop. The pressure difference across the resistive element is measured by means of a sensitive pressure trans-

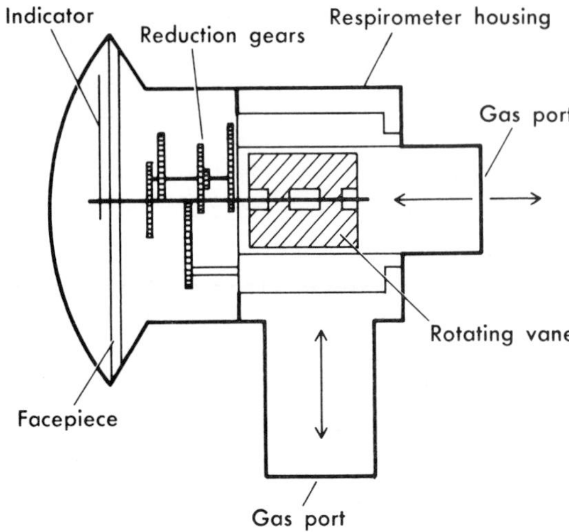

Fig. 9-7 Turbine-type flow sensor. A cutaway diagram of the Wright respirometer. A large rotating vane mounted on jeweled bearings drives reduction gears connected to the main indicator arm. Two gas ports allow flow through the body for measurements of volume; although the vane turns in only one direction, gas can either be inspired through the respirometer or expired into it. Not pictured is a small indicator arm, which marks volumes larger than 1 L on the face, so that accumulated volumes can be measured. The instrument also features controls for engaging or disengaging the vane and for resetting the indicators to zero. (From British Oxygen Co., Ltd.: Operating instructions, Wright respirometer, print No. 630207, Issue 3:6, Aug 1971.)

ducer, with pressure taps on either side of the element. The pressure drop across the resistive element is proportional to the flow of gas as long as the gas flow is laminar (Fig. 9-8, *A*). The flow signal from the pneumotachometer is electronically integrated to derive volume measurements. Turbulent gas flow either upstream or downstream of the resistive element may interfere with the development of true laminar flow. Most pneumotachometers attempt to reduce turbulent flow by tapering the tubes in which the resistive elements are mounted.

Two types of resistive elements are commonly employed. The Fleisch-type pneumotachometer uses a bundle of capillary tubes as the resistive element; laminar flow is generally assured by the capillary tube arrangement. The cross-sectional area of the capillary tubes along with their lengths determine the actual resistance to flow through the Fleisch pneumotachometer. The dynamic range of the Fleisch device must be matched to the range of flows to be measured. Different sizes of pneumotachometers are used to accurately measure high or low flows. The other common variety of pressure differential flow sensor is the Silverman (or Lilly) type. The Silverman pneumotachometer uses one or more screens to act as a resistive

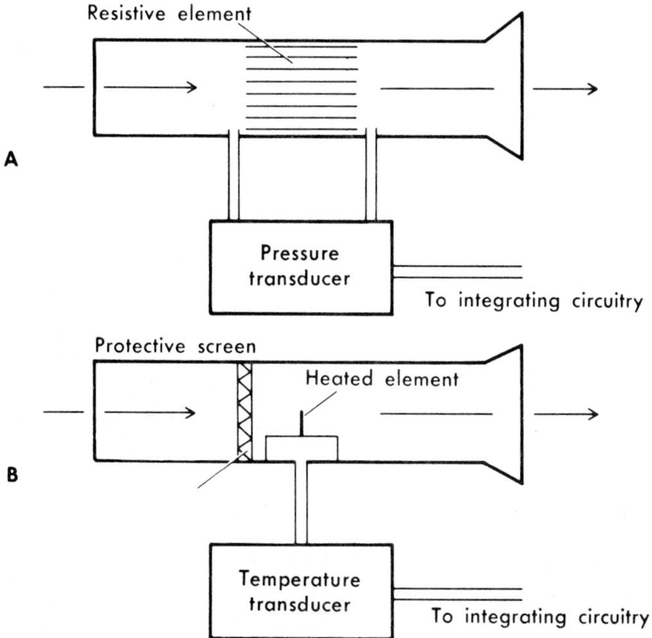

Fig. 9-8 Two common flow-sensing devices (pneumotachometers). **A**, Pressure-differential type pneumotachometer, in which a resistive element causes a pressure drop proportional to the flow of gas through the tube. A sensitive pressure transducer monitors the pressure drop across the resistive element and converts the differential into a signal that varies as the flow changes. The volume passing through the pneumotachometer can be calculated by integrating the flow over the time interval during which the flow occurred; this is usually done by an electronic integrating circuit. **B**, A heated-wire type pneumotachometer in which a heated element of small mass responds to gas flow by heat loss. As the element cools, a greater current is needed to maintain a constant temperature; the current change is proportional to gas flow, and a continuous signal is supplied to an integrating circuit, as for the pressure-differential flow sensor.

element. A typical arrangement has three screens mounted parallel to one another. The middle screen acts as the resistive element with the pressure taps on either side, while the outer screens protect the middle screen and help to assure laminar flow. The Silverman-type pneumotachometer has a somewhat wider dynamic flow range than the Fleisch-type pneumotachometer, making it better suited to measuring varying flows and volumes. Both the Fleisch and Silverman flow sensors employ a heating mechanism to warm the resistive element to 37° C to prevent accumulation of moisture on the element. Condensation or other debris lodging in the resistive element changes the resistance across it and changes the calibration of the device.

Some spirometers use other types of resistive elements, such as porous paper, so that the flow sensor itself is disposable. Typically, these devices have a single pressure tap upstream of the resistive element and the pressure in front of the resistive element is referenced against ambient pressure. The accuracy of these types of spirometers is often dependent on how carefully the disposable resistive elements are manufactured. If the resistance varies widely from sensor to sensor, accurate measurement of flows or volumes requires individual calibration of each unit.

Heated-wire flow sensors. A third commonly used type of flow-sensing spirometer is based on the cooling effect of gas flow. A heated element, usually a platinum wire or small bead of metal called a thermistor, is situated in a laminar flow tube (Fig. 9-8, *B* and Fig. 9-9). Gas flow past the element causes a temperature drop so that more current must be supplied to maintain the preset temperature of the element. The amount of current

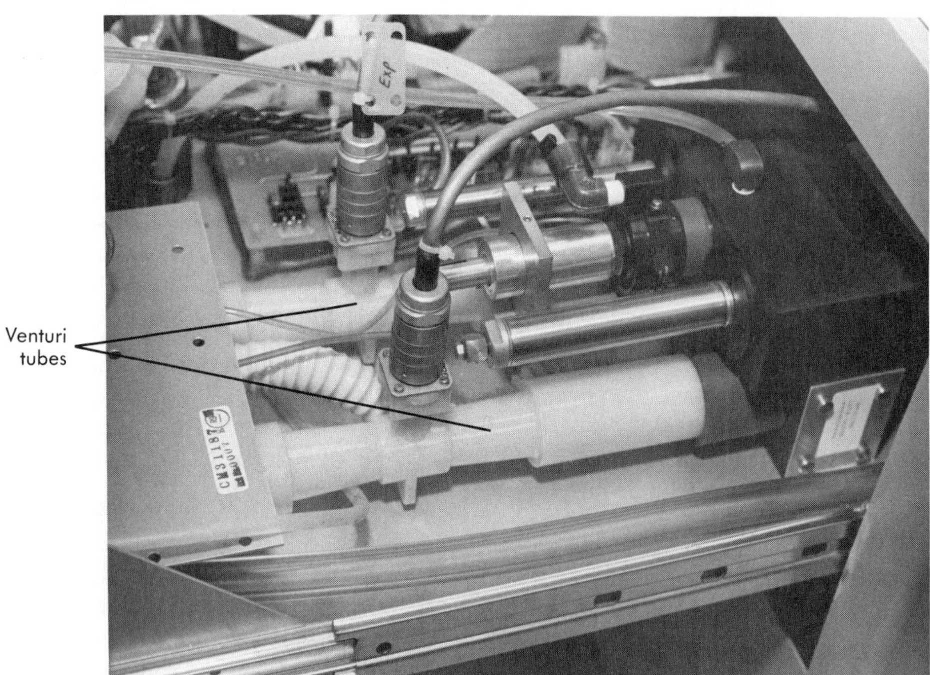

Fig. 9-9 A heated-wire type flow sensor. Venturi tubes contain paired stainless steel probe wires maintained at two different temperatures exceeding body temperature and connected by a Wheatstone bridge. The Venturi tube streamlines gas flow (into laminar flow), and the temperature of the wires is decreased in proportion to the mass of the gas and its flow. Two flow sensors are used; one measures expiratory flow while the other serves as a reference. (Courtesy Gould Medical Instruments, Dayton, Ohio, and Missouri Baptist Hospital, St. Louis, Mo.)

needed to maintain the temperature is proportional to the magnitude of the gas flow. The heated element usually has a small mass so that slight changes in gas flow can be detected. The flow signal is integrated electronically to derive volume measurements. The heated element is normally protected behind a screen to prevent impaction of debris on the element that might change its thermal characteristics. Some systems employ two matched thermistors; one measures gas flow, while the other serves as a reference. Most thermistor-type flow sensors have their elements heated to a temperature well above 37° C so that condensation does not interfere with sensitivity of the element.

Ultrasonic flow sensors. A fourth type of flow-sensing spirometer is designed to use the principle of vortex shedding. A flow tube is constructed with struts placed in the airstream so that gas flowing over the struts is broken up into waves called vortices. An ultrasonic crystal downstream of the strut transmits high-frequency sound waves through the turbulent gas flow to a receiving crystal on the opposite side of the tube (Fig. 9-10). The sizes of the strut and flow tube determine the size of the vortices and allow the device to be calibrated so that each vortex passing through the ultrasonic beam produces a pulse. Each pulse is proportional to specific volume (for example, 1 ml/pulse) and when summed electronically, provides a measurement of volume. The ultrasonic flow-sensing spirometer is relatively insensitive to gas temperature or humidity, although accumulation of moisture on the struts or ultrasonic transducers can cause erroneous readings. The crystals are usually heated to prevent condensation.

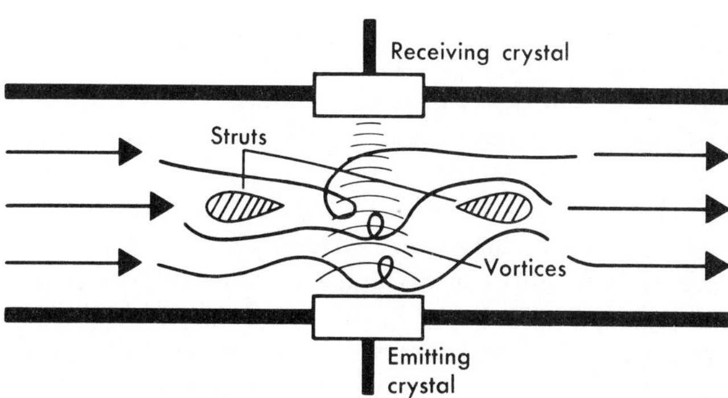

Fig. 9-10 Ultrasonic flow sensor. A beam of ultrasonic waves is emitted by one crystal and received by another crystal on the opposite side of the flow tube. Gas flowing in streamline passes over struts in the tube and forms vortices. This is called *vortex shedding* and changes the frequency of the transmitted ultrasound waves in proportion to the volume of gas forming the vortices. Each vortex causes a "pulse;" the pulses are summed electronically to obtain volume measurements. Volume can be measured for gas moving in either direction.

Pulmonary function testing with the flow-sensing spirometer offers some advantages over volume-displacement spirometry setups. When combined with appropriate gas analyzers and breathing circuits, flow-sensing spirometers can be used to perform lung volume determinations by the open- or closed-circuit methods and to measure diffusing capacity, in addition to standard spirometric measurements. Pressure-differential pneumotachometers are widely used for measurement of flows and volumes in body plethysmographs, exercise testing systems, and metabolic carts. Because of their small size, flow-sensing devices are often incorporated into spirometers designed for portability. Because most of the sensors described require electronic circuitry for integration of the flow signal or summing of volume pulses, flow-based spirometers are usually microprocessor controlled. Some flow-sensing spirometers permit direct connection of the analog signal (i.e., flow, volume, or both) to a strip chart or X-Y recorder, but most use computer-generated graphics to produce volume-time or flow-volume tracings. Most flow sensors can be easily cleaned and disinfected; some sensors can be immersed in a disinfectant without disassembly. As noted previously, many systems use inexpensive, disposable sensors, based on the pressure-differential type, that can be discarded after single-patient use.

There are some disadvantages associated with flow-sensing spirometers. Most of the flow sensors described operate on the premise that a given flow will generate a proportional signal. However, at extremes of flow, either low or high, the signal generated may become nonproportional (i.e., nonlinear). Almost every type of flow-sensing device will display some nonlinearity. Some systems use two separate flow sensors, one for high flows, as in the FVC, and another for low flows, as in V_T excursions. Better accuracy is obtained for flows and volumes by reducing the range of the flow sensor to match the physiologic signal. Most flow-based spirometers "linearize" the flow signal electronically or by means of software corrections before any parameters are measured so that the values will be accurate within acceptable limits.

Turbines, pressure-differential, and heated-wire types of flow-sensing spirometers are particularly affected by the composition of the gas being measured. Changes in gas density or viscosity most often require special corrections to the output of the transducer to obtain accurate volumes. In most systems, these corrections are performed by computer software. A flow-sensing spirometer may be calibrated with air but then be used to analyze mixtures containing helium, neon, oxygen, or other test gases, provided the software is designed to correct for differences in gas composition for each individual test.

Results from any measurement done with a flow-sensing spirometer depend on the electronic circuitry that converts the raw signal into an actual volume or flow. Pulmonary function parameters that are measured on a time base (i.e., FEV_T, MVV, $FEF_{200\text{-}1200}$) require precise timing mechanisms as well as accurate volume or flow measurements. The most common timing mechanism in flow-based spirometers is the detection of the start or end of test by a minimum flow or pressure change. Integration of flow begins when the flow generated through the spirometer has reached a threshold limit, usually around 0.1 to 0.2 L/sec. Instruments that initiate timing in response to volume pulses usually have a similar threshold that must be achieved to begin recording the input signal. Contamination of resistive elements, thermistors, or turbine vanes by moisture or other debris can alter the flow-sensing characteristics of the transducer and interfere with the spirometer's ability to detect the start or end of test. Problems related to electronic "drift" often require flow sensors to be calibrated frequently. Calibration and quality control techniques for volume-displacement and flow-sensing spirometers are included in Chapter 11.

Breathing valves

Several types of valves are commonly used with both volume-displacement and flow-sensing spirometers. These valves allow direction of inspired and expired gas through the measuring transducer as well as sampling for gas analysis.

Free-breathing valves. The simplest type of valve is that which allows the subject to be switched from breathing room air to breathing gas contained in a spirometer or special breathing circuit. Free-breathing valves are routinely employed in both the open- and closed-circuit methods of FRC determination. The free-breathing valve is designed so that the subject can be "switched in" to the system either manually or under computer control at any point in the breathing cycle. Because these types of valves are used mainly for tidal breathing or slow vital capacity maneuvers, resistance to flow is not critical. Most have ports with diameters of 1.5 to 3 cm. For studies involving gas analysis, such as the FRC determination, the valve must be leak free.

Directional (one-way, two-way) valves. Directional valves are used in many types of breathing circuits to ensure gas flow either to the subject or to the measuring device. The simplest type consists of a flap that opens in only one direction. A more common design is that used to separate inspired from expired gas, often referred to as a two-way nonrebreathing valve. This type of directional valve consists of a T-shaped body with three ports and two separate diaphragms (Fig. 9-11). The diaphragms allow gas to flow in only one direction, with the subject connection between the diaphragms, effectively separating inspired and expired gas. These types of devices are commonly used in exercise testing, metabolic studies, or any procedure requiring collection, measurement, or analysis of exhaled gas.

Two variables must be considered in the selection of appropriate two-way directional valves: dead space volume and flow resistance. In the gas collection type of valve just described, the dead space consists of the volume contained between the two diaphragms, along with the volume of any

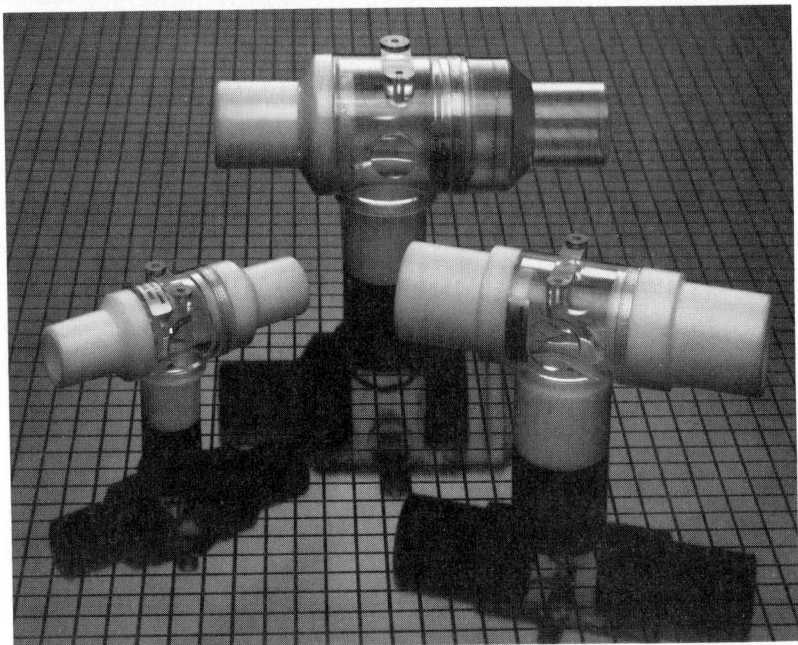

Fig. 9-11 Two-way breathing valves. Three different sizes of two-way valves as employed for studies involving collection or measurement of expired gas. Each valve consists of a T-shaped body containing two diaphragms that separate inspired and expired gas. The smaller valves have less dead space but higher flow resistance, while the large valve has low flow resistance but more dead space. The small- and medium-sized valves are used for studies in which low flows are encountered, such as metabolic measurements. The large valve is appropriate for high flow rates, such as those occurring during maximal exercise testing. (Courtesy Hans Rudolph, Inc., Kansas City, Mo.)

connectors (i.e., mouthpiece). Most manufacturers supply information on the dead space of particular valves, and some have the value printed on the valve body. Unknown dead space can usually be readily determined by blocking two of the three ports and measuring the water volume required to fill the dead space portion of the valve.

Low dead space (i.e., less than 50 ml) valves are required for studies in which the subject's ventilatory status is already compromised, particularly if only normal, tidal breathing is being assessed. Valves with larger dead space volumes may be required to accommodate large-bore ports and low-resistance diaphragms. The valves used during exercise testing to minimize resistance at high flow rates typically have a large dead space volume. The valve dead space should be accurately determined to incorporate corrections in calculations involving gas analysis, such as physiologic dead space measurements. Low resistance to flow is also a critical characteristic of

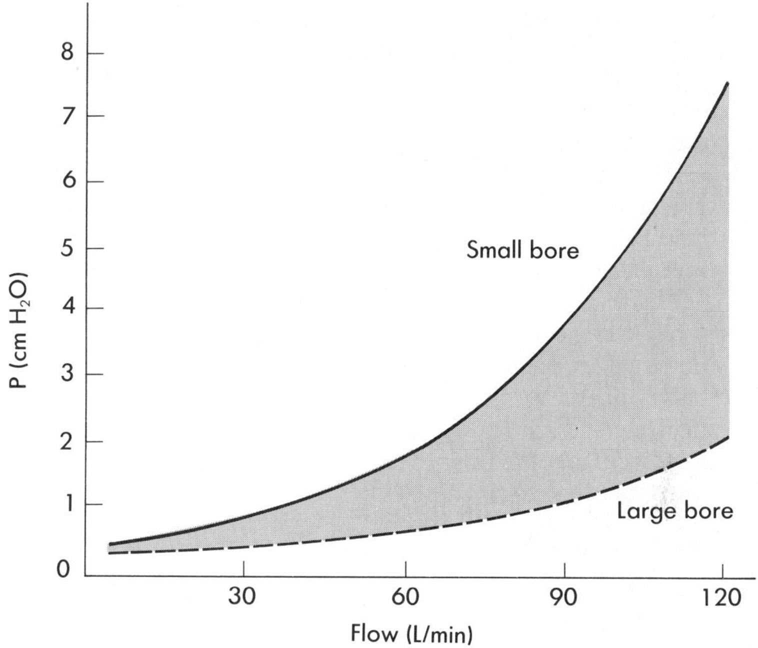

Fig. 9-12 Breathing valve resistance. A graph plotting pressure developed across two different size valves in relation to gas flow through them. For small-bore valves (see Fig. 9-11), pressures less than 1 cm H_2O are generated up to approximately 60 L/min (1 L/sec). Large-bore valves have less resistance (i.e., pressure per unit of flow) and are typically used for studies in which the subject develops high flow rates. Other factors affecting resistance include the design and material used for the diaphragms or leaflets in the valve and whether the diaphragms move freely. Resistance increases nonlinearly in all types of valves, and high resistance can occur even in large-bore valves if extremely high flow rates are attained.

directional valves, whether they are one-way valves or two-way valves, such as those just described. Resistance to flow through most valves is nonlinear and dependent on the cross-sectional area of the valve leaflets or diaphragms (Fig. 9-12). Flow resistance is usually not critical in applications during which flows less than 1 L/sec (60 L/min) are developed, and small-bore directional valves can be selected on the basis of an appropriate dead space volume. Most small-bore nonrebreathing valves have resistances in the range of 1 to 2 cm H_2O/L/sec at flows up to 1 L/sec. If the subject breathes through the valve for long intervals, even small resistances may result in respiratory muscle fatigue and changes in the ventilatory pattern. Applications such as exercise testing typically involve increased flow rates. Large-bore two-way valves are indicated in most situations when the subject can be anticipated to develop flows in excess of 1 L/sec. Pressures of less than 3 cm H_2O can be maintained even at flows of 5 L/sec with large-bore valves. Even appropriately selected valves can cause increased flow resistance if not properly maintained. Rubber, plastic, or silicon leaflets and diaphragms can all stick or become rigid with age. Valves should be disassembled and cleaned according to the manufacturer's directions after each use, and allowed to dry thoroughly before reassembly.

Gas sampling valves. Specialized valves are used to obtain gas samples during procedures such as the single-breath DL_{CO} or CO_2 rebreathing cardiac output. Most gas sampling valves used electrically activated solenoids to rapidly change the direction of gas flow to a spirometer or sample bag. Some devices employ pneumatically powered slide valves that can be triggered manually or by a DC voltage. The primary concern with gas sampling valves is smooth operation with appropriate direction of the gas to be sampled. Electrically activated solenoids may deteriorate with age, particularly if exposed to high humidity conditions such as expired air. Replacement of O-rings or similar types of seals may be necessary to ensure uncontaminated gas samples.

Pulmonary gas analyzers

The types of gas analyzers used in pulmonary function testing are determined by the gases commonly analyzed. O_2 and CO_2 are analyzed as part of patient monitoring, as well as during metabolic studies and exercise testing. Helium analysis is widely employed for closed-circuit FRC determinations and for several types of DL_{CO} tests. N_2 analysis is used in the open-circuit FRC method. CO measurements are integral to all of the diffusion capacity methods currently used.

Table 9-1 lists some of the types of O_2 analyzers available. Most of these are suitable for monitoring purposes, but two types are used for rapid analysis of O_2: the polarographic electrode and the zirconium fuel cell.

Polarographic electrodes. The polarographic electrode is similar to the blood gas O_2 electrode (see Blood Gas Electrodes section of this chapter), except that the platinum cathode is not membraned and a pump draws the sample gas past it at a constant flow. By using special electronic circuitry, a response time of approximately 200 ms can be attained, and continuous analysis of O_2 is possible.

Zirconium fuel cells. An electrode is formed by coating a zirconium element with platinum. The zirconium, when heated to 700° to 800° C, acts as a solid electrolyte between the platinum coating on either side. When the two sides of the electrode are exposed to differing partial pressures of O_2, O_2 traverses the electrode and creates a voltage proportional to the difference in concentrations. Normally, the gas to be sampled is drawn past the element at a constant low flow so that continuous analysis is possible without altering the temperature of the electrode. The temperature must be held constant, so the electrode requires adequate insulation and a warm-up period to reach thermal equilibrium at the elevated temperature. Response times of less than 200 ms are possible with the zirconium fuel

Table 9-1 Oxygen analyzers

Type	Applications	Advantages / disadvantages
Paramagnetic	Monitoring	Discrete sampling only
Polarographic electrode	Monitoring, exercise testing, metabolic studies	Discrete or continuous sampling; requires special electronics for fast response (200 ms)
Galvanic cell (fuel cell)	Monitoring	Continuous sampling; similar to polarographic but does not require polarizing voltage
Zirconium cell	Breath-by-breath exercise and metabolic studies	Heated (700°-800° C) fuel cell; fast response useful for continuous sampling; thermal stabilization required
Gas chromatograph	Exercise testing, monitoring, metabolic measurements	Discrete sampling; response time ≃ 30 seconds; very accurate; multiple gas analysis
Mass spectrometer	Breath-by-breath exercise and metabolic studies, multiple patient monitoring	Discrete or continuous sampling, fast response (< 100 ms); multiple gas analysis; large and complex instrumentation

cell. Both the zirconium fuel cell and the polarographic electrode measure partial pressure of O_2; fluctuations in the pressure in the sampling circuit can affect the concentration measurement. The presence of water vapor in the sample affects both of these electrodes similarly. O_2 concentration is measured accurately but is diluted by water vapor.

Infrared absorption. Several respiratory gas analyzers are based on the principle of absorption of infrared radiation to measure gas concentrations. This technique is most often used in CO analyzers for the DL_{CO} tests, and in CO_2 analyzers for exercise testing, metabolic studies, and bedside monitoring (capnography) in critical care (Fig. 9-13). Two beams of infrared radiation pass through two parallel cells, one containing gas to be sampled and the other containing a reference gas. The two beams converge on a single infrared detector (Fig. 9-14). Between the test cells and the infrared source, an interrupter (chopper) alternates beams to the cells. If the sample gas and reference gas have the same concentration, the radiation reaching the detector is constant; but when a sample gas with a different concentration is introduced, the amount of radiation reaching the detector varies in

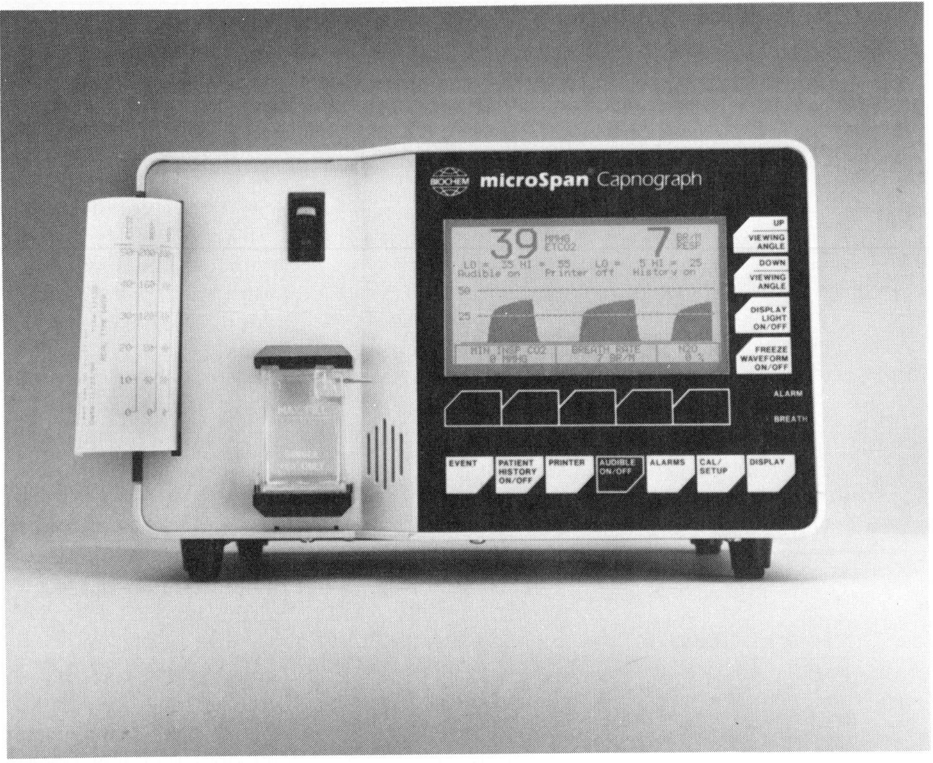

Fig. 9-13 Infrared CO_2 monitor. A microprocessor-controlled infrared CO_2 analyzer, as used for critical care monitoring. A liquid crystal display allows presentation of end-tidal CO_2 values, breathing rate, and CO_2 waveforms. This capnograph includes a printer and alarms, along with a water trap to remove condensation from the sample line. (Courtesy Biochem International Inc., Waukesha, Wis.)

a rhythmic fashion. This causes a vibration in the detector that is translated into a pulsatile signal proportional to the difference between the two beams. Infrared analyzers are readily adaptable to measurements involving small changes in gas concentrations, such as differences between inspired and expired CO in tests of diffusing capacity. Gas can be sampled either continuously or discretely by means of infrared analysis. For continuous sampling, the gas flow rate must be constant and the analyzer must be calibrated at the same flow at which measurements are made. Condensation of water in the sampling circuit can significantly alter the flow rate and affect the accuracy of the measurement. Water vapor in the sample will dilute the gas being analyzed. Water vapor can be removed if speed of response is not critical. If response times are to be kept at a minimum, as during breath-by-breath analysis, the effects of water vapor can be corrected mathematically by assuming that the expired gas is fully saturated.

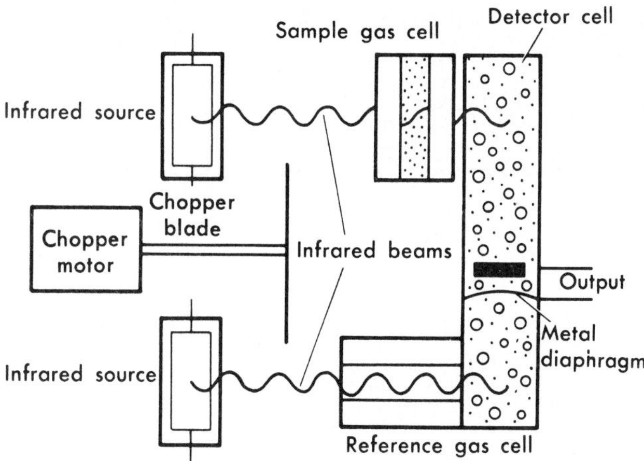

Fig. 9-14 Infrared absorption gas analyzer. Essential components of an infrared gas analyzer, such as is used for determination of CO_2 and CO concentrations. Infrared sources emit beams that pass through parallel cells, one containing a reference gas and the other the sample gas to be analyzed. A rotating blade "chops" the infrared beams in a rhythmic fashion so that when both the reference and sample cells contain the same gas, there is no variation in the radiation reaching either half of the detector cell. When the sample gas is introduced, differing amounts of radiation reach the two halves of the detector cell, causing the diaphragm separating the compartments of the detector to oscillate. This oscillation is transformed into a signal proportional to the difference in gas concentrations. The infrared analyzer is ideal for determination of small concentration changes in gas samples. (From Beckman Instruments, Inc.: Medical gas analyzer LB-2: operating instructions, FM-149997-301, Schiller Park, Ill., 1972.)

Emission spectroscopy. The single-breath and 7-minute N_2 distribution methods, as well as the open-circuit method of determining the FRC (see Chapter 1), require N_2 analysis. A common N_2 analyzer based on the principle of emission spectroscopy is the Giesler tube ionizer (Fig. 9-15). This instrument consists of an enclosed ionization chamber that contains two electrodes and a photocell. A vacuum pump maintains a constant pressure in the ionization chamber by bleeding gas through a needle valve placed in the sample. When a current is supplied to the electrodes, the N_2 between them is ionized and emits light. This light, after being filtered, is collected by a phototube. The intensity of the light is directly related to the concentration of N_2 in the sample, provided that the current, distance between electrodes, and pressure remain constant. The phototube converts the light signal into a DC voltage, which is amplified, linearized, and input to an appropriate meter or computing circuit. The Giesler tube setup allows continuous and rapid analysis of N_2, with response times less than 100 ms. The vacuum pressure must be maintained at a stable level to ensure accuracy and linearity.

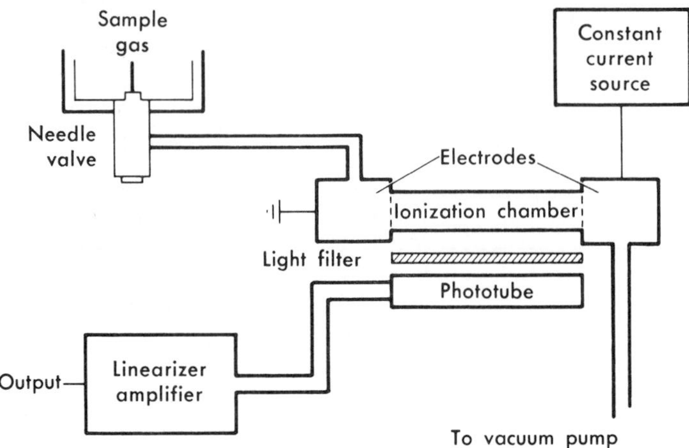

Fig. 9-15 Emission spectroscopy type gas analyzer. The optical emission analyzer (Giesler tube) is commonly used for N_2 analysis. A vacuum pump draws a gas sample into an ionization chamber, where the ionized gas emits light. All light except that from the desired gas is filtered out, and the remaining light is monitored by a phototube. The phototube transmits a signal proportional to the intensity of the light, allowing rapid gas analysis. (From Hewlett-Packard: Application note AN 729, San Diego, 1973.)

Thermal conductivity analyzers. The calculation of FRC by the closed-circuit method and the $DL_{CO}SB$ require He analysis. The thermal conductivity analyzer measures the gas concentrations in the sample by detecting the rate at which different gases conduct heat at varying rates. By placing heated wires or beads in the sample and measuring the change in electrical resistance, the concentration of specific gases can be detected. Two glass-coated thermistor beads serve as sensing elements connected by a Wheatstone bridge circuit (Fig. 9-16). The sensors change temperature, and hence, electrical resistance as a function of the molecular weight of the gases surrounding them. One bead serves as a reference, so that a difference in the concentration of gases at the two sensors can be detected because of the differences in heat conducted away at either of the sensors. Helium analyzers use a reference cell containing no helium. Other gases can be analyzed by means of thermal conductivity as long as other interfering gases are not present. Thermal conductivity analyzers are used in conjunction with gas chromatography (see following paragraph) for this reason. Water vapor and CO_2 are usually scrubbed before analysis when He concentration is being measured. Thermal conductivity analyzers can be used for continuous or discrete measurements, but have a response time of 10 to 20 seconds and cannot be used to detect rapid changes in gas concentration.

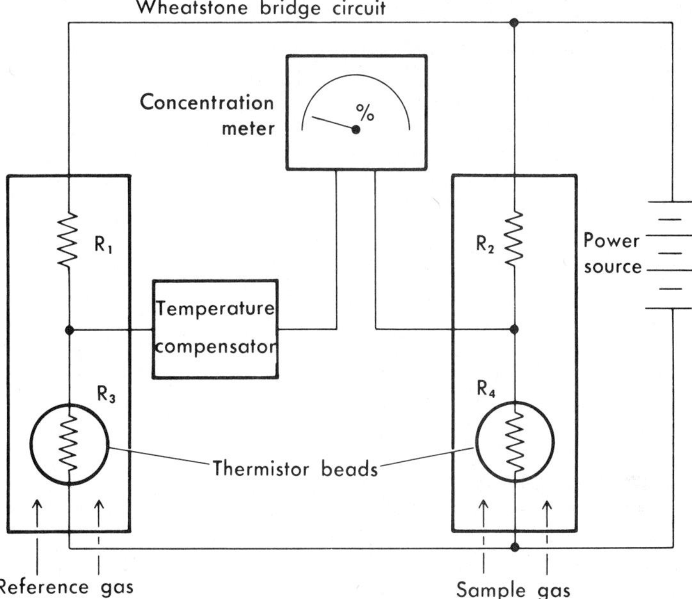

Fig. 9-16 Thermal conductivity analyzer—thermal conductivity gas analyzer such as is used for analysis of He and in conjunction with gas chromatography. Two thermistor beads (i.e., temperature-sensitive electrical resistors) are connected in a Wheatstone bridge circuit. When the thermistors are subjected to the same gas, their electrical resistance decreases equally and the concentration meter registers zero (by calibration). When the sample gas is applied to the sample thermistor (R_4 in this example) and the reference thermistor is submitted to a reference gas, a potential occurs and deflects the concentration meter by a proportional amount. (From Bourns, Inc.: Life systems operations instruction manual, Model LS114-5, Riverside, Calif.)

Gas chromatography. Gas chromatographs combine a means of separating a sample gas into its component gases and a detector, usually the thermal conductivity type described in the previous paragraph. Most chromatographs use the principle of column separation to segregate the component gases of the sample (Fig. 9-17). A column contains material that impedes the movement of gas molecules depending on their size; some columns use materials that combine chemically with certain gases. A combination of columns allows a wide range of gases to be analyzed with a single detector. Helium (He) is used as a "carrier" gas because of its high thermal conductivity. The sample gas with the He carrier is injected into the column. The column allows the component gases to exit at varying rates where they are detected by the thermal conductivity analyzer. The concentrations of various gases can be determined by comparing the output of the thermal conductivity analyzer with a known calibration gas. Since He is

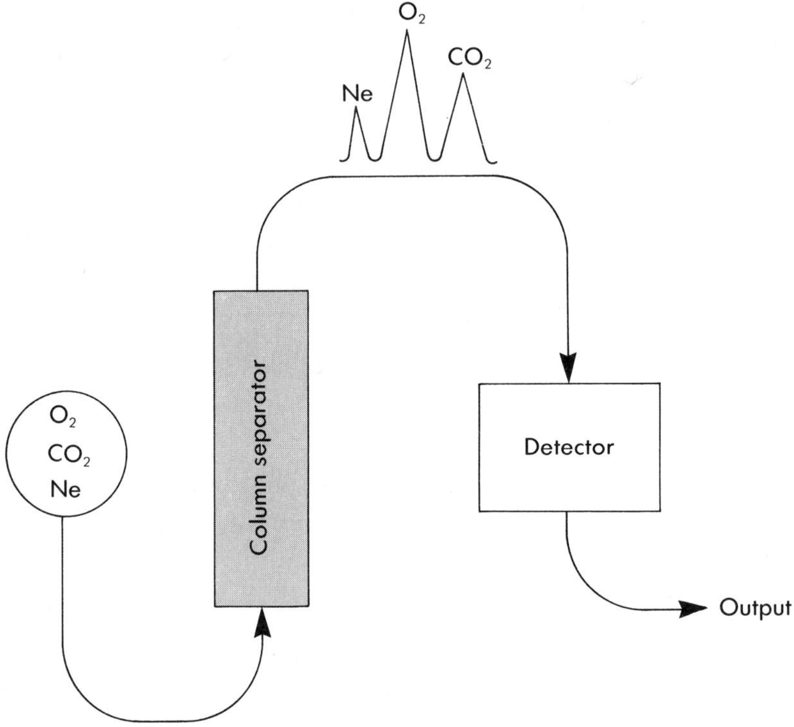

Fig. 9-17 Gas chromatograph. Diagrammatic representation of the components of a gas chromatograph for analysis of respiratory gases. The sample gas moves through a separator column via a carrier gas, usually He. Gases of different molecular sizes pass through the column at different rates and are monitored sequentially by a thermal conductivity type detector. Most gases can be analyzed very accurately by means of appropriate columns.

used as the carrier gas, it cannot be used as an inert indicator for lung volume determinations or diffusing capacity measurements. Neon, which is relatively insoluble, is usually substituted for He. Water vapor and CO_2 are usually scrubbed from the sample to prevent contamination of the separator column. Gas chromatographs are well suited to applications requiring analysis of multiple gases, such as DL_{CO} determinations. Chromatography is very accurate, and it is widely used for analysis of certified reference gases. Gas chromatographs can be used for discrete or continuous measurements, but they require from 15 to 90 seconds for analysis, depending on the gas to be detected.

Mass spectrometry. Perhaps the most sophisticated means of measuring concentrations of respiratory gases is the mass spectrometer. A sample of gas is drawn into a capillary tube by a vacuum pump, which simultaneously reduces the pressure to a preset level. An ionization filament ion-

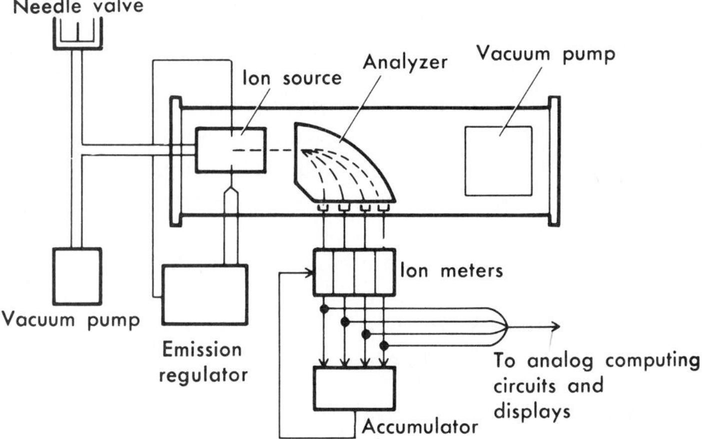

Fig. 9-18 Mass spectrometer. A mass spectrometer in which respiratory gases are analyzed: a vacuum pump draws a small sample of gas into an ionizing chamber, where a current sufficient to ionize the desired gases is supplied; a magnetic analyzer separates the ion beam into constituent gases according to their charge/mass ratio; the separated beams of ions are collected by distinct detectors, and the relative concentration of each gas is determined in comparison to the total output of the detectors. The output signals are usually directed to computing and display circuits. (From Perkin-Elmer Medical Instruments: Advertising brochure for Model 1100, medical gas analyzer, Pomona, Calif.)

izes the sample gases, which are directed into a beam by an electrostatic lens. As the beam passes through a magnetic field, the ions of the various constituent gases separate according to their specific mass and electrical charge (Fig. 9-18). Ion collectors gather the various ions and amplify their charges into a usable signal for monitoring or analog computations. Mass spectrometers have rapid response times (i.e., less than 100 ms) and are capable of detecting multiple gases, making them ideally suited for breath-by-breath measurements. Water vapor does not affect the mass spectrometer itself, but condensation in the sampling circuit can block gas flow or increase the response time. Mass spectrometers are large and require a high degree of maintenance; they are probably better suited to monitoring multiple patients simultaneously rather than being used for a single test. In areas such as exercise testing or anesthesia, where several gases need to be monitored at one time, the mass spectrometer may be the instrument of choice, despite its increased cost and maintenance concerns.

Gas conditioning devices. Interference from water vapor and CO_2 present in expired gas is common to many types of gas analyzers. These two gases are usually removed by chemical "scrubbers." CO_2 may be absorbed by passing the gas through granules containing either barium hydroxide $Ba(OH)_2$ or sodium hydroxide (NaOH). Granules containing NaOH have a light brown appearance that changes to white when saturated with CO_2. The $Ba(OH)_2$ (baralyme) scrubber is usually supplied with an indicator (ethyl violet) that changes from white to purple when saturated with CO_2. NaOH and $Ba(OH)_2$ are mildly corrosive and may generate some heat if exposed to high concentrations of CO_2. Both generate water as a product of combination with CO_2; therefore, they should be placed upstream of the water vapor absorber. Water vapor is commonly absorbed by passing the wet gas over granules of anhydrous calcium sulfate ($CaSO_4$) containing an indicator that changes from blue to pink when exhausted. Failure to adequately scrub water vapor or CO_2 from a gas sample will result in dilution of the remaining gases. Chemical scrubbers should always be used before the manufacturer's expiration date.

BLOOD GAS ELECTRODES, OXIMETERS, AND RELATED DEVICES

Measurements of arterial blood gases routinely include determination of P_{O_2} P_{CO_2}, and pH. Calculation of Sa_{O_2}, HCO_3^-, total CO_2, base excess, and other parameters depend on measurements derived from one or more of the three primary types of electrodes.

Glass pH electrode

The *glass pH electrode* contains a solution of constant pH on one side of the glass membrane. The solution from which pH is to be measured is brought into contact with the other side of the pH-sensitive glass (Fig. 9-19, *A* and *B*). The difference in pH on either side of the glass causes a potential difference, or voltage. To measure this potential, two half-cells are used: one for the constant solution and one for the unknown solution. The constant solution half-cell (i.e., the measuring electrode) is usually a silver-silver chloride wire. The external half-cell that is in contact with the unknown solution is usually a saturated calomel electrode, and is called the reference electrode. These half-cells are connected to a millivolt display that is simply calibrated in pH units. The voltage difference between the two electrodes is proportional to the pH difference of the solutions. Because the pH of one solution is constant, the developed potential is a measure of the pH of the unknown solution. Various means of implementing pH measuring systems are used. The measuring electrode may be constructed as in Fig. 9-19, *B* with the pH-sensitive glass formed into a capillary through which the sample is drawn. Another design features a microelectrode with just the tip exposed to the sample. Electrical contact between the sample and the KCl electrolyte may be formed by a liquid junction or by permeable membrane. Protein contamination of the pH-sensitive glass is a common problem that depends on the number of specimens analyzed. KCl depletion or blockage of the reference junction are also common problems associated with electrode malfunction. Daily, or more often, use of suitable quality control materials can detect these and other problems (see Chapter 11).

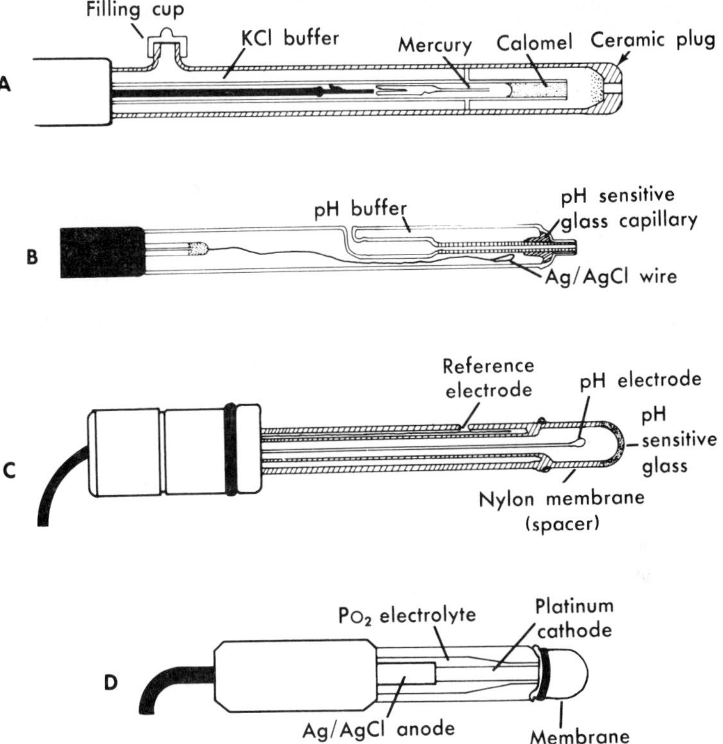

Fig. 9-19 pH, P_{CO_2} and P_{O_2} electrodes. **A**, The reference pH electrode contains a potassium chloride buffer and a porous ceramic plug that allow electrical contact to the exterior; the reference wire develops a constant potential. **B**, The pH-measuring electrode contains a sealed-in buffer and a silver-silver chloride wire. A thin capillary tube, or similar surface, constructed of pH-sensitive glass allows a potential to develop, which varies with the pH of the unknown solution in contact with the glass. The difference between the variable potential and the constant potential of the reference electrode indicates the pH of the sample. **C**, The P_{CO_2} (Severinghaus) electrode is an adaptation of the pH electrode. The pH electrode contains a sealed-in buffer, whereas the reference electrode is the other half-cell and is in communication with a P_{CO_2} electrolyte of aqueous bicarbonate. The entire glass electrode is encased in a Lucite jacket (not shown) containing the electrolyte and capped with a Teflon membrane that is permeable to CO_2. A nylon mesh covers the tip of the internal glass electrode acting as a spacer to keep the electrolyte in contact with the pH-sensitive glass. CO_2 diffuses through the Teflon membrane, is hydrated in the electrolyte, and alters the pH. The pH change is displayed as partial pressure of CO_2. **D**, The P_{O_2} (polarographic) electrode contains a platinum cathode and a silver-silver chloride anode. The electrode is polarized by applying a slightly negative voltage. The tip is protected by a polyethylene or polypropylene membrane, which allows O_2 molecules to diffuse but prevents contamination of the platinum wire. O_2 migrates to the cathode and is reduced by picking up free electrons that have come from the silver-silver chloride anode through the phosphate-potassium chloride buffer. Changes in the current flowing between the anode and cathode result from the amount of O_2 reduced in the electrolyte, and are proportional to partial pressure of O_2.

P_{CO_2} electrode

The *P_{CO_2} electrode* (Severinghaus electrode) measures P_{CO_2} potentiometrically by an adaptation of the pH measurement (Fig. 9-19, *C*). A combined pH glass and reference electrode are placed inside a membrane-tipped plastic jacket that has been filled with a bicarbonate-chloride buffer. The membrane is usually Teflon or a similar material that is permeable to molecules of CO_2. A spacer or wick made of nylon is usually placed between the pH-sensitive glass and the membrane to ensure that bicarbonate electrolyte is in contact with the electrode. When the sample is introduced at the tip of the electrode, CO_2 diffuses across the membrane in proportion to partial pressure until equilibration between the electrolyte and the sample occurs. CO_2 is hydrated in the electrolyte according to the equation:

$$CO_2 + H_2O \Leftrightarrow H_2CO_3 \Leftrightarrow H^+ + HCO_3^-$$

The change in H^+ concentration is proportional to the change in P_{CO_2}. The electrode senses the change in P_{CO_2} as a change in pH of the electrolyte and develops a voltage that is exponentially related to P_{CO_2}, so that a tenfold increase in P_{CO_2} is approximately equal to a decrease of 1 pH unit. By calibrating the pH change when the electrode is exposed to gases with known P_{CO_2} values, partial pressure of CO_2 can be determined. The most common problem with the P_{CO_2} electrode is degradation or contamination of the membrane. Protein or other debris deposited on the membrane slows down the diffusion of CO_2 so that equilibrium may not be achieved during the time the sample is in the measuring chamber. Electrolyte depletion or contamination of the pH-sensitive glass may also occur with extended use. Cleaning and recalibration reduce the variability of repeated measurements.

P_{O_2} electrode

The *P_{O_2} electrode* (Clark electrode) consists of a platinum cathode that is usually a thin wire encased in plastic or glass, together with a silver-silver chloride (Ag-AgCl) anode (Fig. 9-19, *D*). Both the anode and cathode are placed inside a plastic jacket that is tipped with a polypropylene or polyethylene membrane. The membrane is semipermeable and allows diffusion of O_2 molecules. The jacket is filled with phosphate-potassium chloride buffer. A polarizing voltage of -0.7 V is applied to the electrode so that the cathode is slightly negative with respect to the anode, hence the name "polarographic" electrode. O_2 is reduced at the cathode according to the equation:

$$O_2 + 2H_2O + 4e^- \rightarrow 4OH^-$$

Electrons are supplied by the Ag-AgCl anode and flow from the anode to the cathode with a current that is proportional to the number of molecules of O_2 reduced. Each O_2 molecule can take up four electrons, and the greater the number of O_2 molecules present, the greater the current. The membrane causes a diffusion limitation to the number of molecules reaching the electrode. The greater the partial pressure on the sample side of the membrane, the higher the rate of diffusion. The measurement of the current developed within the electrode is therefore proportional to PO_2. As with the PCO_2 electrode, contamination or degradation of the membrane interferes with diffusion of gas and can result in erratic measurements. Most polarographic electrodes use a platinum wire of small diameter to reduce the consumption of O_2 at the tip of the electrode. The exposed surface of the platinum cathode gradually becomes plated with metal ions and must be periodically polished to maintain its sensitivity. Because the membrane causes a diffusion limit to O_2 molecules reaching the cathode, the electrode performs differently when exposed to liquid versus gas samples. Some blood gas systems use gas to calibrate the PO_2 electrode, and noticeable differences may result when the electrode is then used to analyze the tension of O_2 dissolved in a liquid. These differences are usually compensated by correcting the PO_2 by an empirically determined gas-liquid factor (see Chapter 11).

Although the gas measuring (i.e., PO_2 and PCO_2) electrodes and the pH electrode system can each be used separately, all three are usually implemented together in a blood gas analyzer (Fig. 9-20, *A*). Most blood gas analyzers feature some degree of microprocessor control. Such tasks as sample aspiration, rinsing, and calibration can all be done automatically

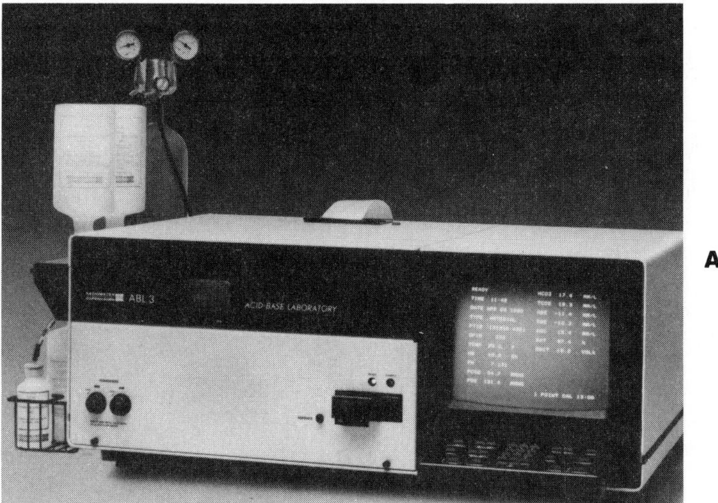

Fig. 9-20 **A**, Automated blood gas analyzer, including automatic flushing and calibration, tonometering of calibrating solutions, and on-line display of results and calibrations using a built-in computer and video display terminal; pH, PCO_2, PO_2 and Hb are measured; HCO_3^-, total CO_2, standard bicarbonate, base excess, and saturation are calculated. (Courtesy Radiometer America, Westlake, Ohio.)

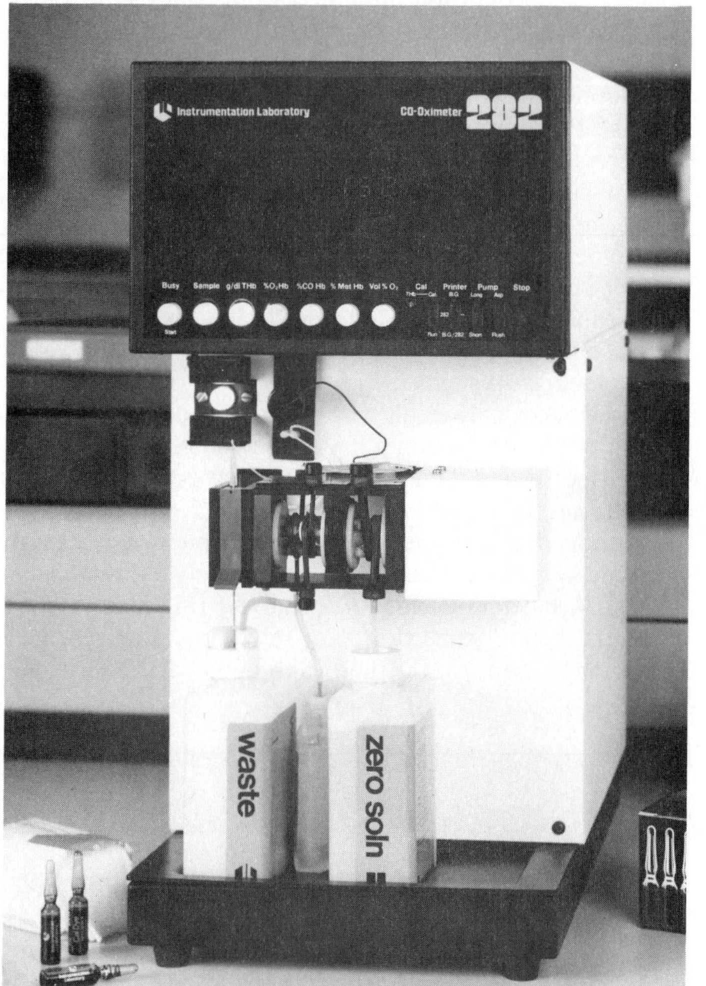

Fig. 9-20 **B**, Automated spectrophotometric oximeter (co-oximeter); a small sample (approximately 0.2 ml) of blood is aspirated, hemolyzed, mixed with diluent, and held in a cuvette while spectrophotometric measurements are made to determine Sa_{O_2}, Vol% O_2, COHb, MetHb, and Total Hb. Flushing and zeroing of the spectrophotometer are performed after each sample. (Courtesy Instrumentation Laboratories, Lexington, Mass.)

under program control. The microprocessor can calculate a wide variety of parameters based on pH, P_{CO_2}, and P_{O_2}, as well as from data input from other instruments. In addition, computerized analyzers can evaluate automated calibrations and track electrode performance to alert the technologist of existing or impending problems.

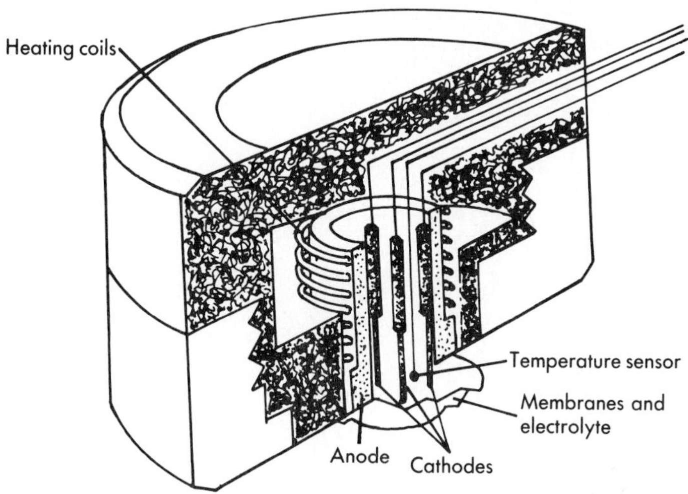

Fig. 9-21 Transcutaneous Po_2 electrode. A cross-sectional diagram of the components of the $tcPo_2$ electrode shows a circular anode around a series of cathodes and a temperature sensor. A heating coil causes local hyperemia so that surface Po_2 more closely resembles Pa_{O_2}. A double membrane separates the electrode proper from the skin.

Transcutaneous Po_2 electrode

The *trancutaneous Po_2 electrode* ($tcPo_2$) operates on a principle similar to that of the polarographic (Clark) electrode. The $tcPo_2$ electrode consists of a ring-shaped silver anode that is heated by a coil to cause hyperemia at the skin placement site. Inside the circular anode is a series of thin platinum cathodes (Fig. 9-21). All of the elements are enclosed in a plastic case, except for the face of the sensor, which is covered by a Teflon membrane. A KCl electrolyte is placed between the membrane and the sensor, then another drop of electrolyte and a cellophane membrane are added to form a double membrane. The flow of current between the silver and platinum electrodes is proportional to the partial pressure of O_2 diffusing through the skin and membrane. A feedback mechanism keeps the temperature constant at the skin site to compensate for changes caused by capillary blood flow, thus stabilizing the measurement. $tcPo_2$ and Pa_{O_2} are not identical, but the gradient between them tends to be relatively constant, so that $tcPo_2$ can be a valuable measurement once the gradient has been established. Conditions that affect perfusion of the skin may alter the gradient between arterial and transcutaneous Po_2 (see Chapters 6 and 8). The transcutaneous Pco_2 electrode ($tcPco_2$) consists of a Severinghaus-type electrode that is mounted in a manner similar to the $tcPo_2$ device. Combination transcutaneous CO_2 and O_2 electrodes are available.

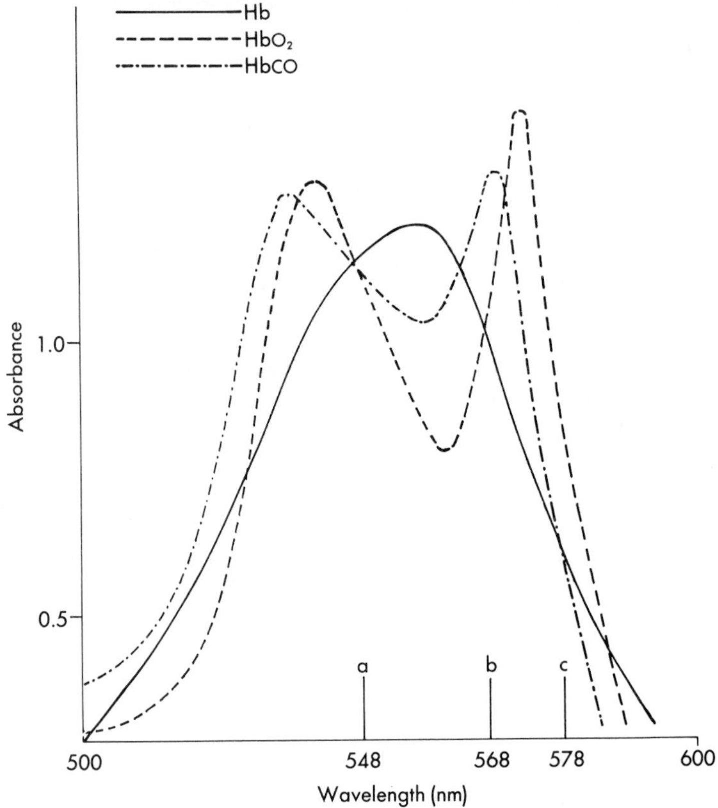

Fig. 9-22 Principle of spectrophotometric oximetry. Absorbance measurements are made at three or more distinct wavelengths (548, 568, 578 nm in this example) as light passes through a blood sample. At 548 nm, all three forms of Hb (Hb, O_2Hb and COHb) have identical absorbances. At 568 nm, only Hb and O_2Hb coincide, whereas at 578 nm, Hb and COHb coincide. The solution of three simultaneous equations provides the relative proportions of each species, as well as the total Hb.

Spectrophotometric oximeter

The *spectrophotometric oximeter* (Fig. 9-20, *B*) uses the principle of light absorption to analyze the saturation of Hb with O_2. In addition, the concentration of carboxyhemoglobin (COHb)—the Hb bound with CO—or other forms of Hb (i.e., methemoglobin and sulfhemoglobin) can be determined; this type of spectrophotometer is sometimes referred to as a co-oximeter. The blood oximeter analyzes the absorption of light at multiple wavelengths; at each wavelength, two or more of the species of Hb have similar absorbances (Fig. 9-22). These common points are termed isobestic points. A wavelength that is isosbestic for oxyhemoglobin (O_2Hb), reduced Hb (RHb), and COHb is 548 nanometers (nm). At this particular wavelength, the absorbance of a mixture of the three pigments is directly proportional to the total concentration of Hb. An isosbestic point for O_2Hb and RHb is 568 nm. The absorbance of COHb at this point is considerably higher; thus, a change in absorbance at 568 nm compared to 548 nm indicates a change in the concentration of COHb relative to the sum of the concentrations of the other two species. 578 nm is the isosbestic point for RHb and COHb, with O_2Hb absorbance being considerably greater. The degree of difference indicates a change in the concentration of O_2Hb relative to the other two pigments. By analyzing the values for absorbance and solving simultaneous equations, the total Hb concentration, O_2Hb, COHb, and MetHb saturation can be determined.

The spectrophotometric oximeter provides essential information regarding the O_2-Hb reaction, particularly in instances when increased concentrations of COHb, MetHb, or other abnormal species of Hb are present. Most automated blood gas analyzers calculate the saturation of Hb using the measured Pa_{O_2} and pH, at normal body temperature (37° C) and assuming that the Hb has a normal P_{50}. Normal adult Hb is 50% saturated at a Po_2 of 26 to 27 mm Hg. These approximations may significantly overestimate the true saturation in the presence of COHb or abnormal hemoglobins, such as methemoglobin. The oximeter provides a more accurate estimate of the actual O_2 saturation of the blood, but may give spuriously low Hb, O_2Hb, and COHb readings if significant amounts of other pigments, such as methemoglobin, are present. Other substances that cause light scattering in the blood specimen, such as lipids resulting from lipid therapy, may also cause false readings. To function properly, the blood oximeter has to hemolyze the sample so that the hemoglobin molecules are evenly suspended in the solution rather than contained within the red cells. Hemolysis is normally accomplished by chemical or mechanical disruption of the red cell membranes. Incomplete hemolysis results in light scattering within the sample rather than in simple absorption. Sickle cells are not easily disrupted, particularly by chemical lysis, and may result in false readings for O_2Hb and COHb.

Some newer co-oximeters feature microprocessor control that allows specific errors such as incomplete hemolysis or abnormal light scattering to be detected and reported. Microprocessor-controlled oximeters also provide corrections so that specific varieties of Hb, such as fetal or animal Hb, can be analyzed. In addition to measurements of O_2Hb, COHb, and MetHb saturations, the blood oximeter can be used to calculate O_2 content and to estimate the P_{50} of the blood. By measuring the actual saturation of a sample of blood (the saturation should be less than 90%) and comparing this value to the calculated saturation, based on the Po_2 and pH of the same blood, a left or right shift of the O_2Hb curve can be determined and the P_{50} can be estimated. This simplified method compares favorably with the classical approach of tonometering the blood sample with a gas of low O_2 concentration and constructing a dissociation curve.

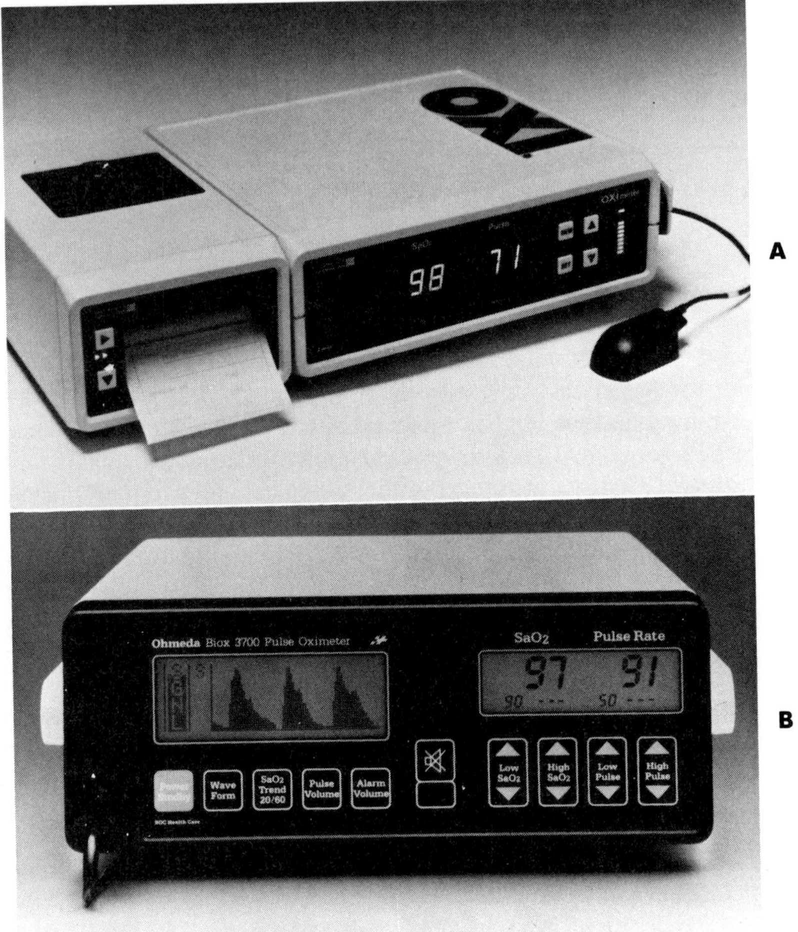

Fig. 9-23 Pulse oximeters. Two representative microprocessor-controlled pulse oximeters. Each provides a digital display of oxygen saturation measured by two-wavelength oximetry along with pulse rate. **A**, Included with this pulse oximeter is a strip chart recorder useful for recording saturation and pulse rate trends. (Courtesy of Radiometer America, Westlake, Ohio.) **B**, A liquid crystal display included with this oximeter allows the operator to visualize the pulse waveform and to monitor signal quality, both of which may be helpful in detecting conditions that interfere with accurate saturation determinations. (Courtesy of Ohmeda, Louisville, Colo.)

Pulse oximeters. *Pulse oximeters* (Fig. 9-23, *A* and *B*) are the most recent development in the effort to assess oxygenation noninvasively. The pulse oximeter's immediate predecessor was a fiberoptic oximeter that passed multiple wavelengths of light through the pinna of the ear and measured the absorption to derive oxygen saturation of Hb. The pulse oximeter treats Hb as a filter that allows only light in the red and near-infrared regions to pass. Beer's law relates the total absorption in a system of absorbers to the sum of their individual absorptions:

$$A_{total} = E_1C_1L_1 + E_2C_2L_2 + \ldots E_nC_nL_n$$

where

A_{total} = The absorbance of a mixture of substances at a specific wavelength
E_n = The extinction of substance *n*
C_n = The concentration of substance *n*
L_n = The length of the light path through substance *n*

In principle, the pulse oximeter measures the absorption of a mixture of two substances, O_2Hb and reduced Hb (RHb); the concentration of either can be determined if their extinction is measured while the path length stays constant.

The wavelengths of light used in pulse oximetry are around 660 nm in the red region of the spectrum and approximately 940 nm in the near-infrared portion. The extinction curves for O_2Hb and RHb show that reduced Hb has an absorption 10 times higher than oxyhemoglobin at 660 nm, while O_2Hb has a higher absorbance (2 to 3 times) at 940 nm. By calculating all of the possible combinations of the two forms of Hb (i.e., varying the saturation from 0% to 100%), the ratio of absorbances at the two wavelengths can be determined, resulting in a calibration curve. The capillary bed does not follow the optical principles exactly as described by Beer's law, so the calibration curve is derived empirically. The ratio of absorbances at the two distinct wavelengths is expressed:

$$R = A_{660\ nm}/A_{940\ nm}$$

A series of R values (i.e., the calibration curve) is determined by relating the ratio to actual saturation measurements. Unlike the spectrophotometric oximeter, which measures absorption in a hemolyzed blood sample, the pulse oximeter measures light passing through living tissue. The transmitted light is not only absorbed but it is also refracted and scattered, so that the absolute accuracy of the pulse oximeter tends to be less than the accuracy of the blood oximeter.

The transmitted light output at each wavelength consists of two components, the *AC and DC components* (Fig. 9-24). The AC component varies with the pulsation of blood. The DC component is much larger than the AC component and is a constant output level; it represents the light passing through the tissue without being absorbed or scattered. The ampli-

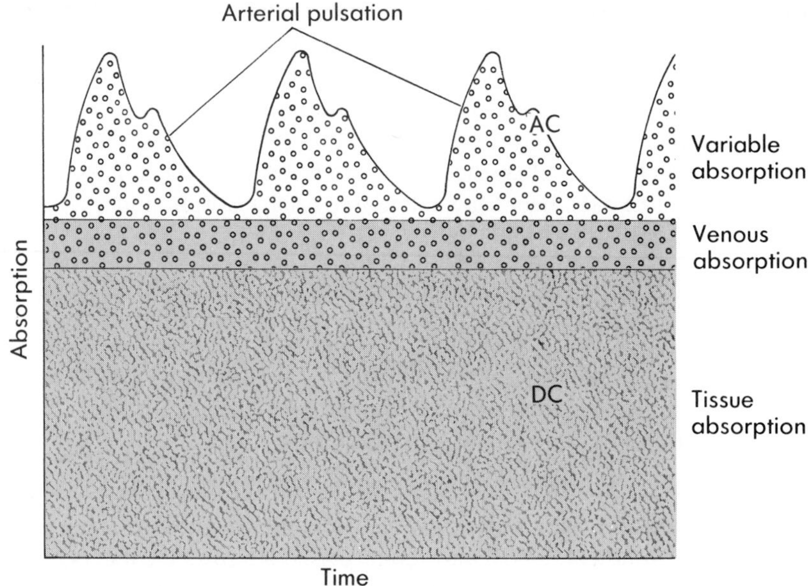

Fig. 9-24 AC and DC components in pulse oximetry. The transmitted light at each of two wavelengths (usually 660 nm and 940 nm) consists of two parts. A larged fixed component, the DC component, represents the light passing through the tissue and venous blood without being absorbed. A second smaller portion is pulsatile in nature and represents the changing absorption as blood pulses through the arterioles; this is represented as the AC component. The pulse oximeter divides the AC signal by the DC signal at each wavelength, effectively cancelling the DC component. The ratio of the AC signals at the two wavelengths is then a function of relative absorptions of O_2Hb and RHb.

tude of both the AC and DC levels depends on the intensity of the incident light. The AC component represents the arterial blood, because it is the arterioles that pulsate in the light path. By dividing the AC level by the DC level at each of the two wavelengths, the AC component is effectively corrected and becomes a function of the extinction of O_2Hb and RHb. The ratio described above then becomes:

$$R = (AC_1/DC_1) / (AC_2/DC_2)$$

where

1 = The red wavelength (660 nm)
2 = The near-infrared wavelength (940 nm)

Correcting the pulsatile component (AC) in this manner allows the pulse oximeter to "ignore" the absorbances caused by venous blood, tissue, and skin pigmentation.

The light source used in the pulse oximeter is the light emitting diode (LED). LEDs are capable of emitting a very bright light near the 660-nm and 940-nm wavelengths required for analysis of Hb saturation. The intensity of light is easily controlled by a feedback circuit that regulates the driving current to the diode. The greater the DC component resulting from pigmentation or venous blood, the greater the current supplied to the LED. A significant drawback to the use of LEDs is that the exact wavelength of light emitted varies with each LED. Each LED has its own "center" wavelength that may differ from 660 or 940 nm by as much as 15 nm. To circumvent this variation, each oximeter must have a series of calibration curves programmed into it, so that it can accommodate different sensors. Because the extinction curves for RHb and O_2Hb are steep and quite different at 660 nm, 10 or more calibration curves are typically required for the red light range. Slight variations in center wavelength are less critical in the 940 nm region, because the extinction characteristics of O_2Hb and RHb are the same from 800 to 1000 nm. A silicon photodiode is the detector for the transmitted light in the pulse oximeter. A single photodiode senses both the red and near-infrared light. The microprocessor that controls the oximeter cycles the LEDs on and off separately 400 to 500 times per second. The oximeter also turns both LEDs off during each cycle so that the photodiode can detect ambient light caused by scattering and can offset the LED signals. By having a short interval when both LEDs are off, the oximeter can measure ambient light levels and subtract them from the levels obtained when the LEDs are on.

Pulse oximeter accuracy tends to decrease at low saturations. Low saturations occur when the concentration of reduced hemoglobin (RHb) increases; because RHb has a much higher absorbance at 660 nm than does O_2Hb, slight variations in the center wavelength of the red LED (as described above) exaggerate the error in measured saturation. This is one reason pulse oximeters exhibit decreasing accuracy at lower saturations.

Because the AC, or pulsatile, component is usually much smaller than the DC component, detecting it can sometimes be problematic. Very low perfusion or poor vascularity can cause the oximeter to be unable to measure the pulsatile component. The oximeter's microprocessor is usually programmed to display a warning message if the photodetector senses inadequate light levels. Motion artifact can also cause inaccuracy with most pulse oximeters. Motion artifact often occurs in the same physiologic frequency range as the signal to be detected (i.e., arterial pulsations). If the motion is consistent and lasts long enough, it introduces a signal of approximately the same amplitude into both the red and infrared channels. The pulse oximeter senses the motion artifact as part of the DC component. This adds a large value to both the numerator and the denominator of the equation for R and forces R toward a value of 1, which equates to a saturation of 85% on the typical oximeter calibration curve.

Most pulse oximeters use the AC signal from one channel, either 660 or 940 nm, to calculate the pulse rate; an algorithm implemented by the microprocessor locates the peaks in the waveform of the AC signal. Some oximeters use this signal to display graphic representations of the pulse waveform. Pulse detection can be enhanced by the addition of a single ECG lead, and the additional input may be necessary to allow the microprocessor to distinguish motion artifact or noise from the true signal.

Reflective spectrophotometers. A specially designed pulmonary artery (Swan-Ganz) catheter that contains fiberoptic bundles makes it possible to continuously monitor mixed venous oxygen saturation ($S\bar{v}_{O_2}$). The catheter has the regular pressure-sensing channels (proximal and distal), a balloon tip for flotation through the right side of the heart, and a thermistor for thermodilution cardiac output determinations. In addition, it contains two fiberoptic bundles (Fig. 9-25). The catheter uses principles similar to both the co-oximeter and the pulse oximeter. The instrument operates on the principle of reflective spectrophotometry, based on the variable reflection of light by O_2Hb and RHb at different wavelengths. Just as the light absorbed by oxygenated and reduced Hb is a function of wavelength, so is the intensity of reflected or back-scattered light. Carefully spaced monofilament optical fibers are used as transmitting and receiving paths for light. Three LEDs, similar to those used in pulse oximeters, illuminate blood flowing past the tip of the catheter via one of the optical fibers. A photodetector receives the reflected light and converts its intensity into a signal. A microprocessor processes the data from the photodetector and calculates two independent ratios of reflected light intensities from the three wave-

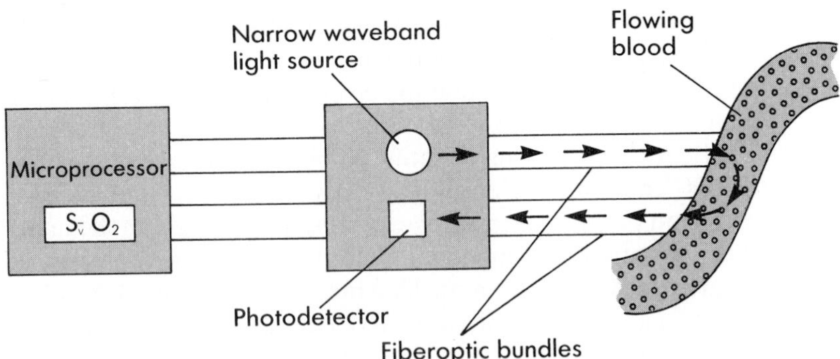

Fig. 9-25 Principle of reflection spectrophotometry. A diagrammatic representation of the components of the optical pulmonary artery catheter used for continuous monitoring of $S\bar{v}_{O_2}$. LEDs provide a narrow waveband light source that is transmitted along one fiberoptic filament to blood flowing past the tip of the catheter. Light reflected from the blood is transmitted back to a photodiode by the second fiberoptic bundle. The light intensity signals are then evaluated by a microprocessor to calculate light intensity ratios (usually two ratios are determined from three wavelengths), which are used to determine the $S\bar{v}_{O_2}$.

lengths. Combining two reflected light intensity ratios reduces the instrument's sensitivity to physiologic phenomena such as pulsatile blood flow or hematocrit, as well as to changes due to light scattering from red cell surfaces and the walls of the blood vessel. The $S\bar{v}_{O_2}$ is calculated from the light ratios using programmed calibration curves, as for the pulse oximeter. As in the pulse oximeter, the saturation measured is the saturation of *functional* Hb (see Chapter 6). The $S\bar{v}_{O_2}$ value derived by this method will be higher than that measured by a co-oximeter, notably in the presence of large amounts of COHb or MetHb. The $S\bar{v}_{O_2}$ is then displayed and charted using a trend recorder (Fig. 9-26). The microprocessor also monitors the absolute intensity levels of the reflected light to allow detection of changes in catheter position or the integrity of the fiberoptics.

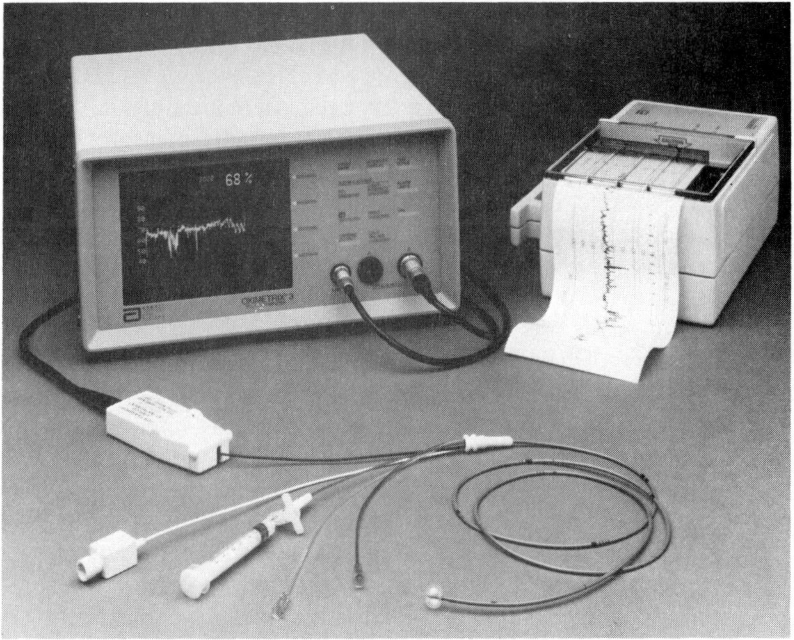

Fig. 9-26 Reflection spectrophotometer and pulmonary artery catheter. A microprocessor-controlled reflection spectrophotometer. The pulmonary artery catheter contains fiberoptic bundles for continuous measurement of the $S\bar{v}_{O_2}$, as well as the usual pressure measuring ports and thermistor for thermodilution cardiac output. The instrument displays mixed venous saturation digitally and by means of a trend graph that can, optionally, be printed. High and low saturation alarms are included along with a "light intensity" alarm to detect artifacts caused by catheter motion or problems with the fiberoptics. (Reprinted with permission from Abbott Laboratories Critical Care Systems, Mountain View, Calif.)

The reflective spectrophotometer has several advantages for monitoring patients in a critical care setting. The $S\bar{v}_{O_2}$ is measured continuously rather than discretely, as occurs when mixed venous samples are withdrawn for routine analysis. Continuous indwelling monitoring allows trending and the use of high and low alarms to detect large changes in mixed venous oxygen saturation. All of the other indices normally available from the pulmonary artery catheter (i.e., pulmonary artery pressures, pulmonary capillary wedge pressures, mixed venous blood samples, and thermodilution cardiac output) can be measured while $S\bar{v}_{O_2}$ is being monitored. A change in mixed venous oxygen saturation, either an increase or a decrease, can result from multiple causes (see Critical Care Monitoring, Chapter 8). The reflective spectrophotometer must be routinely calibrated to ensure that observed changes in $S\bar{v}_{O_2}$ are the result of physiologic phenomena rather than instrument drift. The catheter is usually standardized by calibrating it against an absolute color reference before insertion. After the catheter is in place, calibration is accomplished by comparing the displayed saturation with saturation measured by a co-oximeter and adjusting the output of the indwelling device. This type of calibration is accurate when it is performed but may change if there are shifts in the pH or hematocrit. Because the reflective spectrophotometer measures reflected light in whole blood that is flowing rather than transmitted light in a hemolyzed blood sample, its absolute accuracy tends to be less than that of the co-oximeter. Direct comparison of saturations by the two methods requires correction for COHb and MetHb as measured by the co-oximeter.

BODY PLETHYSMOGRAPHS

Two types of body plethysmographs are in common clinical use: the constant-volume, variable-pressure plethysmograph; and the flow, variable-volume plethysmograph. These are commonly referred to as the pressure and flow plethysmographs, respectively. Both designs are employed for the measurement of VTG (see Chapter 1) and Raw and its derivatives (see Chapter 3).

The pressure plethysmograph is based on the principle that volume changes in a closed container can be determined from measured pressure changes as long as the temperature is constant. A sensitive pressure transducer monitors box pressure changes that are related to volume changes by calibration (see Chapter 11 for calibration techniques). Pressure fluctuations result from the compression and decompression of gas within both the subject's thorax and the box, as well as from thermal changes. The pressure plethysmograph must be relatively free from leaks. A valving mechanism allows the technologist to vent the pressure plethysmograph so that thermal equilibrium can be maintained. By making VTG and Raw measurements at rapid rates (panting), pressure changes caused by thermal drift, leaks, or background noise are minimized. Some plethysmograph systems use a "slow" leak to facilitate thermal equilibrium. This may be accomplished by connecting a long length of small-bore tubing to the box or by connecting the atmospheric side of the box pressure transducer to a glass bottle within the box. Both methods reduce the effect of temperature changes within the box while maintaining good frequency response. Pressure plethysmographs are best suited to maneuvers that measure small volume changes (i.e., 100 ml or less).

The flow plethysmograph employs a flow transducer in the box wall to measure volume changes in the box. Gas in the box is compressed or decompressed and the pressure change is measured as gas flows out of the box through the flow opening. Flow through the wall is integrated, corrections are applied, and the volume change is recorded as the sum of the volume passing through the wall and the volume compressed. In one implementation, the subject breathes through a pneumotachometer that is connected to the room (i.e., transmural breathing). The transmural pneumotachometer allows larger gas volumes (i.e., VC and MEFV curves) to be measured while the subject is enclosed in the plethysmograph. The transmural flow is redirected to the plethysmograph for airway resistance measurements, so that the ratio of flow to box volume can be plotted. For V_{TG} measurements, the flow transducer in the plethysmograph wall is blocked so that the device works as a pressure box. The flow-type plethysmograph requires computerization so that the pressure, volume, and flow signals can be measured in phase. Although thermal changes must be accounted for, the flow plethysmograph does not need to be rigorously airtight.

In each type of plethysmograph (Fig. 9-27), a pneumotachometer is necessary for measuring air flow at the mouth for the Raw maneuver. The flow signal is also used to determine the end-expiratory point for shutter closure in the V_{TG} measurement. The pneumotachometer must be linear across the range of flows typically measured (0 to 2 L/sec) for both spontaneous breathing and panting. Heated Fleisch- or Silverman-types of pneumotachometers (i.e., pressure differential) are usually implemented in the plethysmograph. A mouth pressure transducer is normally coupled to an electronic shutter mechanism. The transducer records mouth pressures, usually in the range of 0 to 20 cm H_2O, when the airway is occluded. Some systems require the technologist to close the shutter by remote control at end-expiration. This is accomplished by observing the tidal breathing maneuver on an oscilloscope and actuating the shutter at end-expiration. Microprocessor-controlled systems allow the shutter to be closed automatically at a preselected point in the breathing cycle. The technologist initiates a sequence in which the computer analyzes the flow signal and closes the shutter when expiratory flow becomes zero.

Recording of the breathing maneuvers may be accomplished by one of several techniques. Some plethysmograph systems use a storage oscilloscope to record the breathing maneuvers. The scope may be erased as often as necessary to obtain acceptable maneuvers. The tracings may then be photographed or transferred to a plotter or X-Y recorder. On computerized

A

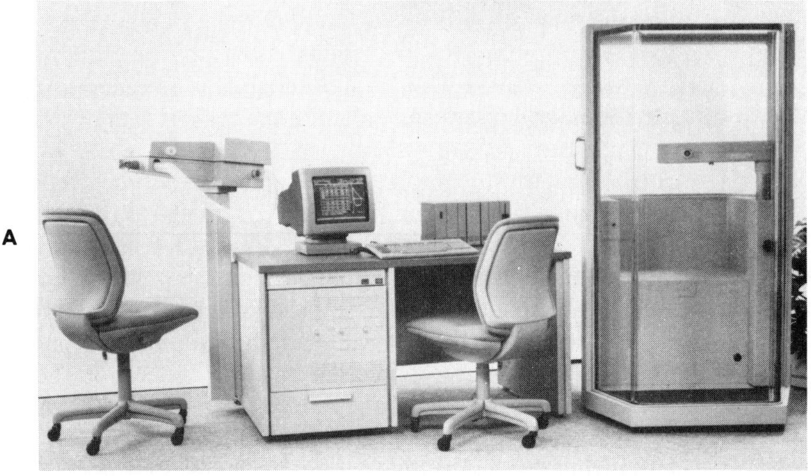

B

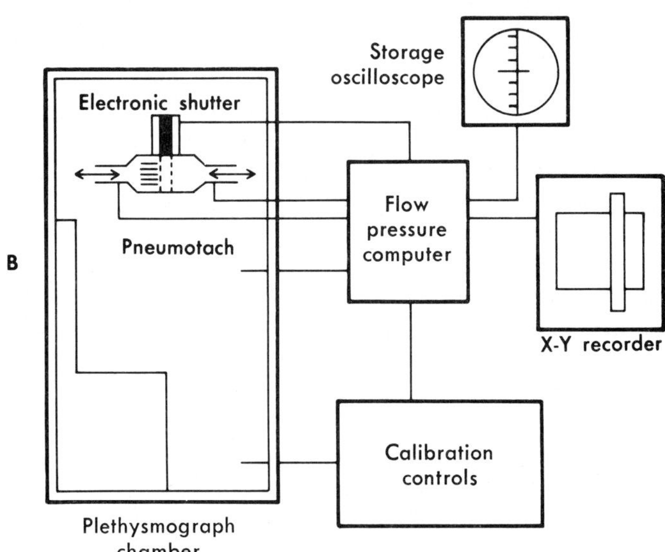

Fig. 9-27 Body plethysmograph. **A**, Modern plethysmograph setup, with a highly transparent box, self-contained calibration equipment, and computerized data reduction and display. (Courtesy Medical Graphics Corporation, St. Paul.) **B**, Diagram of plethysmograph components: pneumotachometer with automatic shutter mechanism; body plethysmograph cabinet; interface/computer for reduction of pressure, flow, and volume signals; storage oscilloscope and X-Y recorder; and calibration instruments with controls.

systems, the breathing maneuvers may be stored in memory, analyzed, then displayed on the video screen. Measurement of tangents or angles from the standard oscilloscope is usually performed by rotating a graticule to align its axes with those of the loop, and then reading the appropriate value. Most computerized systems allow the technologist to select a "best-fit" line drawn by the computer, or to manipulate the tangent via the computer keyboard. Computerized plethysmographs offer the advantage of providing lung volume and airway resistance information immediately upon completion of the maneuver. This aids the technologist in selecting appropriate maneuvers for averaging, as well as in repeating the test as required when spurious values are obtained. Comparison of lung volumes by alternate methods (He dilution or N_2 washout) to plethysmographically determined volumes is easily accomplished with computer-stored data. Computerization also allows panting frequency to be calculated and displayed; measurement made at low frequencies (1 Hz or less) may be more reliable if the subject's breathing is severely obstructed.

Most plethysmographs include the necessary hardware to perform physical calibration (see Chapter 11). These typically include a pressure manometer or U-tube for calibration of the mouth pressure transducer, a flow source and rotameter for pneumotachometer calibration, and a volume-displacement device such as a 30 to 50 ml reciprocating pump for box pressure (flow) calibration. Computerized plethysmograph systems allow automated calibration of transducers using software-generated correction factors, as well as actual physical calibration. A few manufacturers supply quality control devices, such as the isothermal lung analog (see Chapter 11).

The ease with which the subject can enter the plethysmograph and perform the required maneuvers is an important feature of the plethysmograph. Some subjects may experience claustrophobia once inside the plethysmograph. Older boxes relied on solid materials (i.e., plywood) to provide the necessary rigidity for the cabinet so that pressure changes were not damped. Boxes made of durable plastics are largely transparent and less confining for the subject (Fig. 9-27, *A*) while maintaining the necessary rigidity. Equally important is a communication system that allows both voice and visual contact with the subject. Panting against a closed shutter may be difficult for some individuals, and continuous coaching is often necessary to elicit valid maneuvers.

RESPIRATORY INDUCTIVE PLETHYSMOGRAPHS

A noninvasive technique allowing measurement of pulmonary function is based on the principle of inductive plethysmography. The respiratory inductive plethysmograph (RIP) consists of two or more Teflon-insulated coils of wire sewn into elastic bands that are connected to oscillator circuits (Fig. 9-28). The elastic bands are then positioned around the chest and abdomen. Breathing excursions stretch the bands, causing a change in the

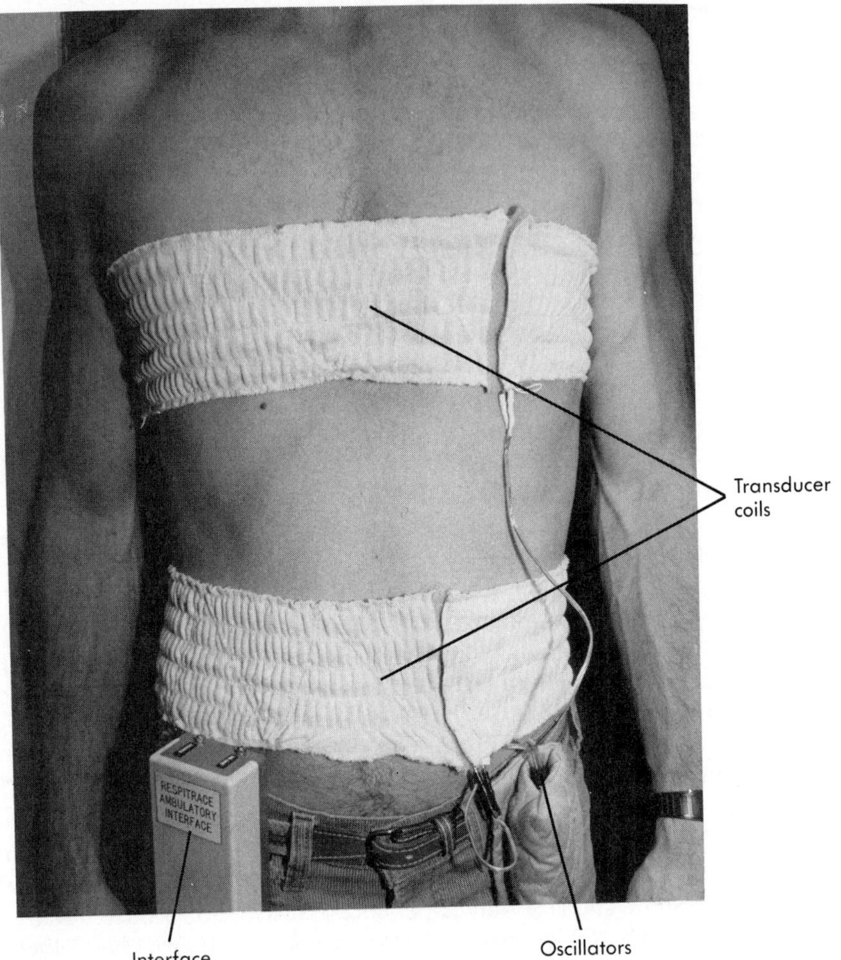

Fig. 9-28 Respiratory inductive plethysmograph (RIP). A typical application of the respiratory inductive plethysmograph—two elastic bands with Teflon-coated coils sewn in are placed around the rib cage and abdomen; oscillators connected to the coils (shown hanging from the belt) monitor changes in the cross-sectional areas of the two compartments as changes in inductance. By calibration, the changes in cross-sectional areas can be converted to volume changes in the two compartments to record V_T, rate, and timing of inspiration and expiration.

inductance in the oscillator circuits. The distension of the coils within the elastic bands is proportional to the change in the cross-sectional areas of the rib cage and abdomen, respectively. Measurement of volumes (i.e., V_T) are accomplished by summing the signals from the two compartments. The validity of this technique is based on the assumption that lung volume change is described with two degrees of freedom—change in thoracic volume plus change in abdominal volume.

The RIP must be calibrated so that changes in rib cage and abdomen cross-sectional areas may be translated into volumes. This is usually accomplished by measuring the relative contribution of the inductances of the two coils as the actual volume change is recorded by means of a spirometer or pneumotachometer. If volumes are measured with two different breathing patterns, a "best fit" line can be generated, which is used to derive calibration factors for each of the transducers. This may be expressed:

$$\frac{RC}{SP} + \frac{AB}{SP} = 1$$

where:

RC = The rib cage contribution to the tidal volume
AB = The abdominal contribution to the tidal volume
SP = The volume as measured by spirometry

The calibration "factors" thus obtained are applied to the output of the two channels as gains, and the RIP may be used to measure V_T, respiratory rate, timing of inspiration (T_I), timing of expiration (T_E), and total respiratory cycle time (T_{total}). Various indices relating the extent of paradoxical and asynchronous movement of the two compartments may also be quantified.

Because calibration is crucial to accurate measurement of volume change, a microprocessor or small dedicated computer is often used to derive calibration factors once the transducer bands have been placed. The computer may also be used to store and process data derived from the plethysmograph and to display graphic representations of the breathing pattern. Changes in body position may affect the calibration factors, so it is important to be able to quickly calibrate the inductive plethysmograph. Once calibration is complete, volume changes can be determined without physical connection to the subject's airway, as is the case with standard methods of assessing ventilation. Respiratory inductive plethysmography is ideally suited to the study of breathing patterns in a variety of disorders, as well as in those subjects in whom connection of a spirometer to the airway is impractical, such as infants and ventilated patients.

RECORDERS AND RELATED DEVICES

An integral part of pulmonary function testing is the recording of volume-time and flow-volume curves, distribution and ventilation tests, lung volumes, and DL_{CO} maneuvers. Many agencies recommend, and some require, inclusion of spirograms as part of the subject's medical record. The American Thoracic Society has published specific guidelines for the presentation of spirometric waveforms according to the test category (see Chapter 11). Graphic representations of measured parameters, such as the MEFV curve, are useful means of displaying a large amount of information in a succinct manner. Quality control of some instrument functions requires recording of analog signals. For example, to check the accuracy of a computerized method of measuring the $FEV_{1.0}$, the volume signal may be recorded using a device for which timing accuracy is known and comparing the manual method with the software-derived value.

The kymograph, a rotating drum carrying chart paper, has been used for recording various respiratory movements (see Fig. 9-1). A kymograph is a mechanical recorder in the strictest sense, because the physical displacement of the bell or bellows is translated into an equivalent movement of the pen as the paper moves beneath it. The accuracy of the kymograph for timed measurements depends almost entirely on the accuracy of the drive motor, which is easily verified. Normally, corrections for BTPS must be made because volume changes in the bell or bellows represent ATPS values. Some systems use calibrated chart paper to allow BTPS values to be read directly from the graph. These systems assume that the subject is at 37° C and the spirometer is at 25° C, which may not always be true. Several commonly used spirometers incorporate the kymograph recording systems.

A second type of device that uses mechanical recording has a constant speed motor to provide paper movement along the time axis (*X*), while the spirometer provides the volume (*Y*) input. This principle is used in many bellows-type spirometers and in some rolling-seal spirometers. For both kymographs and simple chart recorders, the accuracy of the timing motor driving the graph paper is essential for valid measurements of flow. The paper speed should be at least 1 cm/sec for diagnostic purposes; speeds of 2 to 3 cm/sec are preferable if timed volumes are to be manually calculated. The volume axis of the graph should have a scale of at least 5 mm/L, but 10 mm/L is preferable if manual calculations are to be done. To accurately reproduce the "start-of-test," the paper should be moving at a constant speed before recording the volume deflection. Not all recorders fulfill this requirement. The recorder should be able to show at least 10 seconds of volume accumulation after recording begins, and it is preferable to use a little more paper than to prematurely terminate the maneuver.

A second type of device for graphing respiratory maneuvers is the electronic X-Y recorder. In this instance, a two-axis recorder receives electrical input in the form of analog (DC voltage) signals. The signals drive small servo-controlled motors that regulate pen movement (Fig. 9-29). The *X*-axis pen can be driven either by an input voltage or by a built-in timer. The advantage of this type of instrument is that signals can be plotted against one another or against time. The same recorder can be used to plot flow-volume or volume-time curves. The signal generated by a pneumotachometer or other flow-sensing device can be recorded in spirographic form. Gas analyzers coupled to such an instrument allow recording of tests such as the SBN_2 and multiple-breath N_2 washout. The electronic recorder is easy to calibrate; a known voltage can be applied and the recorder gains adjusted to produce an equivalent deflection (i.e., 1 V = 1 cm). Volume transducers that produce analog outputs can then be calibrated against the recorder so that a given volume change in the spirometer causes a proportional deflection on the recorder. Many recorders feature a third dimension for recording in the form of superimposed time measurements, when the main input is not graphed on a time base. A flow-volume loop typically plots flow on the vertical axis and volume on the horizontal axis. An X-Y-T recorder can interpose time marks (tics) on the flow-volume tracing, allowing timed volumes to be obtained as a third dimension. Most electronic X-Y recorders have variable sensitivity on both axes, which allows for greater flexibility than a simple mechanical tracing. Systems equipped with digital displays or computer graphics as well as an electronic recorder allow for easy comparisons of measured values and the spirogram.

Many pulmonary function systems feature both graphic display and recording of spirograms and related tracings by computer (see Chapter 10). Computerized systems typically employ printers capable of printing graphics either by thermal, ink jet, dot matrix, or laser techniques. Many automated pulmonary function systems provide for both computer-generated graphics and an alternate form of recording to allow manual measurements

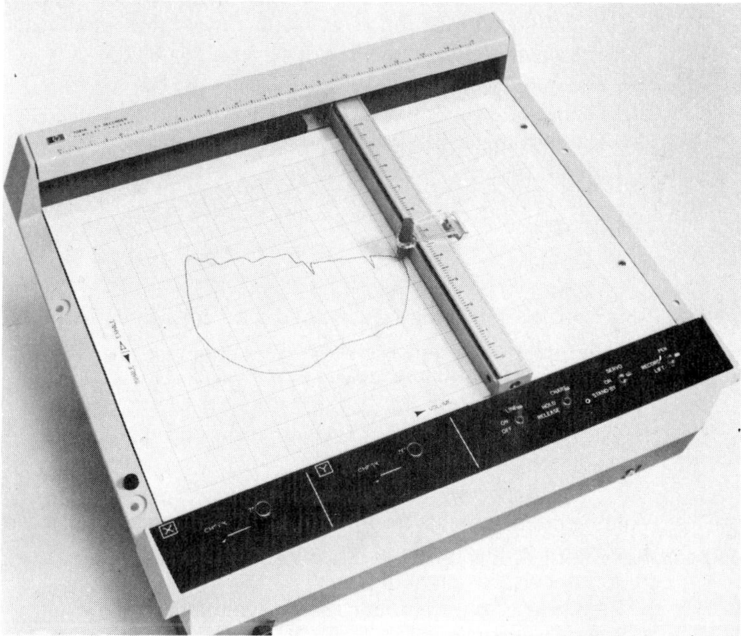

Fig. 9-29 X-Y recorder. An X-Y type of recording device capable of accepting analog inputs for flow, volume, gas concentration, or other typical DC signals, and graphing either against a time base or plotting one input against another (loops). (Courtesy Hewlett-Packard, San Diego.)

for comparison and quality control. A primary advantage of computer-generated graphics is that the data can be manipulated by the computer to provide corrections or linearization before being transformed into a printed tracing. In addition, computer-generated images can be displayed in formats not available with conventional recording devices, such as superimposed flow-volume curves.

SELF-ASSESSMENT QUESTIONS

1. Which of the following are advantages of volume-displacement types of spirometers over flow-sensing devices:
   I. They are easier to clean
   II. Direct mechanical recording of spirograms is possible
   III. They are not affected by the composition of expired gas
   IV. Unlike flow-based spirometers, $DL_{CO}SB$ can be performed
   a. I, II, III, IV
   b. I, III, IV
   c. II, III only
   d. III, IV only

2. A subject has an FVC of 5.2 L measured with a wedge spirometer and 5.1 L measured with a dry rolling-seal spirometer; a subsequent FVC test using a water-sealed spirometer produces values of 4.2, 3.8, and 4.7 L in three attempts. Which of the following might explain these discrepancies:
   I. The water-seal values were not corrected to BTPS
   II. The water-seal spirometer had a leak
   III. The water level was inadequate in the water-seal spirometer
   IV. The spirometer bell was incorrectly positioned
   a. I, II, III, IV
   b. II, III, IV
   c. I, II, III
   d. II, IV only

3. Which of the following factors should be considered in selecting a two-way valve for a test involving gas collection:
   a. Flow resistance characteristics of the valve
   b. Valve dead space
   c. The maximum flow rates likely to occur during the test
   d. All of the above

4. Volume measurements from flow-sensing spirometers are accomplished by:
   a. Electronic integration of the flow signal
   b. Inertial displacement of gas
   c. Summing of pulses proportional to volume
   d. Either a or c

5. Failure to adequately heat the resistive element in a pressure-differential pneumotachometer while performing spirometry will result in:

a. Uncorrected gas volumes
b. Condensation of water on the element
c. Increased flow resistance
d. b and c

6. Which of the following gas analyzers is (are) suitable for breath-by-breath measurement of the fractional concentration of oxygen:
   I. mass spectrometer
   II. gas chromatograph
   III. zirconium fuel cell
   IV. infrared analyzer
   a. I, II, III, IV
   b. I, III
   c. II, III
   d. III, IV

7. Monitoring of expired CO_2 in the critical care setting is usually accomplished using:
   a. A CO_2 gas chromatograph
   b. A thermal conductivity analyzer
   c. An emission spectroscopy type analyzer
   d. An infrared analyzer

8. A membrane covered platinum cathode is commonly used:
   a. In the PO_2 electrode
   b. In the Clark electrode
   c. In the PCO_2 electrode
   d. Both a and b

9. Pulse oximeters sense light transmitted by light emitting diodes as two components, the AC and DC components. The AC component represents:
   a. The constant output resulting from venous absorption and pigmentation
   b. The absorption in the red portion of the spectrum (660 nm)
   c. The absorption in the near-infrared region (800-1000 nm)
   d. The arteriolar pulsation

10. The transcutaneous O_2 electrode ($tcPO_2$) is heated to:
   a. Maintain oxygen reduction within the electrode
   b. Speed up diffusion of oxygen through the membrane
   c. Prevent tissue necrosis at the electrode site
   d. Cause hyperemia to arterialize capillary blood

11. The co-oximeter determines the oxygen saturation of hemoglobin by:
   a. Measuring the absorption of O_2Hb in the infrared spectrum
   b. Comparing the absorbances of O_2Hb, COHb, and MetHb at multiple wavelengths
   c. Titrating whole blood with a weak acid to dissociate oxygen
   d. Both a and b

12. The P_{CO_2} (Severinghaus) electrode measures the partial pressure of CO_2 by:
    a. Chemically extracting CO_2 from HCO_3^-
    b. Measuring the change in H^+ as CO_2 is hydrated within the electrode
    c. Comparing the unknown CO_2 with the CO_2 in a sealed electrode
    d. Ionizing CO_2 molecules between two wires

13. The main difference between a variable-pressure and flow-type plethysmograph is:
    a. The method of measuring mouth pressure
    b. The method of measuring changes in box volume
    c. That the variable pressure type is not airtight
    d. That the flow box utilizes a pneumotachometer

14. If the $FEV_{1.0}$ and $FEF_{25\%-75\%}$ are to be measured manually from a volume-time spirogram, the paper speed of the recorder should be at least:
    a. 1 mm/sec
    b. 1 cm/sec
    c. 2 cm/sec
    d. 10 cm/sec

15. The respiratory inductive plethysmograph monitors changes in lung volumes by measuring changes in the frequency of oscillations from transducers; these changes are proportional to:
    a. The cross-sectional area of the rib cage
    b. The transverse diameter of the thorax
    c. The cross-sectional area of the abdomen
    d. The transdiaphragmatic pressure
    e. The sum of a plus c

16. Which of the following are true concerning the pulmonary artery catheter that uses reflective spectrophotometry for monitoring of $S\bar{v}_{O_2}$?
    I. The saturation of functional Hb is measured
    II. Continuous monitoring is possible
    III. Pulmonary artery pressures can be measured simultaneously
    IV. Thermodilution cardiac output measurements can be made
    a. I, II, III, IV
    b. II, III, IV
    c. I, II only
    d. III, IV only

SELECTED BIBLIOGRAPHY

Spirometers

American Thoracic Society: Standardization of spirometry: 1987 update, Am Rev Respir Dis 136:1285, 1987.

Finucane KE, Egan BA, and Dawson SV: Linearity and frequency response of pneumotachographs, J Appl Physiol 32:121, 1972.

Fitzgerald MX, Smith AA, and Gaensler EA: Evaluation of 'electronic' spirometers, N Engl J Med 289:1283, 1973.

Gardner RM, Hankinson JL, and West BJ: Evaluating commercially available spirometers, Am Rev Respir Dis 121:73, 1980.

Glindmeyer HW et al: A comparison of the Jones and Stead-Wells spirometers, Chest 73:596, 1978.

Hankinson JL: Pulmonary function testing in the screening of workers: guidelines for instrumentation, performance, and interpretation, J Occup Med 28:1081, 1986.

Permutt S: Office spirometry in clinical practice, Chest 74:298, 1978.

Sullivan WJ, Peters GM, and Enright PL: Pneumotachographs: theory and clinical applications, Respir Care 29:736, 1984.

Wells HS et al: Accuracy of an improved spirometer for recording fast breathing, J Appl Physiol 14:451, 1959.

Gas analyzers

Fowler KT: The respiratory mass spectrometer, Phys Med Biol 14:185, 1969.

Norton AC: Accuracy in pulmonary measurements, Respir Care 24:131, 1979.

Rebuck AS and Chapman KR: Measurement and monitoring of exhaled carbon dioxide. In Nochomovitz ML, and Cherniack NS, editors: Non-invasive respiratory monitoring, New York, 1986, Churchill-Livingstone, Inc.

Sodal IE, Bowman RR, and Filley GF: A fast response oxygen analyzer with high accuracy for respiratory gas measurement, J Appl Physiol 25:181, 1968.

Wilson RS and Laver MB: Oxygen analysis: advances in methodology, Anesthesiology 37:112, 1972.

Blood gas electrodes, oximeters, and related devices

Barker SJ and Tremper KK: Pulse oximetry: applications and limitations, In Tremper KK and Barker SJ, editors: International anesthesiology clinics, Boston, 1987, Little, Brown & Co, Inc.

Brown LJ: A new instrument for the simultaneous measurement of total hemoglobin, % oxyhemoglobin, % carboxyhemoglobin, % methemoglobin, and O_2 content, IEEE Trans Biomed Eng 27:132, 1980.

Divertie MB and McMichan JC: Continuous monitoring of mixed venous saturation, Chest 85:423, 1984.

Fahey PJ et al: Clinical evaluation of a new ear oximeter, Am Rev Respir Dis 127 (suppl):129, 1983.

Huch A and Huch R: Transcutaneous, noninvasive monitoring of Po_2, Hosp Pract 11:43, 1976.

Pologue JA: Pulse oximetry: technical aspects of machine design. In Tremper KK and Barker SJ, editors: International anesthesiology clinics, Boston, 1987, Little, Brown & Co, Inc.

Rebuck AS, Chapman KR, and D'urzo A: The accuracy and response characteristics of a simplified ear oximeter, Chest 80:860, 1983.

Severinghaus JW and Astrup PB: History of blood gas analysis, v. oxygen measurement, J Clin Monit 2:174, 1986.

Taylor MB and Whitman JG: The current status of pulse oximetry: clinical value of continuous noninvasive oxygen saturation monitoring, Anaesthesia 41:943, 1986.

Tremper KK and Waxman KS: Transcutaneous monitoring of respiratory gases. In Nochomovitz ML and Cherniack NS, editors: Non-invasive respiratory monitoring, New York, 1986, Churchill-Livingstone, Inc.

Plethysmographs

Bargeton D and Barres G: Time characteristics and frequency response of body plethysmographs, International Symposium on Body Plethysmography, Nijmegen, Prog Respir Res 4:2, 1969.

DuBois AB et al: A rapid plethysmographic method for measuring thoracic gas volume: a comparison with nitrogen washout method for measuring functional residual capacity in normal subjects, J Clin Invest 35:322, 1956.

DuBois AB, Bothello SY, and Comroe JH: A new method for measuring airway resistance in man using a body plethysmograph: values in normal subjects and in patients with respiratory disease, J Clin Invest 35:327, 1956.

Leith DE and Mead J: Principles of body plethysmography, Bethesda, MD 1974, National Heart, Lung, and Blood Institute-Division of Lung Diseases.

Lourenco RV and Chung SYK: Calibration of a body plethysmograph for measurement of lung volume, Am Rev Respir Dis 95:687, 1967.

Respiratory inductive plethysmography

Chadhat TS et al: Validation of respiratory inductive plethysmography using different calibration procedures, Am Rev Respir Dis 125:644, 1982.

Dolfin T et al: Calibration of respiratory inductive plethysmography (Respitrace) in infants, Am Rev Respir Dis 126:577, 1982.

Konno K and Mead J: Measurement of the separate volume changes of rib cage and abdomen during breathing, J Appl Physiol 22:407, 1972.

Sackner MA: Monitoring of ventilation without physical connection to the airway: a review. In Scott FD, Raferty CV, and Goulding L, editors: ISAM Proceedings of the Third International Symposium on Ambulatory Monitoring, London, 1982, Academic Press, Inc.

Recorders

Gardner RM et al: Spirometry: what paper speed? Am Rev Respir Dis 125:89, 1982, (abstract).

U.S. Occupational Safety and Health Administration: Pulmonary function standards for cotton dust, 29 Code of Federal Regulations, 1910.1043 Cotton Dust, Appendix D, Washington, DC, 1980.

10

Computers in the Pulmonary Function Laboratory

Computers have become an integral part of almost every pulmonary function testing system because they can efficiently perform the tasks typically involved in the reduction of pulmonary function data. These tasks include the solution of repetitive calculations, data storage and retrieval, printing of reports and graphs, processing of signals from various transducers, and automated control of the instruments themselves. The advantages of computerization of pulmonary function testing are that fewer errors occur in calculations, calibrations can be performed more consistently, and the variability of repeated measurements is reduced. Test time is often dramatically reduced, for both the subject and the technologist, allowing a wider variety of procedures to be performed. Repetition of effort-dependent tests or tests with questionable results is practical because computerization allows immediate inspection of the measurements. The disadvantages of computerization of pulmonary function testing include decreased understanding and interaction on the part of the technologist, increased complexity of the test equipment, and in many instances, dependence on the computer to produce all measurements.

This chapter examines some of the general components and terminology used with small computer systems, automated data acquisition, important qualities in a pulmonary laboratory system, languages and programming, and some additional practical applications.

Several different levels of computerization are typically found in conjunction with pulmonary function testing systems:

Dedicated microprocessors—Numerous small, portable spirometers use microprocessors to perform calculations and control various instrument functions, such as digital display of data. Many flow-sensing spirometers and some volume-displacement devices use a dedicated microprocessor in conjunction with software stored on ROM chips (see Memory section of this chapter) to perform flow and volume measurements. Other devices, such as pulse oximeters and capnographs, also employ dedicated microprocessors to perform unique sets of instructions. Dedicated microprocessors automate measurements, but they typically allow only minimal user modification. Memory chips capable of retaining a large amount of data permit sophisticated functions such as storage of multiple tests, error checking for reproducibility, and user selection of predicted values.

Microcomputers—The next higher level of computerization is the microcomputer, also referred to as a desktop or personal computer, either incorporated directly into the pulmonary function system or as a standalone instrument interfaced to the spirometer and gas analyzers. The microcomputer-based system usually includes disk storage for programs and data, a high resolution video display, and an external printer. Most pulmonary function laboratory systems are now based on the single-user microcomputer. Microcomputers are also used in conjunction with blood gas analyzers or other laboratory instruments where management of large amounts of data is necessary. Very fast microcomputers can be used in a network for multiple users; the performance of such a network depends on the speed of the computer, the operating system, and the type of user programs being run.

Minicomputers and mainframe computers—Although the microcomputer has replaced the minicomputer to a certain extent, some laboratories interface several instruments or work stations to a central minicomputer. Minicomputers have historically been used to allow multiple users to access data and programs simultaneously. Pulmonary function equipment, exercise testing equipment, and blood gas analyzers can all be interfaced as part of a multiuser system. The selection of a minicomputer versus a mainframe depends on the number of users and the types of tasks to be performed. Minicomputers are commonly employed in laboratory information systems to provide blood gas instrument automation and availability of test results to multiple terminals, but they may be too slow for use with pulmonary function testing equipment.

A great deal of overlap exists between the various levels of computerization commonly found in the laboratory setting. Dedicated microprocessors can be used to collect data (i.e., spirometry parameters) at the bedside, then brought to the laboratory and "dumped" to a microcomputer for permanent storage or printing of results. Microcomputers can be used as intelligent terminals, capable of communicating with minicomputers or mainframe computers, as well as performing specific functions such as pulmonary function tests.

The selection of a computerized pulmonary function system should be based on a careful evaluation of the number and complexity of the tests to be performed, the amount of data to be stored, and the type of reports to be generated. Many applications, such as bedside spirometry, may require only minimal computerization; it may be cost effective to use a system requiring manual measurement of spirograms, particularly if the volume of tests performed is low. In general, choosing a computerized pulmonary function system should follow these guidelines:

1. Define the tasks or types of tests that the system will be expected to

perform. Important questions are:

- What tests are required (spirometry, lung volumes, plethysmography, DL_{CO})?
- How many patients will be tested per day, or per month?
- How much data is to be stored, and for how long?
- What types of reports are to be generated?
- Will the system be used for other purposes, in addition to pulmonary function studies?
- Will the data be transferred to other computer systems or be available to other users?

It is important to identify these tasks in order of importance.

2. Once the tasks have been clearly defined, the software best able to perform the tasks should be selected. Unfortunately, pulmonary function software is often specific to a particular instrument or system. In many cases, both the software and instrument capabilities should be evaluated in reference to the required tasks. Some manufacturers offer various combinations of spirometers, gas analyzers, plethysmographs, and exercise testing equipment, making it possible for the user to select the necessary equipment as well as the software.
3. The actual computer hardware that runs the selected software should be the final element in the selection process. In some instances, there may be little choice as to the computer hardware, as noted previously. Many manufacturers now design software that operates on a range of compatible systems, thus allowing the user to select a computer that meets the present needs and permits future expansion. Compatibility is an important aspect of hardware selection, because computer technology has tended to advance more rapidly than that of spirometers or gas analyzers. Software written with future compatibility in mind allows the user to upgrade the computer hardware to take advantage of faster processors and increased storage capabilities while maintaining consistency in testing methods. Ideally, the computer selected should allow software upgrades as well, rather than requiring a new computer to implement more sophisticated programs. Modular design of the computer system is advantageous in that it permits the user to change part of the system as requirements change or when new technology becomes available. If more than one hardware option is available, the system chosen should maximize functions offered by the software.

Choosing a laboratory computer for purposes other than pulmonary function testing, such as storage of blood gas data and word processing, may differ slightly from the scheme outlined, but the general approach of defining the tasks to be performed before deciding on software or hardware is useful.

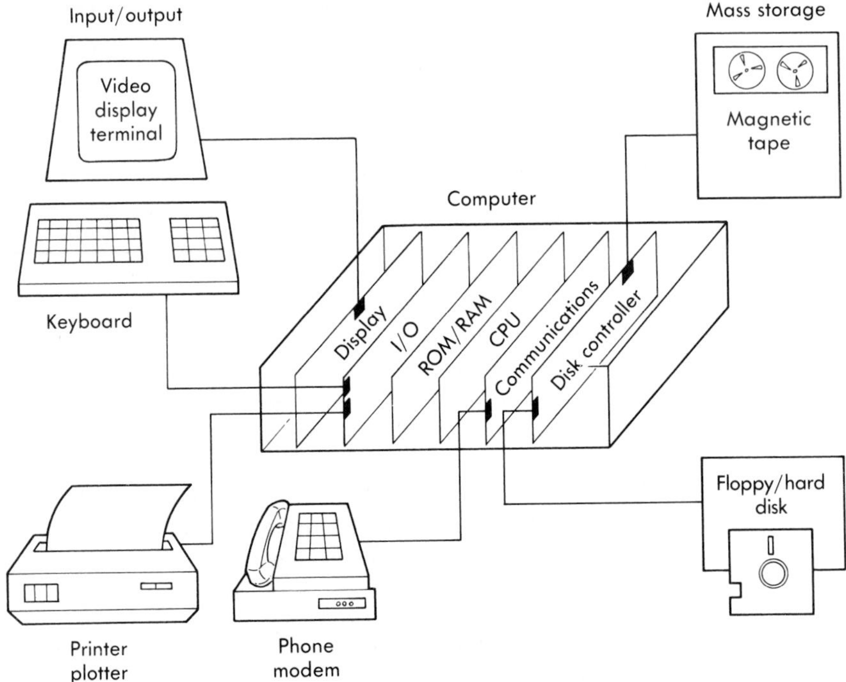

Fig. 10-1 Components of a small computer system. The computer itself includes a central processing unit (CPU, or microprocessor) connected to various divisions of memory (ROM/RAM), input/output processors (I/O boards), and controllers for the video display, disk drives, and communication devices. Typical I/O devices include the video display, the keyboard (the standard input device), and printers or plotters. Communications usually include a serial port and modem for transmission of data over conventional phone lines. Mass storage devices include magnetic tape drives, floppy and hard disk drives, or optical (laser) drives. Many small computer systems allow for addition of various components simply by plugging in different "cards." Not shown is an interface such as might be used with an analog-digital converter (see Fig. 10-2).

COMPUTER SYSTEMS

Most microcomputer and minicomputer systems can be divided into component parts similar to those depicted in Fig. 10-1. These components are typical of small computer systems in general, but they may have functions specific to pulmonary function testing.

Microprocessor or CPU

The *microprocessor, or CPU,* refers to the "brain" of the system. Microprocessors are sometimes referred to as the central processing unit, or CPU. The microprocessor performs most, if not all, of the instructions provided by the software. These instructions typically include calculations, storing and retrieving of data from memory, and controlling of peripheral devices, such as video displays, printers, and disk drives. Microprocessors are classified by the number of "bits" of information that can be handled at one time; a bit is a 0 or 1 in the binary number system. Commonly used in laboratory computer systems are 8-bit, 16-bit, and 32-bit CPUs. Early microcomputers were based on 8-bit processors, capable of addressing 65,536 memory locations. Newer processors (i.e., 16- and 32-bit processors) are capable of addressing as many as 16 million memory addresses. In general, 16- and 32-bit processors can perform calculations more rapidly than smaller microprocessors, both because of their ability to address more memory directly and because they are capable of operating at faster clock speeds. Clock speed refers to the rate at which the microprocessor operates; it is usually quantified in terms of megahertz (millions of cycles per second, or MHz). The fastest microcomputer processors operate at speeds in excess of 30 MHz. The actual speed with which the computer is capable of carrying out a particular task, such as writing a file to disk or retrieving information from memory, is a product of the speed of the individual components as well as the processor speed. Fast microprocessors require equally fast input/output devices (see Input/output devices section of this chapter), which may increase the overall cost of the system. To use very fast microprocessors, some systems rely on special techniques to assist slower components. A common technique is "caching," which places information into a special memory area, or cache, to speed up storage and retrieval from slower devices such as disk drives or regular memory. Special microprocessors, called math co-processors, work in conjunction with the main microprocessor to speed up arithmetic-intensive calculations. Computers with math co-processors typically perform tasks involving calculations much faster than systems without co-processors. Some advanced microprocessors have math co-processor and memory-caching capabilities designed into a single chip. Microprocessors may also be used for highly specific tasks, such as controlling high-resolution video displays or managing large blocks of memory.

In addition to faster clock speeds, 16- and 32-bit processors are capable of multitasking, or running multiple programs simultaneously. The same types of processors, when used with the appropriate operating system, also allow multiple users to share the computer and its peripherals (i.e., printers and disk storage). The combination of multitasking and multiuser capabilities offers numerous possibilities to enhance laboratory data management. Some multitasking systems permit the user to perform diagnostic testing in real time while the computer prints reports or transmits data to another system in the background. A multiuser environment allows pulmonary function testing to be performed at one terminal, while blood gas data is entered at a second terminal, physicians review test results at a third station, and clerical staff print final reports at a fourth work station.

A large proportion of the commercially available computerized pulmonary function testing systems use microcomputers, and most are based on either 16- or 32-bit CPU architecture. While many laboratories do not require multitasking or multiple users, the availability of microprocessors and software that support these functions permits expansion of the system as utilization increases.

Memory

Memory may be classified as read-only memory (ROM) or random access memory (RAM). The computer's ROM usually contains often-used instructions, such as those for controlling the video display or checking RAM when the computer is powered on. Incompatability between certain programs and computers is sometimes caused by differences in the basic input/output system (BIOS), which makes up a large portion of ROM. ROM cannot be changed by a user program, but it can be altered if the chip containing the instructions is replaced. Programmable ROM chips (PROMs) or erasable programmable ROM chips (EPROMS) are often used in just this way in some pulmonary function testing systems. By placing instructions to communicate with a particular piece of equipment on a PROM, it becomes quite easy to change to different equipment, by simply installing a new PROM.

The RAM available in a computer refers to the amount of memory that is available for user programs. RAM is normally occupied by the computer's operating system (see Operating systems section of this chapter) and the user's application programs, which are loaded from an external source, such as a disk or tape. Many microcomputers maximize their use of available memory by breaking the application program into modules and then loading only those segments that are required for a certain test; this technique conserves RAM but may slow down overall program execution if many modules are loaded and unloaded. Advances in chip technology have made large amounts of RAM relatively inexpensive, so that even microcomputers can manage extremely large and complicated programs.

Both RAM and ROM are quantified in terms of memory units or bytes; each byte contains 8 bits (either 0 or 1). A byte can take on 256 distinct values. Two bytes taken together form a *word,* which contains a 16-bit number. Each memory byte or word can be used to store data or instructions. A kilobyte is the equivalent of 1024 bytes, and most small computer systems use from 256K to 1024K. In general, an 8-bit microprocessor can address only 64K of memory without special adaptations; early 16-bit CPUs were able to address up to 1024K by combining two 16-bit numbers to derive a 20-bit address. 1024K is usually referred to as a megabyte (M), approximately 1 million bytes. Newer 16- and 32-bit microprocessors have address spaces of 16M. Although these microprocessors can physically address 16M, most systems use a more manageable 1M to 6M.

In addition to the ability to accommodate large amounts of real working memory, or RAM, many advanced microprocessors, such as the Intel* 80286, 80386, and 80486 can also provide as many as 1024 megabytes (i.e., a gigabyte) of virtual memory. Virtual memory is mapped into the computer's physical memory; when more memory is needed, the contents of the physical memory are swapped out to a disk drive or other storage device. The computer's operating system has to manage the swapping of actual and virtual memory contents.

Another means of increasing the amount of memory available in the microcomputer is use of bank-switched memory. A special memory board that contains banks of RAM chips is typically added to the computer. Bank-switching, also referred to as expanded memory, allows more memory to be installed in the computer than can actually be addressed by the microprocessor. A special memory manager program then interacts with the user application program to use the extra memory banks. Bank-switched memory is very fast, but in some operating systems, the added RAM can only be used for program data, not for the program itself.

Most pulmonary function application programs do not require large amounts of memory to run, but more data can be held in memory at one time and sophisticated calculations can be performed with more available RAM. Storage and graphical display of the raw data from multiple spirometry efforts (i.e., flow-volume curves) may require considerable amounts of RAM.

The storage capacity of devices such as tapes, floppy diskettes, and hard disks (see Mass storage devices section of this chapter) are often classified in terms of megabytes (M) of memory, as well as in kilobytes (K).

Input/output devices

Input/output (I/O) devices are parts of the computer system through which data are either entered or displayed. These include the monitor or CRT, the keyboard, mass storage devices such as disk or tape drives, printers, modems for communications over telephone lines, as well as special interfaces between the computer and analog output instruments (see Data Acquisition and Instrument Control section of this chapter). Some I/O devices, such as disk drives, modems, and special interfaces, perform both input and output. Other I/O devices are for input only, such as the keyboard, or output only, such as the monitor and printer. Because most of these peripheral devices are quite complex, they often employ highly specialized integrated circuits (chips), or even their own microprocessor, to carry out various tasks. Many small computer systems are modular (see Fig. 10-1), using a main circuit board (motherboard) into which various I/O cards may be plugged. This open architecture design is quite flexible and allows systems to be tailored to very specific needs, such as are found in the pulmonary function laboratory. The ability to upgrade a computer sys-

*Intel is a registered trademark of Intel Corporation.

tem, such as by adding a larger disk drive or more memory, is also enhanced by being able to replace an individual component rather than the entire system. Advanced chip technologies now allow many of the functions previously assigned to specific I/O cards to be placed directly on the motherboard. While this limits the flexibility of the system somewhat, the overall size of the computer can be reduced dramatically.

Mass storage devices

Mass storage devices include magnetic tape systems, "floppy" and "hard" disks, and optical disks. *Magnetic tape systems* are usually employed on larger multiuser systems (i.e., mainframe computers) in which a large amount of data must be maintained. Smaller tape drive units are sometimes used for data storage when a large volume of data is recorded but does not require rapid or random retrieval. Some tape units are employed as inexpensive backups to floppy or hard-disk systems.

On microcomputer-based pulmonary function testing systems, *floppy disk drives,* or a combination of floppy disk and and hard drive, are most commonly used. Several sizes of floppy disk drives are widely available; common diskette sizes include 5¼ inches and 3½ inches. The volume of data that can be stored on a disk is described by the number of tracks available and the density with which the data is recorded. The 5¼-inch diskettes hold either 360K or, in the high-density version, 1.2M of data. The 3½-inch diskettes also come in two capacities, 720K and 1.44M. Many microcomputers are supplied with one size of floppy disk drive, but some systems use both to facilitate transfer of data between computers. The chief advantages of floppy disks for program and data storage are that they are inexpensive, lightweight, and portable. The primary disadvantages of floppy diskettes are that they can be damaged rather easily, they are relatively slow compared to hard disks, and they eventually wear out.

The *hard disk,* or *fixed drive,* uses a technology similar to that of the floppy disk, except that instead of a flexible plastic disk, a solid metal platter is employed. The hard drive allows a much greater amount of data to be stored in approximately the same space as a floppy drive and to be accessed much more quickly. Hard disks are commonly described by the total storage space provided, with 20- to 40-megabyte disks being widely used for small laboratory systems, and 40- to 600-megabyte disks being employed in some of the more sophisticated designs. The advantages of the fixed disk over floppy drives are the large amount of data all contained on a single device and the speed with which the data can be accessed. Some disadvantages of the hard disk include the necessity of backing up large amounts of information, usually on floppy disks or tape, and keeping track of hundreds or even thousands of files on a single drive. Advances in hard-disk technology have reduced the rate of mechanical failures as well as the cost to store a megabyte of information. Sophisticated software tools are available, and usually required, to manage hard disks; most of these programs feature file management, diagnostics, and back-up features. Several manufacturers offer removable hard disks that allow large amounts of information to physically be moved from one computer to another or to be removed for security purposes.

The *optical drive,* or laser drive, is a high-capacity storage device that uses a laser to write information on a plastic disk. The simplest type of optical disk is not erasable; i.e., data can only be written to the disk once. These types of device are commonly referred to as Write Once Read Many (WORM) drives. A more sophisticated type of optical drive uses a combination of laser and magnetic pulses to write data on the plastic disk; the data may then be erased or modified by altering the state of the magnetic pulses. Either type of optical disk is ideally suited for storage of large amounts of data, such as flow-volume or other physiologic waveforms. Optical drives are very useful for storage of reference information or for archiving data that must be retained for later retrieval, such as ECG or pulmonary function data. Optical disks are capable of holding approximately 800 megabytes of data, so that several thousands of routine pulmonary function tests can be archived on a single volume. The drive itself is approximately the size of a conventional hard drive, and the laser disk is about the size of a 5¼-inch floppy disk.

A related type of pseudo-storage device is the electronic disk, or RAM disk. The RAM disk is a disk drive defined in the memory of the computer; it has no physical parts, but it acts just like a very fast disk drive. Because they are so fast, RAM disks are ideal for programs that access the disk often for data manipulation or creation of temporary files. However, because the RAM disk is not a permanent storage device, any data contained on it must be transferred to a floppy or hard disk before powering down the computer.

Software

Software refers to all of the instructions contained in the memory, both ROM and RAM, of the computer. These sets of instructions are referred to as *programs.* Most microcomputer-based systems use an operating system that controls the computer's various functions and application programs that perform the specific tasks that the user selects (i.e., pulmonary function testing, word processing, data base management). Most application programs are loaded into the computer from disk or tape, but many basic functions are contained on ROM chips. This is particularly true of many portable spirometry units that feature a dedicated microprocessor. In these devices, all software is contained on chips, either PROMs or EPROMs, and is immediately available when the unit is powered on.

DATA ACQUISITION AND INSTRUMENT CONTROL

One of the primary advantages of computerized pulmonary function systems is the ability to process analog signals from various transducers (i.e., spirometers, pneumotachometers, gas analyzers) to perform automated acquisition of data. Equally important is the computer's capacity for controlling certain instrument functions (i.e., valve switching, recording) to allow the technologist to easily manage complex test maneuvers. Both data acquisition and instrument control are implemented by means of an interface (Fig. 10-2) that permits the computer to communicate with various types of pulmonary function equipment.

One of the primary devices employed in interfacing pulmonary function equipment with computers is the analog-to-digital (A/D) converter. The A/D converter accepts an analog signal, usually a DC voltage in the range of 0 to 10 volts, or −5 to +5 volts, and transforms the signal into a digital value. A/D converters are classified by the number of bits (i.e., binary digits) into which they convert the signal; the greater the number of bits, the greater the resolution of the input signal by the resulting digital value. A "12-bit" converter can transform a voltage into a number represented by 000000000000 to 111111111111 as a binary number. In the dec-

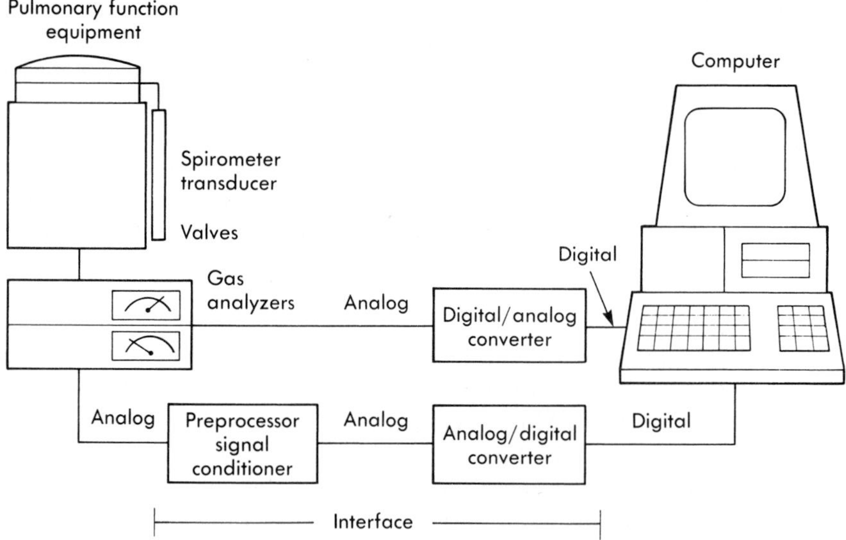

Fig. 10-2 Computer interface for pulmonary function testing. Components of a typical interface between a spirometer, gas analyzers, and a small computer are represented. Analog signals from the pulmonary function equipment are preprocessed so that the analog-to-digital (A/D) converter can manage them. The A/D converter then transforms a voltage, usually DC, into digital data in the form of a binary or hexadecimal number. The digital data is then processed by the computer for calculations, display, and storage. For the computer to control various instrument functions, a digital-to-analog converter transforms digital data into appropriate analog signals to control various system components.

imal numbering system, this corresponds to a range of 0 to 4,096 (2^{12}). If a 10-L spirometer that produces an analog signal ranging from 0 to 10 V (equal to 1 V/L) is connected to a 12-bit converter, the signal is divided into 4,096 parts, with a resolution of about 0.0024 volts, or a 2.4 ml over the 10-L volume range. In effect, the smallest volume change that could be detected by the computer for this spirometer system would be 2.4 ml. Sampling from a transducer that has a voltage range of ±5 volts, as might be found in a flow sensor measuring bidirectional flow, with a 12-bit converter would have a similar resolution of 0.0024 volts, because the full scale input range is still 10 V. In this case, the actual flow resolution would depend on the sensitivity of the transducer or what range of flows would cause a full-scale deflection. 12-bit converters are used for most volume and flow sampling applications; 8-bit and 10-bit converters are sometimes used for functions that do not require high resolution.

In addition to the resolution of the A/D converter, the rate at which data are sampled is important to the accuracy of the data gathered. Most A/D converter systems consist of between 8 and 16 distinct channels, each of which is capable of accepting a separate analog input. The highest sampling rates are usually attained when conversions are done on only one or two channels. For tests in which a great deal of accuracy is required and in which the signal changes very rapidly, such as a forced expiration, conversions may be performed on a single channel. The Nyquist sampling theorem indicates that the sampling rate (i.e., the number of samples taken per second) should be at least twice the frequency of the sampled waveform. The highest frequency components of a typical peak flow signal are within 0 to 12 Hz, or cycles per second, and the high-frequency components of a forced vital capacity volume are somewhat less. High-speed converters can perform more than 20,000 conversions per second on a single channel; as more channels are included in the conversion scheme, the rate for each channel is typically reduced. Most computerized pulmonary function systems sample data on multiple channels at rates of 100 Hz or greater, usually exceeding the frequency bandwidth by more than a factor of 2. The maximum accuracy is attained by matching the output of a particular transducer (i.e., spirometer) to a particular A/D converter with the appropriate sampling rate and voltage resolution. High sampling rates and high-resolution conversion require very fast microprocessors and increased memory for storing the extra data. In general, the lowest sampling rate that will allow acceptable resolution of the signal also allows the greatest flexibility in terms of processing times and computations on the data. Another approach to sampling, for volumes and flow signals, is to measure the time required for a predetermined volume or flow change. For example, the number of clock ticks that occur for a volume change of 100 ml can be measured, and flow can then be calculated. This technique typically requires a spirometer that includes a position encoder or that generates pulses for each volume increment. The accuracy of such a system depends on the resolution of the clock during rapid flow and the size of the volume increment.

Some analog signals require special handling before A/D conversion, as well as computations on the digital data after conversion. These signal-conditioning functions are often included in the interface between the test instrument and the computer, and they are referred to as "preprocessing." Most transducers include amplifiers that allow setting of offsets and gains; these are primitive forms of signal preprocessing. A common example of signal preprocessing would include transforming a resistance into a voltage so that A/D conversion would be possible. Other preprocessing functions of the interface might include such devices as peak signal detection and counting or timing circuits. Many A/D converter systems have the capacity to process and store data in their own RAM memory until the computer requests it; this allows high-speed data acquisition by the interface and provides flexibility in programming the computer. The "smart" interface performs data acquisition and holds the information so that the computer can retrieve the data at a slower rate, making computations and corrections as required. The use of a "smart" interface permits the data to be transmitted in any one of several formats, such as ASCII codes.* Standardized formats allow modification of the software that reads the data as well as upgrading of the computer without replacing the entire testing system.

Many instruments, such as pulse oximeters and capnographs, use their own microprocessor and A/D board to display data and have a communication port so that an external computer or printer can be interfaced. The RS-232 serial port is typically used, but other faster types, such as the RS-422 and RS-485, are becoming common. The "serial" port transmits data one bit at a time, usually in a fixed pattern. The speed at which the transmission occurs is termed the baud rate, expressed in bits/second, and may vary from 300 to more than 19,000, depending on the type of connection and equipment involved. The pattern of bits needed to transmit a byte of data may range from 8 to 10, including the data bits and extra bits to signal the beginning or end of a byte. Most computers that have a serial port can be interfaced to the instrument using one of these standardized protocols. Some laboratory instruments support parallel ports that transmit bytes of data at one time, rather than bits as in the serial port. Parallel ports are typically used for interconnection with printers, and the test instrument contains software that formats the data to be printed.

Another function of the interface between the computer and the testing instrument is the conversion of digital information from the computer into analog signals. This is accomplished by the digital-to-analog (D/A) converter, which can be viewed as the complement to the A/D converter described previously. In this case, a digital input results in an analog output voltage proportional to the value of the input byte. In its simplest form,

---

*(*A*merican *S*tandard *C*ode for *I*nterchange of *I*nformation)

the D/A converter acts as a relay switch between the computer and the instrument, and it is commonly referred to as digital I/O or digital expansion. A nonzero value sent from the computer can be used to activate an electrically operated valve or solenoid, after the converter generates the required voltage (typically 5 VDC). D/A conversion allows the computer to perform tasks such as activating kymographs or recorders, switching valves in automated circuits, and opening solenoids to add oxygen, helium, or other gases. Other common uses of D/A signal conversion are to allow the user to check various instrument functions that are normally under software control or to perform automatic calibration. Built-in diagnostic procedures permit the technologist to track down equipment problems, and specifically to isolate those attributable to the transducers (i.e., spirometer, gas analyzers) from those that may be due to failure of the computer hardware or software.

Many pulmonary function systems provide alternate means of controlling various functions that are normally computer controlled. Manual controls allow use of the spirometer, gas analyzers, and associated equipment, even if the computer becomes unavailable.

COMPUTERIZED PULMONARY FUNCTION TESTING SYSTEMS

The interdependence of pulmonary function testing equipment and computers makes the capabilities of the computer system especially important. Because the technology of small computers and their peripherals advances so rapidly, users cannot anticipate all of the possible applications that the computer may have in the future. If a particular system presently meets specific testing needs, it should be able to continue to perform the same functions. An important consideration is whether the system (hardware and software) is both upwardly and downwardly compatible. Upwardly compatible hardware means that the computer itself can be enhanced and still perform tests with the same spirometer or gas analyzers. Very often this level of compatibility is determined by the type of interface employed, as described earlier in this chapter. A related concern is whether the computer system can accommodate enhancements to the testing system, such as the addition of equipment to perform DL_{CO} tests, body plethysmography, or exercise/metabolic studies. Upward and downward compatibility in the area of software means that improvements to a particular program ("upward" changes) do not invalidate or render unusable previously generated data. If a program enhancement allows new or more accurate data to be generated while at the same time it accommodates old data, the program can be considered "downwardly" compatible. This type of compatibility is especially important for longitudinal studies in which subjects may be tested over a period of years.

Accuracy and dependability

The first and most important quality of any computerized pulmonary function system is its ability to perform the required measurements, and to do so dependably with acceptable accuracy. In addition to required accuracy of the transducers (i.e., spirometer, gas analyzers), both the computer hardware and software must be designed in such a way that overall accuracy is not compromised by the automated acquisition of data. Careful selection and implementation of data acquisition hardware (see Data Acquisition and Instrument Control section earlier in this chapter), appropriate sampling rates, and controlling software are typically the responsibility of the equipment manufacturer. The simplest means of assessing the accuracy of a computerized system for individual users is to compare computer-generated results to those obtained by manual calculation. A means of recording raw signals from spirometers and gas analyzers, as well as complete documentation of all equations used by the software, is required for this type of comparison. Testing normal subjects, such as lab personnel, is typically easier than using a test simulator, although devices that furnish reproducible flow signals (see Chapter 11) provide controlled inputs for repeated testing. If the accuracy of any component test cannot be easily verified, the system may be difficult to maintain in day-to-day use. Because the software required for data acquisition in spirometry, lung volume determination, diffusing capacity, and plethysmography is complex, it is relatively rare that a program is completely free of errors. This high level of complexity requires that the program developer offer continuing program upgrades and support, as well as ongoing software development. A system for documentation of hardware or program modifications and validation of measurements should be maintained.

Computerized pulmonary function testing allows enhancements that assess the quality of the data obtained. Most pulmonary function software does some checking for errors both during data acquisition and after results have been calculated. Examples of this include calculation of the back-extrapolated volume during spirometry and analysis of the reproducibility of the FVC and $FEV_{1.0}$ (see Chapter 11). Digitized spirometry waveforms may be used to simulate the forced vital capacity maneuver using a computer-controlled syringe, or simply to check the accuracy of the software that reduces the data obtained. Although not practical for most laboratories, the use of standardized waveforms is recommended by the American Thoracic Society for the validation of spirometers and spirometry software.

Computerized and manual testing

A second important quality of any automated system is its ability to also perform nonautomated tests. As noted previously, manual calculations of component tests are normally the best means of assessing the accuracy of the measurements, for both the input devices and for the software. Because of the complexity of even small computers and the number of peripherals (i.e., disk drives, printers) commonly used, the failure of a single component can often disable a computer-dependent pulmonary function testing system. In a high-volume laboratory, a computer failure may cause cancellation of many procedures. A serious shortcoming of many computerized systems is that both graphic and tabular data are computer generated; that is, no analog recording system is available. A computer malfunction under these circumstances often means that no data can be recorded. A similar consideration is that, in some circumstances, the technologist may need to alter the exact method or sequence that the automated system normally requires. A valuable asset is a computer system that allows user intervention for data verification or modification of the test maneuver sequence.

Software design

The ease with which a computerized pulmonary function system can be used is one of the most desirable qualities of any automated testing system. In general, use of the computer should speed up the test routine while enhancing both the quality and the accuracy of the data obtained. The software should allow the necessary repetition of maneuvers required for obtaining valid data. Typically, the program should be able to hold three to eight FVC maneuvers in memory for comparison and selection. Additionally, the software should accommodate two to four slow VC maneuvers, two to four MVV efforts, one or more lung volume determinations, two to four DL_{CO} tests, and multiple panting maneuvers if plethysmography is implemented.

Carefully designed software makes allowances for various degrees of cooperation by the subject tested; in effect, the software must handle unusual occurrences, such as the subject interrupting the sequence of the test, without loss of data or system lockup. Computerization of spirometry (i.e., FVC, $FEV_{1.0}$) requires pattern recognition algorithms for determining the start and end of test, and back-extrapolated volumes. Automation of lung volume determinations or DL_{CO} typically requires computer control of breathing circuits, valves, and gas analyzers, and presents an array of problems somewhat different than those encountered in automated spirometry.

The capacity for user modification is perhaps the most important aspect of appropriately designed software. The simplest means of customizing software is to build modifiable parameters into the program, then allow the user to select the desired options and save them in a configuration-type of file. User-selected program options allow the software to meet a wide variety of laboratory needs. Conversely, poorly designed software may require the technologist or the subject to perform many more steps than the same procedure used manually; this typically occurs for lung volume or DL_{CO} tests in which operator intervention is required for setting up special circuits or gas analyzers. Many systems employ a "turnkey" approach in software design; i.e., the program is written so that the operator may perform tests with little or no knowledge of what the computer is doing. Such systems function best for simple maneuvers that do not require operator intervention; they also allow the technologist to concentrate on eliciting the best possible effort from the subject. In most instances, however, the turnkey approach does not completely eliminate the need for the technologist to perform some computer-related procedures, such as preparing new storage disks or backing up patient data. Another drawback of some turnkey types of systems is lack of flexibility in the choice of options that the operator may have. Perhaps the most widely used means of providing an easy-to-use software package is to employ menu-driven programs. Menu-driven programs are those that prompt the operator as to the sequence of steps that the computer will accept; the prompts are typically always displayed somewhere on the video display and can usually be selected by a single keyboard entry. A well designed menu-driven program allows the technologist to perform even complex tasks quickly, without a great deal of orientation, and to concentrate on obtaining adequate subject cooperation. In addition, menu-driven applications typically require only single-key entries for most functions or provide a means of pointing a moving cursor at specific menu items; in either format, the program can easily check for invalid input. A popular implementaton of the menu-driven approach incorporates the use of window-based applications. As the user navigates among different menu options, a series of windows open on the video display, either side-by-side or overlaying one another. Each window contains a related set of options, so that the user can intuitively deduce how selections are made as well as understand the relationship between the choices in various windows.

Hardware and software documentation

Perhaps as important as any of the previously described attributes of computerized pulmonary function systems is the documentation provided by the manufacturer and/or programmer. The complexity of data acquisition programs such as those used in pulmonary function testing, and of the operating systems typically required for even small computers, necessitates thorough documentation. Appropriate documentation of computer programs includes all the information necessary to get the system up and running, even for the novice pulmonary function computer user. Information should be included that describes the interconnection of all peripheral devices, as well as any initialization or installation programs that must be run. If the system is provided in several different configurations (i.e., different computers) each should be clearly described, and separate instructions should be provided for each component.

Every segment of the application program (i.e., pulmonary function testing software) should be carefully outlined, including diagrams of sample screen displays and printouts and a description of the user input that is required. Examples, either in text format or via sample data from the computer itself, are invaluable for training new users on complicated systems. Many commercially available pulmonary function systems use generic operating systems (i.e., MS-DOS*, OS/2*, UNIX†), while other manufacturers support their own proprietary operating systems. In either case, the functions of the operating system (i.e., file handling, backing up of data) should be fully documented along with the pulmonary function application programs. An extremely useful adjunct is the "on-line" or context-sensitive type of "help" function. These types of programmed assistance usually consist of one or more screens of text that the operator can access from within the pulmonary function testing program, or which the program displays when an error occurs. On-line help functions greatly speed up orientation to a new system, as well as the use of functions that may not be performed on a routine basis. A glossary of computer terms is helpful, particularly if the applications program redefines commonly used terms or keys on the computer keyboard. An explanation of error messages is important in tracking down software problems versus operator errors.

The potential for problems arising from computational errors in either the hardware or software dictates that special precautions be taken in regard to documenting how an automated testing system arrives at the reported results. Manufacturer-supplied operation manuals should include detailed descriptions of all formulas that the software uses in its calculations, both for tests and for predicted values. All formulas should be adequately referenced to the scientific literature. Software source code may be furnished by the programmer, but it may be less useful than a detailed description of software functions, depending on the programming expertise of the user. The user should be able to manually calculate all values for comparison with the software-generated results. Manual calculations require that the testing equipment provide all necessary raw data, as described previously, and that tracings (i.e., spirograms, flow-volume curves) be standardized so as to allow manual measurement of flows and volumes. Changes in computational methods, pattern recognition algorithms, or formulas themselves that are made when a particular software version is "upgraded" should be detailed by the programmer. If test results change significantly because of software upgrades, such as when an upgrade corrects a software problem, modification of previously derived results may be necessary. Maintenance of patient results in a data base format (see following Data Management section) permits such "corrections" to be applied.

User-generated documentation should include a log or data base of validation routines and related measures, such as testing of normal subjects or the use of simulators.

---

*MS-DOS and OS/2 are registered trademarks of Microsoft, Inc.

†UNIX is a registered trademark of AT & T.

Data management

The format in which test data is stored by a computerized laboratory system is the attribute that may require the most careful consideration. Essential elements to consider in selecting a system to manage patient data are the complexity of the raw and reduced data to be saved, how many tests will be done per month or year, and what type of access to the data is required. Three general approaches to data management are typically implemented in automated pulmonary function equipment:

Temporary or no data storage. Many portable spirometers and most manual laboratory spirometers provide either temporary storage of patient data or none at all. Some spirometers that use a dedicated microprocessor often use battery-powered RAM, allowing multiple patient tests to be stored in memory for inspection and printing. Many of these instruments permit temporary storage so that the data can be recalled after the microprocessor is powered down, and the stored information can be transferred (dumped) to another computer or to a printer. Some monitoring devices, such as pulse oximeters, also provide for limited data storage with interfaces for communicating with external computers or printers.

Permanent patient data files. Because many automated pulmonary function test systems use microcomputers, permanent storage of patient data is usually accomplished by creating files on either floppy or hard disks. The simplest design for this type of storage is to assign all of the patient data to one or two conventional computer files that are named with a unique identifier, such as a Social Security Number. The amount of data that can be stored in files of this type is usually limited by the operating system that the computer uses and the physical capacity (kilobytes or megabytes) of the storage device. A commonly used format is one in which patient demographic data and individual test results are stored in defined fields within each file. Specific test data can be retrieved by extracting the value located in a particular position within the file. Graphic data (i.e., raw data for reconstructing spirograms or flow-volume curves) is usually stored in a format that allows the data to be read into the computer sequentially. Because several hundred to several thousand raw data values may be required to draw a spirogram, graphic data typically take more space than tabular data on the storage device.

Data base storage. A more highly organized method of computerized storage for pulmonary function data used a relational data base format. In this model, similar tests, such as spirometry, lung volumes, and DL_{CO}, from different subjects are stored in files that are linked to form a data base. Each set of test data forms a record within an individual file. The results of a particular study are linked across files by a common index, such as a unique patient number. This structure allows data base functions such as sorting, selecting, searching, editing, and reporting of various combinations of patient data. Some practical applications of a data base system for management of pulmonary function data include:

1. Serial comparisons of multiple tests on a single subject and longitudinal studies on groups of subjects
2. The ability to perform specialized queries relating any of the stored data fields for purposes of research or laboratory management
3. The ability to generate highly specialized reports
4. Use of multiple sets of predicted values stored in a data base format, and input of user-defined coefficients for predicting normal values

Most relational data base systems support a special command language, such as Structured Query Language (SQL), which allows the user to access the data base for data entry and retrieval, report generation, and maintenance functions such as importing or exporting records.

No matter what type of data storage is used, it is usually not realistic to store all raw data, except in a research setting, because of the large amount of raw data generated from multiple spirometric efforts, lung volume determinations, and DL_{CO} maneuvers. Most systems reduce the data load by limiting the amount of graphic information stored. Because of the importance of volume-time and flow-volume tracings in a pulmonary function laboratory, a completely "paperless" filing system may not be practical if all patient efforts must be maintained. Computer storage of the interpretation text may use more storage space than the test results if lengthy interpretations are commonly made.

A common limitation to the amount of patient data that can be managed from a practical standpoint is the storage media that a particular system uses. The high-density (1.2 to 1.44 M) floppy diskette can typically store the data from several hundred subjects, depending on the types of tests performed and the graphic data saved. Hard disk systems of 20 Mb or more can obviously store much more data; however, they also typically require a more sophisticated operating system to keep track of the files created, and they must periodically be backed up to prevent loss of a large amount of information should the drive fail. These considerations are magnified as the capacity of the hard disk system is increased. Individual laboratories must carefully decide on the most appropriate means of maintaining subject data files, including scheduled backups and security of computer stored information. Other important attributes of a computerized data filing system for pulmonary function studies include some means of editing stored data easily and transferring the data to other computers for use with other programs. Most commercially available pulmonary function software allows for user selection of the actual data to be saved, in addition to providing algorithms to assist in choosing valid data (see Chapter 11). If the software controls the data stored for each component (i.e., patient information, spirometry, lung volumes) a file editor is useful for correcting erroneous user input or for manually entering data obtained by an independent means.

Printers and plotters

One of the most noticeable advancements in computerized pulmonary function testing in recent years is the capability of generating high-quality, high-resolution graphic representations of volume-time spirograms, flow-volume curves, and plethysmograph tangents in addition to tabular data. Peripherals used for printing graphic images and reports include the dot matrix printer, ink-jet printers, thermal printers, laser printers and the digital plotter.

Dot matrix printers. These printers use a series of between 9 and 24 pins to generate both alphanumeric characters and graphics. The fastest dot matrix printers, which print more than 200 characters per second, use fewer pins to achieve high speed, and the text characters are not fully formed. Most dot matrix printers, using various combinations of pins, can produce near letter-quality characters at lower speeds or draft-quality characters when a quick report is needed. Dot matrix printers are relatively fast and have the ability to generate high-resolution graphic images, but usually at rates significantly less than for text printing. Some dot matrix printers, especially high-speed models, may be somewhat noisy in the testing area. Some printers use multicolor ribbons so that color graphics and text can be generated.

Thermal transfer printers. These printers are extremely quiet but require heat-sensitive paper, which may discolor with time. Thermal printers are used on many portable spirometers to generate reports that include text and graphics. Their small size, paper widths may vary from only 2 to 8 inches, makes them practical for transportable units. The text characters resemble those produced by dot matrix printers, and the speeds are somewhat less than fast dot matrix printers.

Ink-jet printers. These printers apply a small jet of ink directly to the paper to form both characters and graphic images; they are very quiet and relatively fast. Text quality equals that of most 24-pin dot matrix printers and is close to the high-quality characters produced by laser printers. Color ink-jet printers allow text and graphics to be printed.

Laser printers. These printers offer the highest quality text and graphics. Laser printers use a laser beam to form the images of letters and graphs on a drum, which then transfers toner to paper, printing an entire page at one time. The speed of laser printers is described by the number of pages of text that can be printed per minute, which usually ranges from 6 to 10 pages. Graphic images are more complex and require longer to print than text, but the speed usually equals that of the dot matrix printer. Laser printers are very quiet and relatively easy to maintain. The high-quality text and graphic images that the laser printer can produce are not inexpensive; laser printers can cost two to three times as much as a good quality dot matrix printer, and the cost per page is also somewhat higher. Laser printers are large and heavy, often occupying more space than the microcomputer itself. Laser printers contain their own microprocessor and RAM memory. Increased memory, of more than 1 megabyte, or special interface cards are usually required if full-page graphic images are to be printed routinely.

Digital plotters. These plotters interface directly to many computers, and with appropriate software to drive them, they can be used to produce high-quality, multicolor representations of almost any figures that can be generated on the video display. Plotters are generally slower than dot matrix printers when producing alphanumeric characters, but they produce graphs rapidly. However, they are usually quiet, which may be an important consideration in a busy laboratory.

To speed up the generation of graphic images, and to allow the computer to be used while the printer is working, many systems use a hardware printer buffer or a software spooling program. The hardware buffer is a memory device placed between the computer and printer or plotter that accepts data much faster than the printer alone. The data are then fed to the printer/plotter at a slower rate while the computer is freed to perform other tasks. Many printers have built-in memory that functions as a buffer. A software spooler is a program that resides in memory along with the pulmonary function testing programs and functions much like the hardware buffer. The spooler accepts data, then "spools" it to the output device at an appropriate rate. Dumping graphic images, even with a buffer or spooler, is usually slow because of the large number of bytes required for high resolution graphics. Spoolers are somewhat less efficient than hardware buffers because the computer's microprocessor must control the spooler, while the hardware buffer has its own processor. High-speed microprocessors that support multitasking can perform printing as a background process with little or no loss of speed.

Hardware and software compatibility

One of the benefits of a computerized pulmonary function laboratory is the availability of the computer for tasks other than performing automated testing. This perhaps explains the trend that many manufacturers are following of interfacing existing pulmonary function equipment with generic microcomputers and peripherals (Fig. 10-3). Two important considerations, if the computer is to be used for additional tasks, are whether the system will run commercial (off-the-shelf) software, and whether the pulmonary function software can be used in conjunction with other programs.

Compatibility with commercial software depends largely on the microprocessor and operating system that the computer employs. Because of the large variety of microcomputers available, determination of software compatibility may require actual testing on the system in question. In addition, the user must have a basic familiarity with specific programs to ascertain if the hardware that is incorporated into the pulmonary function testing system supports the commercial program (see Additional Applications section of this chapter). For example, a pulmonary function testing system

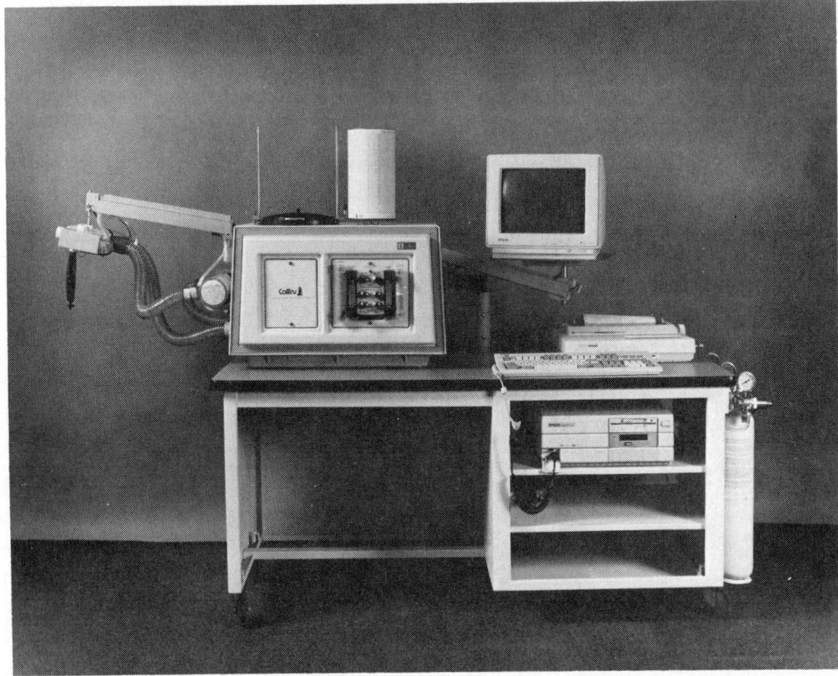

Fig. 10-3 Computerized pulmonary function system. An automated pulmonary function system, including Stead-Wells spirometer, kymograph, and gas analyzers for performing lung volumes and DL_{CO}, is interfaced to a generic microcomputer. The microcomputer allows rapid processing of data, including calculation of test variables, BTPS corrections, display of tabular and graphic information, and data storage on floppy or hard disk. The computer can also be used for other tasks. (Courtesy Warren E. Collins, Inc., Braintree, Mass.)

that uses an ink-jet printer may not function with a word processing program unless the program specifically supports that printer.

The use of other programs as adjuncts to the pulmonary function software may be quite easy or it may require rather high-level programming, if it is possible at all. Two typical applications would be running a separate program simultaneously with the pulmonary software and transferring data (i.e., test results) from the pulmonary software to another program, such as a data base or spreadsheet. The function of the pulmonary function application can often be enhanced by using it with programs such as an operating system shell; memory resident utilities, such as calculators, notetakers, and help files; print spoolers; or RAM disks. Compatibility with these types of programs usually requires testing, and may depend on whether the pulmonary function software was designed to operate with other programs in memory. The ability to transfer data between the pulmonary function software and other applications is also very useful. For example, if the pulmonary function program creates standard text files, then a simple text editor or word processor can be used to modify them or generate customized reports. Most data base and spreadsheet programs (see Data bases and Spreadsheet sections of this chapter) have functions that allow them to import data, if the data are in a format that is widely used. Similarly, if the pulmonary function software is well documented or the source code is available, then application programs in a higher-level language such as BASIC, C, or PASCAL can be developed to access data generated by the program. Some manufacturers provide this type of customization as part of the original purchase, while others provide source code and documentation so that customization can be provided by the user.

Communications

An application of pulmonary function testing that is becoming increasingly widespread is the "outreach" type of testing facility. Typically, this consists of pulmonary function test equipment located at a remote site, which then communicates with a central laboratory computer via standard phone lines. The remote or satellite laboratory may be miles away or within the same building. The telecommunications supporting this type of system are usually implemented by means of a modem at both locations. The modem translates digital data from the computer into tones for phone line transmission that can then be decoded back into digital data by the receiving computer's modem. Many computers have an RS-232—more or less an industry standard for communications—or similar port built in. The communications port allows data to be transmitted serially, (i.e., one bit at a time) very rapidly either to a modem, for remote devices, or to another local device, such as a computer, or printer. The combination of the RS-232C port and modem allows a small computer at a remote site to transmit and receive data from a centrally located host. The host system supports specially designed software that allows communications with several remote terminals. In this way, computerized tests are performed at the remote site, and a copy of the data is transmitted to the host system where it can be evaluated and interpreted.

A related type of system is the multiuser computer, in which a centrally located computer communicates with smaller computers or simple terminals to share programs and data. This type of setup is referred to as a *local area network.* Although multiuser systems have previously required a minicomputer, faster and more powerful microprocessors can support multiple users with the appropriate operating system. Multiuser systems are ideal for large laboratories in which computerized pulmonary function testing, exercise testing, and blood gas analysis are all performed. A multiuser computer permits stations to be "dedicated" to particular tasks, while sharing programs that are needed in several areas and transferring data from one location to another. Multiuser systems are complex and somewhat difficult to implement, but they may save time and money in a high-volume laboratory if they are properly designed.

System maintenance

In a large, automated pulmonary function testing system that includes various input devices along with monitors, disk drives, printers, plotters, and modems, system maintenance may become involved. In addition to the service to spirometers and gas analyzers, the computer and its peripherals also require preventive and sometimes corrective maintenance.

Perhaps the most common source of problems is the software itself; programs may load improperly or fail while accessing data from a storage device or other peripheral. Most operating systems and languages provide ample error messages to assist in tracking down software problems. Good application programs report full error messages; some systems report only error codes, which must then be looked up in a manual. Careful evaluation of error codes or messages often provides an indication of the source of the error. Programs often fail when attempting to communicate with a peripheral device that is not ready or that is operating incorrectly. For example, if the program expects data from the analog-to-digital converter, but the converter is not functioning, the program may try to process incorrect data or simply lock up. Well-designed software contains error traps to handle most types of input or communication errors, but not every problem can be anticipated. A troubleshooting guide is invaluable in tracking down computer problems, and should be keyed to the error messages that the program displays. Many systems contain diagnostic programs that allow memory checks, disk drive checks, and related hardware evaluation. Such diagnostics allow the user to determine if the error is software- or hardware-based. A large number of utility programs are available for microcomputers and peripherals that allow testing of disk drives, file integrity, and system performance.

Because most application programs use disk or tape drives for data and program storage, errors arising from problems with the storage device are rather common. Because hard drives are capable of holding large amounts of data, a device failure may mean the loss of significant information. The most direct solution to these errors is to maintain adequate backups of all programs and data, and to rotate backup disks or tapes at regular intervals. For hardware malfunctions, such as printer breakdowns and disk drive failures, the usual course of action is to replace the suspected component. Many systems use components that are relatively easy, although not always inexpensive, to replace. Dirt, dust, smoke, and humidity quite often interfere with sensitive electronics, but they can be managed with a minimum of preventive care. Cabling and connectors between components are another source of hardware errors that should be evaluated whenever a peripheral begins functioning erratically or suddenly stops functioning.

Because of the number of computerized systems available, not every capability can be adequately described. Those discussed herein include many of the important aspects related to automated data handling in the pulmonary function laboratory and may be considerations in the selection of a computerized testing system.

LANGUAGES AND PROGRAMMING

The majority of pulmonary function technologists may use computerized pulmonary function testing systems without programming expertise. However, to fully understand the process of data acquisition and processing, some background in programming concepts and computer languages is helpful. A sound understanding of how the computer controls various peripheral devices is useful for tracking down both hardware and software malfunctions. Some programming skill may allow the development of utility routines to supplement a full-scale testing package. Many application programs, such as data bases, use their own "command" languages to allow programming of often-used functions. Understanding the operating system that controls most computer functions is a valuable tool for the technologist, because it allows him or her to manage not only the pulmonary function software, but various utility programs as well.

Computer languages

Each microprocessor recognizes a set of instructions that are referred to as "machine language." These instructions are usually in binary form (0 or 1) and represent the lowest-level language for controlling the computer. Because it is difficult to program using binary numbers, a special "assembly" language is used that applies mnemonics to each command. An assembly language program may be written using a text editor or word processor. This code is then processed by an assembler, which converts the mnemonics into machine language instructions. The resulting low-level program is usually stored in the form of hexadecimal bytes; hexadecimal refers to the number system with a base equal to 16 decimal. Assembly language programs are extremely fast and usually do not require a great deal of RAM. However, writing large programs in assembly language is a task that requires a great deal of programming expertise; the programmer must not only understand the machine language instructions but also must be familiar with the specific hardware that the microprocessor will address. Many commercially available general purpose programs (i.e., word processors, spreadsheet) as well as some pulmonary function packages are written in assembly language.

BASIC (Beginner's All-purpose Symbolic Instructional Code) has been used for more than 20 years, and it has gained a lot of popularity with the scientific and technical community because of the ease with which it can be learned. High-level mathematic and text handling functions as well as file management are all possible in BASIC. Although it is relatively easy to write complex programs in BASIC, the language functions through an interpreter, which significantly slows execution. The BASIC interpreter translates each program line as the program is running into code that the microprocessor can then execute. BASIC is often too slow for many applications, such as communicating with fast devices such as A/D converters. Two solutions to the slow execution problem with BASIC programs are widely applied. The first is to use a combination of machine language subroutines and BASIC code to speed up critical portions of the program. A machine language routine might be used to access the A/D converter and then pass the numeric values back to the BASIC program that called the subroutine. The second solution is to "compile" the BASIC program code into a form that is quite similar to native machine language. With careful programming, a speedup of tenfold or more is often possible using compiled BASIC. One problem with this technique is that some BASIC commands cannot be compiled easily, particularly those that allow BASIC to function through the computer's operating system. Similarly, the compiled BASIC program cannot be easily modified without recompiling the source code. Nonetheless, some pulmonary function software packages use one or more of these techniques and support BASIC as the primary program language. For relatively short programs, especially when execution time is not critical, BASIC functions well because of its ease of use and ability for rapid modification.

FORTRAN (FORmula TRANslation) has been the high-level language implemented for most scientific and technical applications, particularly on minicomputers. FORTRAN is a compiled language. The source program is coded according to a structured format and then compiled before the program is actually run. In general, compiled programs execute much faster than interpreted programs, as in BASIC, because error checking is carried out during the compilation phase. FORTRAN supports calls to machine language subroutines so that it can be used as high-level language and still manage tasks such as reading data from A/D converters or other instruments. FORTRAN was designed primarily for numeric manipulations and does not allow for easy handling of text characters. The large number of programs and subroutines already written and the fact that FORTRAN is available for most microprocessors may make it attractive for laboratories developing their own software.

A third high-level language with increased implementations in pulmonary function laboratories is PASCAL. PASCAL is a compiled language that requires a highly structured source program. The source program is compiled into an intermediate form called p-code, which is then interpreted at the time the program is run. PASCAL supports a number of functions that allow complex programs to be written easily, much like BASIC, but with the advantage of greater speed of execution. Because PASCAL is highly structured, PASCAL programs can be written in small parts, and then the parts can be linked together as a series of procedures or used repeatedly as necessary. Another advantage of the highly structured nature of PASCAL is the ability to create libraries of routines that can be incorporated into programs.

The high-level language that has assumed a leading place in the development of many commercial software packages as well as pulmonary function software is C. C has a block structure similar to PASCAL, but it is more concise and efficient. By design, C is a simple language, and is often categorized as the lowest of the high-level languages. The flexibility of C allows it to duplicate many assembly language functions, while programs can be written in more understandable and maintainable code. Because C is capable of relatively low-level operations, C programs can achieve levels of speed and efficiency comparable to assembly language programs. C programs are built around functions, with one function, always called *main,* as the entry point into the program. Functions can call other functions, including themselves, and can retrieve values from the called routine. C has been widely used for development of operating systems (see next section) as well as application programs. UNIX, the popular multiuser, multitasking operating system, is written almost entirely in C. C is also well suited for applications running under the MS-DOS or OS/2 operating systems. The simplicity and flexibility of C allows C programs to be highly transportable. As long as the program does not use hardware-specific features, applications developed for one microprocessor can easily be adapted to run on another microprocessor.

Many language systems support interaction between languages; this allows one high-level language to call subroutines or functions written in another language, either high- or low-level. New high-level languages provide facilities to define new and complex data structures, called objects. Programs written using these structures are called object-oriented programs (OOPs). Object-oriented programming adds more structure to languages such as PASCAL and C by binding data together with routines (i.e., procedures and functions) that act on it. Object-oriented programs are highly modular, making it easy to replace or enhance parts of a program without affecting the rest of it.

Operating systems

Perhaps the "language" most often used in pulmonary function laboratories is the operating system (OS) or disk operating system (DOS). The OS is primarily responsible for supervising input/output functions of the computer, such as file management, controlling information sent to the video display, and accepting input from the keyboard or other devices. The OS also coordinates many functions from the application programs running on the computer, no matter what language they use. The technologist may use the operating system for several important functions: copying files or programs, backing up data files, calling a directory of files on a particular device, sorting files, as well as for running specific application programs. Most operating systems support an automatic mode of control; this allows the user to perform multiple procedures by executing a single program. Commands normally entered from the keyboard are stored in a special file called a "batch" or "job control" file. By calling the batch file, the same steps can be repeated as often as needed. Batch files are extremely helpful for initializing small computer systems; programs for controlling printers, screen displays, and other devices can be loaded automatically so that the main program functions correctly. Batch files can also be used for tedious tasks, such as backing up selected data files on a routine basis. Other utilities offered by most operating systems include programs for formatting storage media (i.e., disks), editing files, protecting files with passwords, deleting files, and defining parameters for the operation of the video display and the printer. Most OS functions are initiated by entering commands at the keyboard. "Shell" programs provide an alternate interface so that the user does not have to remember the system's commands or type them. Sophisticated interfaces allow the user to indicate the desired function with a special pointing device, such as a mouse or touch screen, by opening windows on the display in response to various choices.

Several operating systems are in use on minicomputers and microcomputers, but a few are quite common—MS-DOS, OS/2, UNIX. While a few pulmonary function systems support their own operating systems, most use one or more of the "off-the-shelf" systems to provide compatibility with other commercially available software. MS/DOS has a large base of application programs, but it is limited to providing single-user microcomputer functions. OS/2 provides multitasking capabilities on advanced 16- or 32-bit processors. UNIX supports both multitasking and multiple users, and can be run on both minicomputers and microcomputers. Many hybrid operating systems are available that allow programs designed to run under one operating system to be used in different operating environments, or to enhance program capabilities by allowing access to more sophisticated operating system functions.

While most pulmonary function laboratories use computers for performing tests, relatively few do extensive programming. Development of a comprehensive pulmonary function testing package, complete with interfacing to all necessary laboratory instruments, is an involved task. Most laboratories developing their own software find it useful to engage professional programmers and consultants. The cost, in time and money, of producing a custom testing program is usually prohibitive, unless special computer resources (i.e., programmers and facilities) are available. However, programming skills using languages such as C, PASCAL, BASIC, FORTRAN, or ASSEMBLY can allow in-house development of utilities and supplementary programs to enhance or extend commercially available software. A working knowledge of the operating system used by a particular computer can greatly enhance day-to-day functions of the laboratory.

Skill in using other application programs, such as spreadsheet and word processors, can increase the productivity of a system designed primarily for pulmonary function testing.

ADDITIONAL APPLICATIONS

In addition to software for automating pulmonary function testing, several other types of application programs lend themselves to use in the pulmonary function laboratory. These include interpretation programs for pulmonary function tests, blood gas data, and quality control programs; spreadsheets; data base managers; word processing programs; and educational applications.

Pulmonary function interpretation programs

Many pulmonary function software packages include an interpretation program as an option. Most interpretation programs are based on one or more sets of algorithms for defining the presence of obstructive, restrictive, combined, or normal patterns on standard spirometry, lung volumes, and DL_{CO}. These interpretive programs analyze the results measured during standard pulmonary function studies, comparing the values attained by the subject to predicted normal values. Most algorithms are based on the same logic that a clinical interpreter might use. The computerized interpreter, however, does not have the benefit of including the subject's clinical history or other laboratory findings in the interpretation process. Depending on the sohistication of the program, computerized interpreters generally manage to point out the presence or absence of obstruction or restriction. Incorrect computerized interpretations may occur if test results are invalid because of inadequate effort or nonreproducible data. Computerized interpretation in no way substitutes for evaluation by a qualified interpreter, but it is helpful in situations in which an immediate report of gross abnormalities is necessary, or for teaching purposes. If a computerized interpretation is included in the report to become part of the medical record, it should be clearly labelled as such. Computerized interpretations should never be used as the only interpretation, and they should always be reviewed by a qualified reader.

Blood gas programs

Computerization in the blood gas laboratory includes several different categories of programs. Blood gas interpretation by computer is implemented by applying algorithms to evaluate acid-base status and oxygenation. Computerized blood gas interpretation can be useful in situations in which immediate interpretation to rule out gross abnormalities is required. Because the computer can routinely evaluate all of the measured and calculated blood gas parameters, it may often suggest abnormalities that the casual interpreter might overlook. As with computerized pulmonary function interpretation, blood gas interpretations should always be held as preliminary and formally verified by a qualified interpreter. Other contexts in which computerization is useful in the blood gas laboratory are quality control and data reporting. Because evaluation of multiple levels of controls requires statistical manipulation of large amounts of data (see Chapter 11), the computer is ideally suited to maintaining a quality assurance program. Most quality control programs require the calculation of means and standard deviations for each level of each component control material (i.e., pH, $P\text{CO}_2$, PO_2). Because controls are usually run daily or more frequently, often on multiple instruments, computerization of data files greatly reduces the record-keeping functions in a busy laboratory. A second advantage is that the computer can be used to interpret the results of quality control runs in real time, so that the technologist can immediately determine the status of each individual blood gas electrode (see also Chapter 11). Quality assurance programs that are compatible with a variety of microcomputers are available from several professional organizations.

Data reporting lends itself to computerization because many patients receive multiple blood gas analyses. Most automated or semi-automated analyzers can be interfaced via the standard RS-232 (see Data Acquisition and Instrument Control section of this chapter) or similar communication port so that blood gas data can be stored on disk or tape, with reports generated as required. Interfacing of the blood gas analyzer directly to a hospital information system allows blood gas data to be available wherever a terminal is located, and tends to reduce transcription errors and lost results.

Data bases

Data base management programs are available for almost every small computer. Most allow the user to design what information will be stored and how it will be arranged. Computer data bases permit the user to save information in much the same manner as a conventional file, but the computer can rapidly sort the information, search for records meeting specific criteria, and generate reports as required. A common application in an area such as pulmonary function testing is maintaining records of tests performed, patient demographics, diagnoses, and referral sources. Other uses include records of departmental inventory, expenditures, and similar operational information. As noted previously, some pulmonary function software packages use a relational data base for storing test results from pulmonary function or blood gas studies. The combination of a relational data base and a large-capacity hard disk makes it possible to maintain a large number of patient studies that can be retrieved using typical data base queries. Reference lists and bibliographies can be maintained as a data base. A number of free-form data bases are available that allow disparate types of data, such as memos, reports, references, and test results) to be accessed in a manner similar to the records and fields of a conventional data base.

Many commercially available data base management programs can be integrated so that information from spreadsheets, word processing programs, or even pulmonary function data can be easily exchanged.

Spreadsheets

Electronic spreadsheets were originally designed as financial planning tools, replacing the ledger book. However, their ability to organize numeric data and perform repetitive calculations make them ideal for many scientific and technical purposes. Spreadsheets use matrix arithmetic; numbers or formulas are placed in the cells of a two-dimensional matrix. A value or the result of an equation can then be accessed by referring to its location (i.e., row and column). By adding math and logic functions, rows or columns of numbers can be added, subtracted, averaged, or otherwise evaluated. The spreadsheet is quite useful for statistical calculations, such as computation of means and standard deviations for blood gas quality control. Many spreadsheets have basic statistical functions built in. Reducing data from procedures such as exercise tests, in which the same calculations are performed repetitively (i.e., at each exercise work load), can be quickly performed via the spreadsheet. A formula can be entered in one cell and then replicated to additional cells, with the variables in the formula being adjusted relative to the position of the cell in the spreadsheet. If a formula sums the two cells immediately above it, a copy of the formula that will always add the two cells above it may be made anywhere on the sheet. Any data that are normally reduced using a calculator can be managed by a spreadsheet. Most spreadsheets can also be used for storing and editing numeric data, and for generating customized reports. Typical spreadsheet applications include conventional data base functions, importing data from and exporting data to other applications, and generating graphic representations of numeric data.

Word processing

Text handling or processing is one of the most widespread uses of small computer systems. In conjunction with an appropriate printer, a word processor can be used to generate almost any type of document that normally would require typing or printing. In addition, the document is stored on magnetic media so that revisions or copies can be made as needed. In the laboratory environment, word processors are ideal for maintaining documents, such as procedure manuals, that typically require constant updating. In addition, word processors can be used to generate customized reports; in many instances, data can be transferred directly from another program (i.e., spreadsheet, data base) and incorporated into the report. Pulmonary function software that stores data in text files can usually be interfaced to a word processing program for custom report generation. Some pulmonary function software packages include a simple editor for inserting comments or adding an interpreation to the stored report. While not a full-fledged word processor, these editors permit text data to be stored and retrieved along with the usual tabular data.

Educational programs

Computer-assisted instruction has several potential applications in the pulmonary function laboratory. Information that is normally taught by repetitive drill can usually be administered via computer. Many programs are available to allow multiple choice and other types of questions to be administered via the computer; because the computer can easily score the results of a test taken, it becomes both an educational and evaluation instrument for certain types of material. Computerized simulations are another teaching tool that can be adapted for laboratory personnel, particularly for interpreting the results of pulmonary function studies or blood gas analyses.

Libraries of reference material covering a variety of subjects are available on laser disks, called CD-ROM disks. Although somewhat slow, these devices allow huge amounts of reference data to be available via the computer and they may replace conventional reference texts for information that does not change often.

SELF-ASSESSMENT QUESTIONS

1. Computer memory that contains a fixed set of instructions that cannot be changed by a user program is (are):
   a. RAM
   b. ROM
   c. PROM
   d. EPROM
   e. b, c, and d

2. The optical disk (laser disk) differs from conventional floppy diskettes in that:
   a. It is much smaller in size
   b. It can store many times more data
   c. It can only be used to store numeric data
   d. All of the above

3. The smallest volume that can be measured by a "12-bit" analog-to-digital converter interfaced to a 10-L spirometer is:
   a. 83 ml
   b. 12 ml
   c. 4.096 ml
   d. 2.4 ml

4. Microprocessor-controlled laboratory instruments can communicate with an external computer by means of:
   a. A preprocessor
   b. A D/A converter
   c. An expanded memory board
   d. A serial port

5. The best means of determining the accuracy of software used to reduce pulmonary function data is:
   a. Performing frequent calibration checks
   b. Performing duplicate tests on a random basis
   c. Checking results against the same data calculated manually
   d. Both a and b

6. Documentation of a microcomputer-based pulmonary function system should include:
   I. Directions for the operating system of the computer
   II. Formulas used by the software
   III. Explanations of error codes generated by the computer
   IV. Instructions for installing peripheral devices
   a. I, II, III, IV
   b. II, III, IV
   c. II, III only
   d. II, IV only

7. A program can be considered downward-compatible if:
   a. It can be upgraded by laboratory personnel
   b. It can be transferred to a smaller microprocessor
   c. It can accept data from previous versions of the program
   d. It can be run on either a floppy or hard disk system

8. Which of the following devices are capable of printing graphs:
   I. Laser printers
   II. Dot matrix printers
   III. Thermal transfer printers
   IV. Digital plotters
   a. I, II, III, IV
   b. I, II, IV
   c. II, III, IV
   d. I, III only

9. A "shell" program is often used to:
   a. Provide multitasking capabilities to an operating system
   b. Provide multiple users access to the same file
   c. Provide an interface to the operating system
   d. Enhance the compatibility between application programs

10. Comptuerized interpretation of blood gas analysis:
   I. May be used if a qualified interpreter is not available
   II. May be useful in detecting gross abnormalities
   III. May suggest subtle abnormalities that might have been overlooked
   IV. Uses a series of algorithms to evaluate acid-base and oxygenation status
   a. I, II, III, IV
   b. I, III, IV
   c. II, III, IV
   d. II, III only

SELECTED BIBLIOGRAPHY

Computerized pulmonary function testing

American Thoracic Society, Committee on Proficiency Standards for Clinical Pulmonary Laboratories: Computer guidelines for pulmonary laboratories, Am Rev Respir Dis 134:628, 1986.

Black KH, Petusevsky ML, and Gaensler EA: A general purpose microprocessor for spirometry, Chest 78:605, 1980.

Crapo RO et al: Automation of pulmonary function equipment—user beware!, Chest 90:1, 1986, (editorial).

Dickman ML et al: On-line computerized spirometry in 738 normal adults, Am Rev Respir Dis 100:780, 1969.

Gardner RM et al: Computerized decision-making in the pulmonary function laboratory, Respir Care 27(7):799, 1982.

Jones NL: Clinical exercise testing, ed 3, Philadelphia, 1988, WB Saunders Co.

Computer data acquisition

Engleman B and Abraham M: Personal computer signal processing, Byte 4:94, 1984.

Mellichamp D, editor: Real-time computing—with applications to data acquisition and control, New York: 1983, Van Nostrand Reinhold.

Tompkins WJ and Webster JG, edtiors: Design of microcomputer-based medical instrumentation, New Jersey, 1981, Prentice Hall.

Wyss CR: Planning a computerized measurement system, Byte 4:114, 1985.

Computer applications

Byers RA: Everyman's database primer, Culver City, Calif, 1984, Ashton-Tate.

Cohn JD, Engler RC, and DelGuercio RL: The automated physiologic profile, Crit Care Med 3:51, 1975.

Ellis JH, Perera SP, and Levin DC: A computer program for the interpretation of pulmonary function studies, Chest 68:209, 1975.

Gardner RM et al: Computerized blood gas interpretation and reporting system, Computer 8(1):39, 1975.

Miller H: Introduction to spreadsheets, PC World 2:66, 1984.

Silage DA and Maxwell C: A spirometry/interpretation program for hand-held computers, Respir Care 28:62, 1983.

Languages and programming

Duncan R: Advanced OS/2, Bellevue, Wash, 1988, Microsoft Press.

Kernigham BW and Ritchie DM: The C programming language, ed 2, Englewood Cliffs, N.J., 1988, Prentice Hall.

Norton P: Inside the IBM-PC, New York, 1986, Brady Books.

Waite M, Martin D, and Prata S: Unix primer plus, Indianapolis, 1983, Howard W Sams & Co, Publishers.

Wolverton V: Running MS-DOS , ed 2, Bellevue, Wash, 1988 Microsoft Press.

11

Quality Assurance in the Pulmonary Function Laboratory

ELEMENTS OF LABORATORY QUALITY CONTROL

Quality control is essential to the operation of the pulmonary function laboratory in order to obtain valid and reproducible data. Four main components are necessary for a quality assurance program:

1. *Methodology.* The type of equipment used (i.e., spirometer, gas analyzer, recorder) determines to a certain extent the procedures required for calibration and quality control, and how often such procedures must be performed. The particular methods used for spirometry, lung volumes, $D_{L_{CO}}$, blood gases and exercise testing are usually determined by the needs of physicians using the laboratory, as well as by the number and complexity of the tests performed. Methods and equipment that have been validated in the scientific literature are typically easier to maintain and control than those that have never been evaluated, or which, after evaluation, have failed to meet minimum standards.
2. *Instrument maintenance.* As with the particular methodology employed, the type and complexity of the instrumentation for a specific test will determine the extent of day-to-day maintenance that will be required. Preventive maintenance is that which is scheduled in anticipation of equipment malfunction, to reduce the possibility of equipment failure. Corrective maintenance or repair is unscheduled service required to correct equipment failure that is signaled by quality control procedures or extreme results during testing. Familiarity with the operating characteristics of spirometers, gas analyzers, plethysmographs, and computers is best accomplished by manufacturer support and thorough documentation. A procedure manual (see box on p. 288) and accurate records are essential to an ongoing maintenance program, and are required by most accrediting organizations.
3. *Control methods.* Test signals appropriate to each particular instrument (spirometers, gas analyzers, blood gas analyzers) are necessary to determine both the accuracy and the precision of the data reported. Because many laboratories use computerized pulmonary

function or blood gas analyzers, control signals are required to ensure that both software and hardware are functioning within acceptable limits. Control methods may vary from mechanical flow generators (for spirometers) to tonometered blood (for blood gas analyzers).

4. *Testing (sampling) technique.* A primary means of ensuring quality data is to rigidly control the methods and procedures by which data are obtained. In pulmonary function testing, "sampling technique" refers to the ability of the technician to perform the test procedure and the subject's ability to cooperate in the test maneuvers. Technician and subject performance, as well as proper equipment function, must be evaluated on a test-by-test basis, by applying appropriate criteria to determine the acceptability of the results.

This chapter deals primarily with the appropriate control signals for instrument maintenance and calibration, and with criteria for acceptability for various categories of pulmonary function tests (i.e., spirometry, lung volumes, DL_{CO}). The operating characteristics (methodologies) of various types of pulmonary function testing equipment were discussed in Chapter 9.

PULMONARY FUNCTION PROCEDURE MANUAL

Items to be included in a typical procedure manual for a pulmonary function laboratory. For each procedure performed the following should be present:

1. Description of the test, and its purpose
2. Indications for ordering the test and contraindications, if any
3. Description of the general method(s) and any specific equipment required
4. Calibration of equipment required before testing, referencing manufacturer's documentation as needed
5. Patient preparation for the test, if any (i.e., withholding medication)
6. Step-by-step procedure for both computerized and manual measurement/calculation of results
7. Quality control guidelines with acceptable limits of performance and corrective actions to be taken
8. Safety precautions related to the procedure (i.e., infection control, hazards), and alert values that require physician notification
9. References for all equations used for calculating results and predicted normal values, including a bibliography
10. Documentaiton of computer protocols for calculations and data storage; guidelines for computer downtime
11. Dated signatures of the medical and technical directors

Each laboratory should have a written quality assurance program that includes descriptions of the methods employed for specific tests, the limitations of the procedure (if any), indications or schedules for maintenance, quality controls to be used, action to be taken if controls exceed specified limits, and specific guidelines as to how tests are to be performed. The quality assurance program should be included as part of the laboratory procedure manual (see box on p. 288).

Two concepts that are central to quality assurance are the definitions of *accuracy* and *precision.* Accuracy may be defined as the extent to which measurement of a known quantity results in a value approximating that quantity. In most laboratory settings, this is accomplished by taking repeated measurements and calculating the mean (or average) for the data. If the mean value approximates the known, then the instrument is considered to be accurate. Precision may be defined as the extent to which repeated measurements of the same quantity can be reproduced. If the same parameter is measured repeatedly and the resulting values are similar, the instrument may be considered precise. Accuracy and precision are not always present concurrently in the same instrument. A spirometer that consistently measures a 3-L test volume as 2.5 L is precise, but not very accurate. A spirometer that evaluates a 3-L test volume as 2.5, 3.0, and 3.5 L on repeated maneuvers shows an accurate mean of 3.0 L, but the individual measurements are not precise. Determination of the accuracy *and* precision of instruments such as spirometers is particularly important because many common pulmonary function tests are "effort dependent." The largest value observed, rather than the mean, is often reported as the "best test" (see the Criteria for Acceptability of Spirometry section of this chapter), based on the premise that the subject cannot overshoot the effort-dependent variable.

CALIBRATION AND QUALITY CONTROL OF SPIROMETERS

Calibration of spirometric devices is accomplished by one or more of several different methods:

1. Adjustment of the analog output signal from the primary transducer (i.e., bell, bellows, flow sensor)
2. Adjustment of the sensitivity of the recording device
3. Software correction (compensation)

Spirometers that produce a voltage signal by means of a potentiometer (see Chapter 9) normally allow some form of gain adjustment so that the analog output can be matched to a known input of either volume or flow. A related technique is the adjustment of the sensitivity of the recording device (such as an X-Y plotter or strip chart recorder) so that a known input produces a given deflection on the recording device. This method is appropriate when the recorded tracing is to be measured manually. Because of the widespread use of computerized data reduction, the signal produced by the spirometer is often corrected by applying a compensation factor in the software. A known volume (or flow) is injected into the spirometer using a large-volume syringe (3 L or more), and then a correction factor is calculated based on the measured versus expected values:

$$\text{Correction factor} = \frac{\text{Expected Volume}}{\text{Measured Volume}}$$

The correction factor derived by this method is then stored by the software and applied to the subsequent volume measurements. For example, if a syringe volume of 3 L is injected into a spirometer and a volume of 2.97 L is recorded, the correction factor would be:

$$1.010 = \frac{3.00}{2.97}$$

The correction factor 1.010 would then be used to adjust subsequent volume measurements. This method assumes that the spirometer output is linear, so that the correction factor would be correct for any volume, large or small. Many computerized systems allow the correction factor to be "verified" by re-injecting a known volume, not necessarily 3 L, and checking the input against the output. Care should be taken that the ATPS syringe volume is not automatically "temperature corrected" by the software, as this would produce an erroneously high measured value and a low correction factor. Other factors that might influence establishment of the software correction value include the accuracy of the large-volume syringe and the speed with which the injection is performed. An inaccurate syringe or leaks in the connection to the spirometer will produce faulty software corrections. Some systems, particularly flow-based spirometers, require that the syringe volume be injected within certain flow limits so that the software can generate correction factors based on a series of injections.

Quality control of spirometric devices is closely related to calibration, and the two are sometimes confused. An important distinction is that calibration (adjustment) may or may not be needed, but quality control must be applied on a routine basis. Calibration, whether it includes the output of the spirometer, recorder sensitivity, or generation of a software correction factor, involves adjusting the device to perform within certain limits. Quality control is a test performed to determine the accuracy and/or precision of the device using a known standard or signal. Various control methods (signal generators) are available for spirometers:

1. *Simple large-volume syringe.* A syringe of at least 3-L volume (Fig. 11-1,*A*) should be used to generate control signal for checking the volume deflection of volume-displacement spirometers and the associated deflection of the recording device. A large-volume syringe may also be used to check the volume accuracy of flow-sensing devices. Spirometer quality control should be performed at least once each day that the device is to be used. For field studies, such as industrial applications or epidemiologic research, in which the spirometer is moved about or used for a large number of tests,

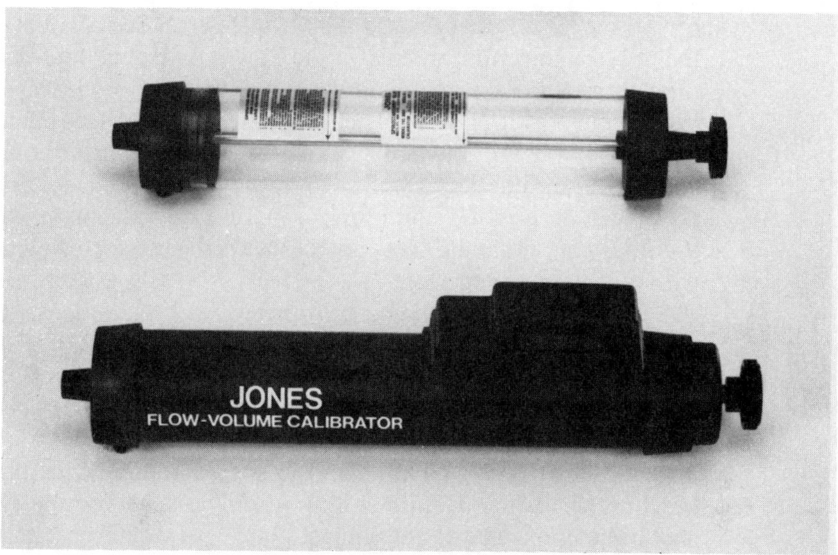

Fig. 11-1 Equipment for spirometer calibration. **A,** 3-L syringe used for simple volume calibration. A 3-L syringe is recommended for both calibration and quality control. **B,** Computerized FVC simulator that uses a microprocessor to measure $FEV_{1.0}$ and other flows during injection of a 3-L volume. The volumes and flows delivered can be compared with those that the spirometer reports. (Courtesy Jones Medical Instrument Co., Oakbrook, Ill.)

checks of accuracy should be performed several times daily to prevent reporting of erroneous values. A wide range of volumes should be used to access the accuracy of the spirometer across its volume range (i.e. the spirometer should record 1 L, 3 L, and 5 L with equal accuracy). For volume-displacement spirometers, accuracy should be checked across the volume range at least quarterly. A 3-L syringe injection performed when the spirometer is nearly empty or nearly full should yield comparable results. The volume accuracy of a spirometer over a range of flows should also be tested. Although a range of flows can be generated by varying the speed at which the syringe is emptied, it is impossible to reproduce those flows to check the precision of the spirometer. However, applying different flows and measuring the resulting volumes may provide insight as to whether the device and the software remain accurate at low and high flows. At least three different injection times (0.5 to 1.0 seconds, 1.0 to 1.5 seconds, and 5.0 to 5.5 seconds) may be used with a 3-L syringe to simulate a wide range of flows.

Computerized syringes (Fig. 11-1,*B*) are available for assessing the accuracy of commonly measured parameters such as $FEV_{1.0}$ and

$FEF_{25\%-75\%}$. These syringes use a built-in microprocessor that times the volume injection, calculates the flow parameters, and displays the volumes and flows for comparison with those produced by the instrument being tested. The computerized syringe offers the advantage of being able to deliver a 3-L volume for calibration and simple volume checks, as well as for testing the accuracy of the software that derives the commonly reported flows. Simple volume accuracy checks should be applied as if a subject were being tested, with a few exceptions.

For volume-displacement spirometers, a check for leaks should be performed daily before assessing volume accuracy. The device should be filled with air to approximately half of its volume range, and a constant pressure should be applied, by means of a weight or spring. No change in the volume tracing should be noted while the pressure is applied, and the volume should return to its original baseline when the pressure is removed. The large-volume syringe should be connected to the subject port, with whatever circuitry is employed for the actual test. To prevent automatic correction to BTPS, the spirometer temperature correction should be set at 37° C, unless a specific routine for volume checks (or calibration) is provided within the software. In some systems, temperature correction cannot be overridden; injection of a 3-L volume (at ATPS) will typically result in a reading greater than 3 L because the system attempts to "correct" the volume to body temperature (BTPS). For water-sealed spirometers, the syringe should be filled and emptied several times to allow equilibration with the humidified air of the device. For some flow-sensing instruments, a length of tubing must be connected to the flow sensor (particularly those in which the flow transducer is close to the mouth) to avoid artifact caused by the flow generated via the syringe. The accuracy of any spirometer can be calculated:

$$\% \text{ Error} = \frac{\text{Expected Volume} - \text{Measured Volume}}{\text{Expected Volume}} \times 100$$

where:

Expected Volume = The actual volume of the syringe
Measured Volume = The result recorded for the test

The maximum acceptable error, according to the American Thoracic Society recommendations (see Table 11-1), is ±3% or ±50 ml, whichever is larger. If the percentage error exceeds 3%, a careful examination of the spirometer, recording device, software, most recent calibration, and testing technique should be carried out.

2. *Sine wave rotary pumps.* A second method of checking volume accuracy of spirometers is the volumetric syringe or piston driven

via a rotary drive motor. This type of device produces a biphasic volume signal, which is useful for checking accuracy as the volume and flow simulate both inspiration and expiration. Although this type of device is of limited use for assessing the accuracy of a spirometer for most flow measurements, it is ideal for checking the frequency response, particularly at higher flow rates. This type of signal is necessary to evaluate a spirometer's ability to adequately record tests such as the MVV. The American Thoracic Society (ATS) recommends that spirometers that measure MVV record a 2-L sine wave within 5% from 0 to 250 L/min. Although such tests are impractical for most clinical laboratories, they should be available from manufacturers when necessary. Sine wave pumps are also commonly used in the calibration of body plethysmographs.

3. *Automated syringes.* These devices are similar to the simple large-volume syringes that are used manually, but they have some combination of computer-controlled motor drive or electronic output. For the most part, computerized syringes are restricted to equipment manufacturers and to research applications centering on testing available clinical equipment. Other commercially available devices use sensors (magnetic) coupled to microprocessors to cal-

Table 11-1 Minimal spirometry standards*

Test	Range/accuracy BTPS (L)	Flow range (L/sec)	Time (sec)	Resistance/back pressure	Test signals
VC	7 L ± 3% or 50 ml, whichever is greater	0-12	30		3-L calibrated syringe
FVC	7 L ± 3% or 50 ml, whichever is greater	0-12	15		24 standard waveforms
FEV_T	7 L ± 3% or 50 ml, whichever is greater	0-12	T	Less than 1.5 cm H_2O/L/sec at 12.0 L/sec flow	24 standard waveforms
Time zero	Time point from which all FEV_T measurements are taken			Determined by back-extrapolation	
$FEF_{25\%-75\%}$	7 L ± 5% or 0.2 L/sec, whichever is greater	0-12	15	Same as FEV_T	24 standard waveforms
$\dot{V}$	12 L/sec ± 5% or 0.2 L/sec whichever is greater	0-12	15	Same as FEV_T	Manufacturer proof
MVV	Sine wave 250 L/min at 2-L tidal volume to ±5% of reading	0-12 ±5%	12-15 ±3%	Less than ±10 cm H_2O at 2 L V_T at 2.0 Hz	Sine wave pump 0.4 Hz ± 10% at 12 L/sec

*Summarized from Standardization of spirometry—1987 update, Am Rev Respir Dis 136:1285, 1987.

culate various flows, such as $FEV_{1.0}$ and $FEF_{25\%-75\%}$ as described previously in this chapter (see Fig. 11-1,*B*).

4. *Explosive decompression devices.* Explosive decompression simulates the exponential flow pattern of a forced expiratory maneuver. Such devices use a known volume of gas compressed to a fixed pressure, then released through an orifice. Some devices use air, while others use CO_2 as the compressed gas. The primary advantage of this type of device is that it allows measurement of flows as well as volumes to be reproduced, thus allowing quality assurance checks on most spirometric parameters, for both hardware and software. In addition, the fact that the test signal can be reproduced as often as necessary allows not only accuracy but precision as well to be assessed. Explosive decompression devices may be limited for use with automated systems that require a particular pattern of respiration to trigger recording, such as inspiration-expiration-inspiration. Another potential limitation is the use of CO_2 as the compressed gas. Flow-sensing spirometers that use a physical principle that is affected by the gas composition may yield unacceptable values (See Chapter 9).
5. *Known subjects.* A semi-quantitative means of assessing the accuracy and precison of spirometric devices is the repeated measurement of known subjects. All routine spirometric measurements may be performed on subjects who will be available for future comparison, such as laboratory personnel. Although individual signals for FVC, $FEV_{1.0}$ and $FEF_{25\%-75\%}$ show a good deal of variability when test subjects are used, all aspects of the testing protocol are evaluated, including hardware, software, and testing procedure. This allows for a readily available check of the overall function of the spirometer; it does not, however, replace the checking of accuracy by means of a known-volume syringe. To provide meaningful comparisons, the mean and standard deviation of five to ten spirometric measurements for each reported parameter should be recorded for at least three known subjects. These subjects should have repeat tests at least quarterly, or whenever questionable test results are observed. The control subjects should reflect the patient population routinely tested (i.e., adults, children). Interlaboratory testing of known subjects in two or more laboratories allows a form of proficiency testing, so that the accuracy of an individual laboratory can be assessed. Testing of healthy known subjects (usually 10 or more) can be useful in assessing the appropriateness of the reference value equations used for predicting normal values (see Selecting and Using Predicted Values in the Appendix).

In addition to checking the volume and flow accuracy of spirometers, there are several other important aspects of quality control that require routine evaluation:

1. *Flow resistance.* Normally the "back pressure" from a spirometer should be less than 1.5 cm H_2O at 12 L/sec flow. Resistance to flow is measured by placing an accurate manometer or pressure transducer at the subject connection and applying a known flow. This is easily accomplished with flow-sensing devices, but it is somewhat difficult with volume-displacement devices, and such measurement is normally performed only when there is some reason to suspect that the spirometer is causing undue resistance.
2. *Frequency response.* The ability of the spirometer to produce accurate volume (and flow) determinations across a wide range of frequencies. This applies most notably to the MVV, because the frequency varies with the individual subject. Frequency response is usually evaluated by means of a sine wave pump, and testing is performed only if the spirometer is suspect.
3. *Flow.* Because flow-sensing spirometers directly measure flow and indirectly calculate volume (by integration or counting volume pulses), it is sometimes useful to assess the flow accuracy of such devices. Inaccurate measurement of flow almost always results in inaccurate volume determinations. A rotameter may be used in conjunction with an adjustable compressed gas source to apply gas at a known flow to the device. A weighted volume-displacement spirometer (water-sealed) can also be used to generate a known flow. Many flow-sensing spirometers use a volume signal to perform software calibration (correction), as described previously in the Calibration and Quality Control of Spirometers section of this chapter. However, it may be useful to check the flow output of the device at several different known flows if the volume accuracy of the device seems to vary with flow.
4. *Recorders.* Recording devices are perhaps as important as the volume/flow transducers themselves in providing accurate spirometric tracings. The ATS has recommended that a recorder be required for all spirometers, with slightly different recorder standards depending on the intended application of the spirometer. For diagnostic functions (i.e., recognition of disease patterns or unacceptable maneuvers) the recorder must have a sensitivity on the volume axis of at least 5 mm/L (BTPS) and a time base of at least 1 cm/second. For manual measurements (or for instrument validation studies), the recorder must have a volume sensitivity of at least 10 mm/L (BTPS), and a time base of at least 2 cm/second. Hard copy recordings of volume-time or flow-volume tracings should be made as part of all spirometric measurements. Flow-volume curves should be plotted with expired flow upwards on the vertical axis and expired volume from left to right on the horizontal axis. A 2:1 ratio of the flow to volume scales should be maintained. For diagnostic purposes, the flow sensitivity of the flow-volume display should be at

least 2.5 mm/L/sec, while for manual measurements or validation, the flow sensitivity should be at least 5 mm/L/sec. Sensitivity on the volume axis of flow-volume displays should be the same as for volume-time curves. A standard flow-volume curve for manual measurement would then have a flow sensitivity of 2 L/sec equal to 10 mm, and a volume sensitivity of 1 L equal to 10 mm. Accurate recorder speed and volume sensitivity are particularly important when the results to be reported are obtained by manual calculation. Recorder accuracy should be checked at least quarterly. Paper speed can be easily checked with a stopwatch. With the paper or recording pen moving, a volume signal is applied at regular intervals so that deflections are placed on the tracing. The intervals between the deflections are then measured and compared with the speed of the recorder. Electronic or strip chart recorders can usually have their speed adjusted; kymographs and similar mechanical recording devices may require more sophisticated repair.

Common problems

Some of the common problems detected by routine quality control of spirometers include:

- Cracks or leaks (in volume-displacement spirometers)
- Low water level (in water-sealed spirometers)
- Sticking or worn bellows
- Inaccurate or erratic potentiometers
- Obstructed or dirty flow tubes (flow-sensors)
- Mechanical resistance (in volume-displacement spirometers)
- Leaks in tubes and connectors
- Faulty recorder timing
- Inappropriate signal correction (BTPS)
- Improper software calibration (corrections)
- Defective software or computer interface

CALIBRATION AND QUALITY CONTROL OF GAS ANALYZERS

Accurate analysis of both inspired and expired gases is required for measurements of lung volume (gas dilution techniques), $D_{L_{CO}}$, and gas exchange during exercise or metabolic testing. In most instances, the accuracy of the final results of these tests depends on the accuracy of both the volume transducer and the gas analyzers used. Although various types of gas analyzers are commonly used in pulmonary function testing, some general principles apply to both their calibration and quality control. As noted prevously in this chapter, calibration refers to the process of adjusting the output of the instrument to meet certain specifications, while quality control refers to a method of routine checking of the accuracy and precision of the device.

Calibration techniques for gas analyzers include the following:

1. *Physiologic range.* Because many analyzers are not linear or may exhibit poor accuracy over a wide range, it is important to calibrate the device to match the physiologic range over which measurements are to be performed. O_2 analyzers may be used to measure fractional concentrations from 0.21 to 1.00, representing a wide physiologic range. However, if the O_2 analyzer is to be used for exercise testing of subjects breathing room air, it should be calibrated over the range from 0.12 to 0.21, as this represents the typical physiologic range of expired O_2 likely to be encountered. Reducing the physiologic range of the analyzers generally allows greater accuracy and precision. Some types of analyzers provide range adjustments just for this purpose, as well as user-selectable amplification. Test gases used for calibration should represent the extremes of the physiologic range.
2. *Sampling conditions.* Generally, gas analyzers must be calibrated under the same conditions that will be encountered during the actual testing procedure. Analyzers that are sensitive to the partial pressure of the test gas (see Chapter 9) may be affected by the sample flow rate. For tests in which gas is sampled continuously by pumping it from the breathing circuit, the sampling flow rate *must* be adjusted before calibration and left unchanged during sampling. If gas flow is stopped before the measurement is actually performed, the sampling flow rate is not critical, but the analyzer must be calibrated under conditions of no flow. A common problem is to calibrate the analyzer, then change the configuration of the sampling circuit (i.e., add tubing, three-way stopcocks). Any absorber circuits (CO_2, H_2O, dust filters) should be in place during calibration as well.
3. *Two-point calibration.* The most common technique for analyzer calibration involves exposing the device to two known gases. If the test involves a gas that is not normally present in expired gas, (such as He, CO, or Ne) room air may be used to zero the analyzer, and a test gas representing the upper end of the physiologic range may be used to span the analyzer. The He dilution FRC and $DL_{CO}SB$ are examples of such maneuvers; both the He and CO analyzers are "zeroed" by drawing room air into the sensor cells, assuming that He and CO are not present in the atmosphere. Then a test gas containing a known concentration of the gas to be analyzed is admitted to the sensor. The analyzer gain is adjusted to match the known concentration. The test gas approximates the concentration to be analyzed during the test. The analyzer may then be re-zeroed, and the entire process is repeated to verify the calibration. A similar technique may be employed using two gases of known concentration if the expirate normally contains varying concentrations of the gas. For example, room air and 12% oxygen might be used to perform a two-point calibration for an O_2 analyzer for exercise testing.

Depending on the stability of the analyzer, calibration may have to be repeated before each test application. Regardless of the methodology employed, gas analyzers should be calibrated before each patient for lung volume determinations, DL_{CO}, exercise tests, and metabolic studies. Gas analyzers used for monitoring (capnographs) should be calibrated on a schedule commensurate with the extent of use (usually daily or more often), and in accordance with the manufacturer's recommendations. The accuracy of the calibration gas should reflect the necessary accuracy of the measurements involved. For the analyses such as those involved in exercise or metabolic studies, calibration gases should be accurate to at least two decimal places (i.e., hundredth of a percent). Calibration gases may require verification by an independent method.

4. *Multiple-point (linearity) calibration.* An assumption made by the simple two-point technique is that the output of the analyzer is linear between the points used for calibration. To verify linearity or to determine the pattern of nonlinearity, three or more calibration points must be determined (Fig. 11-2). The multiple-point calibra-

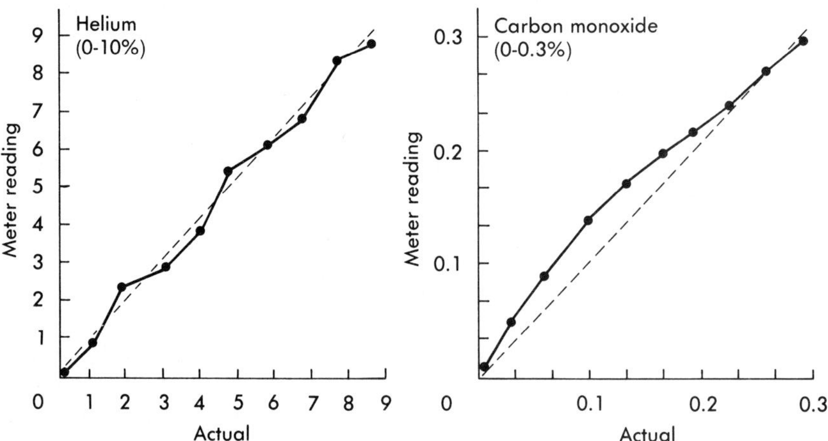

Fig. 11-2 Calibration/linearity check of gas analyzers—typical plots of varying gas concentrations in relation to the meter readings of the analyzers for two gases (He and CO). In each case, different dilutions of a known gas are prepared and submitted to the analyzer. The meter reading is then compared to the actual (calculated) value. In the example, the He analyzer shows good linearity in the comparison of measured versus expected concentrations. The CO analyzer shows a nonlinear pattern, as expected for an infrared CO analyzer. If enough points are determined, a "calibration" curve can be generated for correction of the meter readings; by mathematically fitting the curve, an equation can be generated for subsequent correction of meter readings.

tion is performed in a manner similar to the two-point, except that the concentrations of known gases across the range to be analyzed are checked and then plotted. If multiple points are determined, a linear regression may be calculated to determine the slope of the line relating the measured gas concentrations to the expected gas concentrations. Most statistics textbooks describe the calculation of simple linear regression. If the analyzer is indeed linear, the points plotted fall in a straight line; if the analyzer is nonlinear, a calibration curve may be constructed to correct analyzed samples. In most instances, an equation describing the nonlinear curve can be generated and then used either manually or by software to correct meter readings. Many nonlinear analyzers incorporate electronic circuitry that linearizes the output. Linearity of analyzers used for DL_{CO}, lung volume determinations, exercise testing, and metabolic studies should be reevaluated at least once every 6 months. Some analyzers may require more frequent checks, depending on the extent of use.

Quality control of gas analyzers can be performed by submitting various concentrations of known test gases to the analyzer, and by testing a lung analog or known subject. Multiple test gases with concentrations in the range of the analyzer can be maintained, but may be a rather complex quality control method for most clinical laboratories. A simpler technique is to prepare serial dilutions of a known gas using a large-volume calibrated syringe, such as the type used for simple volume calibration. For example, 100 ml of He and 900 ml of air may be mixed in a 1-L syringe to produce a 10% He gas mixture, and then be injected into the analyzer. Subsequently, 100 ml of He might be diluted in 1000 ml, then 1100 ml, and so on, with the expected concentrations calculated:

$$\text{Expected \% Test Gas} = \frac{\text{Volume of Test Gas}}{\text{Total Volume of Gas}} \times 100$$

where:

$$\text{Total Volume of Gas} = \text{Test Gas} + \text{added air}$$

As each dilution is analyzed, the meter reading is recorded and plotted against the expected percentage (see Fig. 11-2). This method is simple and available to most labs. Care must be taken when preparing samples in this way so that air does not leak into the syringe and further dilute the test gas. The volume of air in the syringe connnectors should be considered when calculating the dilution of the test gas; some calibrated syringes account for the connector volume.

A second method of verifying analyzer performance involves simulating either lung volume or DL_{CO} maneuvers. This may be accomplished using a fixed- or variable-volume lung analog, which is simply an airtight container of known volume (Fig. 11-3). The lung volume simulator is con-

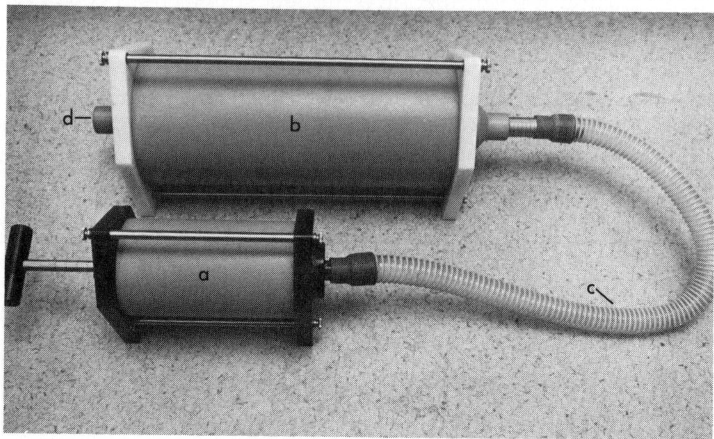

Fig. 11-3 FRC/DL_{CO} calibrator. A typical setup for checking the calibration of either an open- or closed-circuit FRC system, or a $DL_{CO}SB$ system. **A,** Large-volume syringe; **B,** variable-volume closed container (the volume is varied by setting the internal piston); **C,** connective tubing so that the syringe can be used to "ventilate" the closed container; **D,** system connection for attachment to the subject port. The system volume is determined by adding the volume set on b plus the volume of c (determined by filling with water and measuring), plus any dead space contained in the connections. The large-volume syringe is then used to simulate breathing for the specific test being checked.

nected at the subject connection, with the system prepared for lung volume or DL_{CO} determination. A large-volume syringe may then be used to "ventilate" the lung analog, mimicking the procedure as it would be performed by a subject. A calibrated syringe alone may also be used to simulate the maneuver, by starting with a volume of air in the syringe and applying a method similar to that described on p. 299 for serial dilutions. At the end of the test, the resulting lung volume is compared with the known volume of the analog system. Simulation of the $DL_{CO}SB$ maneuver in this way should produce values very near zero, because both He and CO are diluted in the simulator, and their relative concentrations should be identical. If the two analyzers are not linear in relation to one another, the resulting gas concentrations will vary (i.e., their ratio will not equal 1.0) and the calculated $DL_{CO}SB$ will be either above or below zero. This method tests not only the gas analyzer(s), but also the volume transducer, breathing circuit, and software as well. Temperature or gas corrections should be overridden or not performed. If the volume of the lung analog can be varied, a linearity check at several different dilutions can be performed. Some computerized systems do not allow lung analog simulators to be readily used because the software is designed to make all necessary corections for human subjects. However, if the software reports gas analyzer values directly, the accuracy and linearity of various dilutions can be checked.

Testing known subjects is a third means of quality checking gas analyzers, but it may not detect small changes in performance, because the entire lung volume, DL_{CO}, or exercise system (analzyers, volume transducer) is used. Despite the natural variability (as much as 10% in DL_{CO} or exercise parameters) occurring with testing of known subjects, gross malfunctions of systems involving gas analyzers can be detected. Known-subject tests on at least three subjects should be performed quarterly or whenever questionable values are obtained. The known-subject method may be the most useful for checking automated exercise testing and metabolic measurement systems.

Common problems

Some of the common problems occurring with gas analyzers that may be detected by routine quality control checks include:

- Leaks in sampling tubes or connectors
- Blockage of sampling tubes
- Exhausted water vapor or CO_2 absorbers
- Contamination of photocells or electrodes
- Improper mechanical zeroing (taut band display)
- Inadequate warm-up time
- Deterioration or contamination of column packing material (gas chromatographs)
- Poor vacuum pump performance (mass spectrometer or N_2 analyzers)
- Chopper motor malfunction (infrared analyzers)
- Electrolyte or fuel cell exhaustion (O_2 analyzers)
- Aging of detector cells (infrared analyzers)
- Poor optical balance (infrared analyzers)

CALIBRATION AND QUALITY CONTROL OF PLETHYSMOGRAPHS

The calibration techniques described here apply primarily to a variable-pressure, constant-volume plethysmograph. Users of flow-based plethysmographs should perform the calibration procedure for the box transducer according to the manufacturer's instructions; the mouth pressure and pneumotachometer calibration will be similar for both types of plethysmographs.

1. *Mouth pressure transducer.* Physical calibration can be done by directly connecting it to a water (or mercury) manometer that includes the range of pressures normally measured (± 25 cm H_2O). Air is injected into one port of the manometer to cause a deflection of 5 cm (for example), thus creating a difference of 10 cm between the two columns of the manometer. The gain of the mouth pressure amplifier is then adjusted so that the signal appearing on the display device (oscilloscope, recorder, or computer screen) deflects by an amount equivalent to 10 cm H_2O per centimeter. This deflection then becomes the calibration factor for the mouth pressure trans-

ducer (in this example, 10 cm H_2O/cm). For computerized systems, the output voltage of the transducers (mouth, box, and flow) is typically measured and a software correction factor (offset) is determined. This correction factor is then applied by the software as the signals are acquired.

2. *Box pressure transducer.* Physical calibration is accomplished by closing the box and applying a volume signal comparable to that which occurs during subject testing. In a 500-L plethysmograph, a volume signal of 25 to 50 ml is typical. A sine wave pump connected to a small syringe is ideal because the same volume can be added and removed from the box, at varying frequencies. With the pump operating, the gain of the box pressure transducer is adjusted so that the volume change in the box causes a specific deflection on the display device. For example, the pressure signal generated by a 30-ml syringe might be adjusted to cause a 2-cm deflection on an oscilloscope; the box pressure calibration factor would then be 15 ml/cm. This procedure can be repeated at varying frequencies from 0.5 to 5.0 cycles/second (Hz) to verify an appropriate frequency response; the deflection should not change with different frequencies. Flow-based plethysmographs may be calibrated similarly, except that the output of the box flow transducer is adjusted, rather than that of a pressure transducer. The plethysmograph is normally calibrated empty, then a volume correction for the subject is applied during the final calculation (see Appendix).
3. *Flow transducer.* The pneumotachometer is physically calibrated by applying a known flow of gas via a rotameter or other calibrated flow device. The gain of the pressure transducer connected to the pneumotachometer is adjusted in a manner similar to that used for the mouth and box pressure transducers, so that a known flow causes a specific deflection on the display. For example, a flow of 2 L/s may be set to cause a 2-cm deflection, resulting in a flow calibration factor of 1 L/sec/cm. If an adjustable rotameter is used, the linearity of the pneumotachometer can be verified by checking the deflections at various flows. A weighted spirometer may also be used to generate a known flow. Some computerized systems avoid the necessity of a constant-flow generator by using a fixed volume from a calibrated syringe. A 3-L volume can be injected and the flow integrated; the gain of the flow signal is then adjusted until the output of the integrator produces the known volume.

As described previously in this section, some computerized plethysmograph systems provide for electronic or software adjustment of the transducers. The known physical signals are similarly applied, but gain adjustments are done electronically or by generating a software correction factor. Another check provided by some systems is a calibrated voltage signal applied to the display device; this should not be confused with the actual physical calibration described previously in this section, but may be used to check the oscilloscope or recorder after physical calibration.

Quality control of the body plethysmograph is usually accomplished by use of an isothermal lung analog, a known subject, or comparison with gas dilution or radiologic lung volumes.

An isothermal volume analog can be constructed from a 4- to 5-L glass bottle that has been filled with metal wool (usually copper) to act as a heat sink (Fig. 11-4). The mouth of the bottle is fitted with two connectors, one to be attached to the subject connection of the mouth shutter, the other to

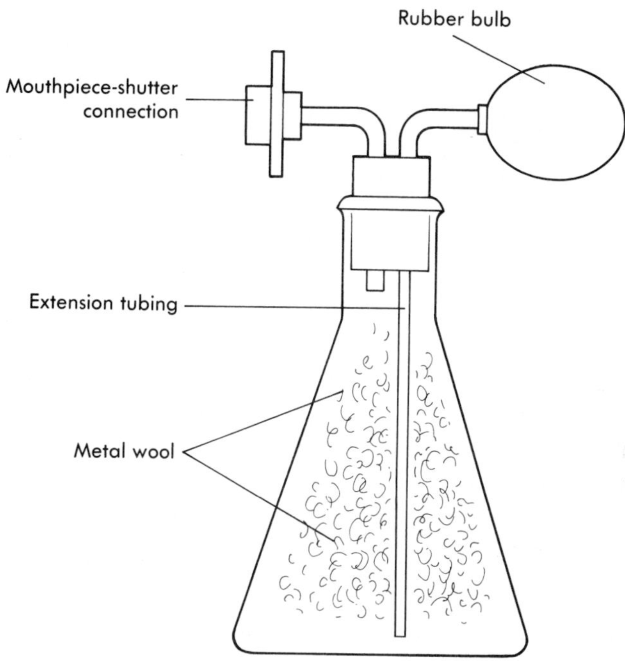

Fig. 11-4 Isothermal lung analog—A schematic of the isothermal lung analog for quality control of the body plethysmograph. A large (approximately 4-L) jar is fitted with a stopper with two openings. One opening connects to the mouthpiece shutter apparatus of the plethysmograph, and the other is connected to a rubber hand bulb with an extension deep into the bottle. Metal wool (copper) is used to fill the container and acts as a heat sink so that pressure changes in the bottle cause only minimal changes in gas temperature. By having a subject in the plethysmograph squeeze the bulb (while breath-holding) the V_{TG} maneuver is simulated. A P_{mouth}/P_{box} tangent may be recorded and the volume of the container calculated. The calculated volume should compare to within 5% of the volume of the device. The true volume may be determined by filling the container with water and subtracting the volume of the metal wool. The volumes of the connectors and rubber bulb should be considered as well.

a rubber bulb of 50- to 100-ml volume. The actual volume of the device can be determined by subtracting the volume of the metal wool (calculated from its weight times density) from the volume of the bottle, or by filling the device with water from a volumetric source. The dead space of the connector and rubber bulb should also be added to the total volume. The check is performed by a subject seated in the sealed box with the isothermal volume device connected and the mouth shutter closed. While breath-holding, the subject squeezes the bulb; a P_{mouth}/P_{box} tangent is recorded and the volume is calculated as usual, except that the P_{H_2O} is not subtracted. The measured volume should equal the volume of the isothermal lung analog (as derived above) $\pm$ 5%. The correction for the subject volume, normally based on the subject's body weight, should include the subject plus the known volume of the isothermal lung analog. The entire procedure may be repeated at various frequencies from 0.5 to 5.0 cycles/second to check the frequency response of the box; the tangents or angles should not change as the bulb is compressed at different rates.

The accuracy of the pneumotachometer can be assessed by the use of known resistances. Resistors can be made using fixed orifices or from capillary tubes placed in a flow tube. In either case, the resistance across the device is measured at a known flow rate. The resistor may then be added in front of the pneumotachometer while a subject breathes (or a known flow is applied), and the increased resistance should equal that of the resistor.

A second means of checking the accuracy of the plethysmograph is to measure parameters from a known subject (a series of 10 measurements provides an adequate mean value with which subsequent results may be compared). Despite day-to-day variability in subjects, this method allows checking of the VTG, airway resistance and conductance, as well as evaluating the box itself, the transducers, the recording devices, and the software. Unfortunately, discrepancies between the mean of previous measurements and an individual quality control trial often do not indicate which section of the equipment may be causing the problem. Routine application of controls, in conjunction with checks of the calibrations performed, may demonstrate which transducer or component is responsible for the problem.

A third method of checking the accuracy of the plethysmograph is to compare the VTG with lung volumes from a normal subject determined by gas dilution or radiologic techniques. Good correlations (greater than 0.90) have been demonstrated between gas dilution, radiologic, and plethysmographically determined lung volumes in normal subjects. Large differences (i.e., differences greater than 10%) in volumes measured by plethysmograph and one of the other methods are nonspecific but may serve as an indicator of equipment malfunction. Because this method and the known-subject technique described previously in this chapter are based on measurements of individuals, it is important that the subject performs the breathing maneuvers correctly (see Criteria for Acceptability of Lung Volumes and Plethysmography section of this chapter).

Common problems

Some common problems that may be identified by routine quality control of body plethysmographs include:

- Leaks in door seals or connectors (pressure boxes)
- Improperly calibrated pressure transducers
- Obstructed or perforated pneumotachometers
- Excessive thermal drift
- Poor frequency response
- Excessive vibration (poorly mounted transducers)

CALIBRATION AND QUALITY CONTROL OF BLOOD GAS ANALYZERS

Blood gas analyzer systems may be divided into two categories on the basis of the type of calibration employed—manual or automatic. Although the principles involved in both automatic and manual calibrations are similar, some important differences exist, particularly in the technologist's role in instrument maintenance.

Manual calibration of the blood gas electrodes involves exposing the gas measuring electrodes (Po_2, Pco_2) to two or more gases with know partial pressures of oxygen and carbon dioxide, and bringing two or more known buffers into contact with the pH measuring electrode. Calibration gases spanning the physiologic ranges of the Po_2 and Pco_2 electrodes are used in much the same fashion as for gas analzyers described in the Calibration and Quality Control of Gas Analyzers section, previously in this chapter. Typical combinations would include one calibration gas with a fractional O_2 concentration of 0.20 (20%), and a fractional CO_2 concentration of 0.05 (5%); a second calibration gas would have a CO_2 concentration of 0.10 (10%) with an O_2 concentration close to zero. If blood specimens with very high or very low partial pressures of oxygen are to be analyzed, the analyzer can be calibrated with a gas of corresponding fractional concentration. For shunt studies in which the subject breathes 100% oxygen, the analyzer may be calibrated with 100% gas. After bubbling the gases through water at 37° C to saturate them with water vapor, they are allowed to flow into the measuring chamber. The partial pressures of the calibration gases are dependent on the ambient barometric pressure; for each calibration gas, the partial pressure is calculated:

$$P_{gas} = F_{gas} \times (P_B - 47)$$

where:

P_{gas} = Partial pressure of calibration gas
F_{gas} = Fractional concentration of the same gas
P_B = Ambient barometric pressure
47 = partial pressure of water vapor at 37° C

Each calibration gas is allowed to remain in the measuring chamber until equilibrium is reached. Once the partial pressure reading has stabilized, the appropriate control is adjusted to match the electrode to the calculated pressure. As with expired gas analyzers, a "low" gas is used to zero (balance) the electrode; a "high" gas is used to adjust the gain (slope) of the electrode. Zeroing the electrode does not necessarily mean using a gas with a partial pressure of zero, but rather setting the low range of the electrode. As noted previously, two-point calibrations are commonly used to calibrate gas analysis devices; more than two calibration gases, however, must be used to prove the linearity of the electrode system. On most blood gas systems, a combination of calibration gases is used so that the PO_2 is calibrated over a range of 0 to 150 mm Hg and the PCO_2 is calibrated from approximately 40 to 80 mm Hg.

Because some systems use precision gases to calibrate the gas electrodes but measure gas tensions in a liquid (blood), some difference may exist between analysis of the same partial pressure in gas or liquid. The reduction of O_2 at the tip of the polarographic electrode occurs more rapidly in a gaseous medium than in a liquid. If the electrode is calibrated with a gas, its response when measuring a liquid will be to read slightly low. This difference is termed the gas-liquid factor. A correction factor can be derived by calibrating the electrode using a liquid that has been tonometered (see discussion of tonometry later in this chapter) with the calibration gas, and then measuring the calibration gas itself and deriving a ratio based on the difference between the two. Gas-liquid corrections may be clinically important when measuring high partial pressures of oxygen, particularly above 400 mm Hg. Some systems use tonometered solutions for routine calibration of the gas electrodes, thus avoiding the necessity of determining the gas to liquid ratio. Some liquid-liquid difference may exist depending on the solutions used (i.e., whole blood versus an aqueous buffer).

Manual calibration of the pH electrode system is performed by exposing the measuring electrode to two (or more) known buffers. The "low" buffer typically has a pH of 6.840 (similar to the sealed-in buffer used in the measuring electrode), with a "high" buffer in the range of 7.38 (close to normal adult blood pH). The zero and gain of the pH voltmeter is adjusted to match these known points.

Automatic calibration of blood gas analyzers differs slightly from manual calibration, not in the gases or reagents involved, but in the role of the technologist in ensuring that the procedure achieves the desired outcome. In general, the gas tension electrodes are balanced and sloped using two (or more) gases of known fractional concentrations or tonometered solutions. Adjustment of the output of each electrode's amplifier is performed by a microprocessor. The computer controls bringing the calibration gases or buffers into contact with the electrodes and then stores the calibration values. The microprocessor compares the calibration values to expected values that are derived from the partial pressure of the calibration gases. The microprocessor then adjusts the zero and gain (for a two-point calibration) to correct for the observed differences between the measured and expected values. Most computerized blood gas analyzers store the results of the calibration for comparison with the subsequent calibration. The amount of drift that occurs between calibrations can then be used as a check on the electrode's stability.

Automatic calibration of the pH system is performed similarly, with the microprocessor adjusting the electrode output to match two or more known buffers. Most automated systems include checks of the various other parameters that are fundamental to accurate blood gas analysis, such as barometric pressure and the temperature of the measuring chamber. Some computerized systems tonometer solutions for calibration of the gas and pH electrodes. The microprocessor calculates the partial pressures of the calibration gases based on its reading of an internal barometer. Once the P_{CO_2} of the tonometered solution is calculated, the pH can be determined, because the buffers are usually a bicarbonate-based solution. The built-in tonometer allows expected values for all three electrodes to be determined.

Because automatic calibration occurs at predetermined intervals, and because adjustments are performed based on the response of the electrodes, all of the necessary conditions for an acceptable calibration must be met before the procedure actually begins. During the automatic calibration, inadequate buffer or calibration gas may cause the microprocessor to make excessive adjustments to the electrode(s) output. A similar problem can arise when blood or protein contaminates the tip of the electrode, altering its sensitivity. If an automatic calibration occurs, the microprocessor adjusts the electrode's output in an attempt to bring it into range. Although this process may work well for minor changes in electrode sensitivity, it cannot adequately calibrate the electrode if the buildup of debris at the measuring surface is excessive. The technologist must maintain the buffers, gases, and electrodes themselves so that automatic calibration can occur successfully. Inappropriate adjustments may be detected easily by routine checks of calibration results.

Manual and automatic calibration of blood gas analyzers each have advantages and disadvantages. Manual instruments allow complete control over the analysis, including determination of the endpoint of the measurement. Manual calibration with gases of high or low partial pressures (notably O_2) permit adjustment of the measuring range of the instrument to accommodate special tests such as shunt determinations. Manually calibrated instruments tend to be less precise than automated analyzers because of the variability introduced by the technique of the technologist. The chief advantage of instruments that calibrate automatically is the precision that is possible. The microprocessor controls sample size, timing, rinsing, and most other aspects of calibration and sample analysis. The apparent simplicity of the automated calibration is often a disadvantage. Although less attention may be required on the part of personnel performing analyses, those same technologists must be even more proficient in identifying electrode malfunctions. Some computerized instruments provide error flags or warnings whenever an automatic calibration senses unacceptable electrode performance, but the technologist is responsible for assessing and correcting the problem. Systematic errors can sometimes be masked by instruments that calibrate themselves. Contamination of the calibrating gases or buffers is a common example. If the microprocessor adjusts electrodes to match a contaminated calibration standard, the calibrations appear normal but analysis of control samples will show differences. Detection of these types of systematic errors usually requires proficiency testing, as described later in this section.

Two general methods of quality control for blood gas analysis are in widespread use: (1) tonometry, and (2) commercially prepared controls. The interpretation of blood gas quality control is the same with either of these methods, with a few minor differences:

1. *Tonometry.* A tonometer is a device that allows precision gas mixtures to be equilibrated with either whole blood or a suitable buffer. One commonly used tonometer creates a thin film of blood or buffer by spinning the sample in a chamber that is flooded with the precision gas. A second type bubbles the gas through the sample to create a large surface for gas exchange. In either design, the tonometer is maintained at 37° C and the gas is humidified. After an equilibration period determined by the gas flow rate and the volume of the control sample being prepared, a portion of the sample is transferred to the blood gas analyzer. The expected gas tensions are calculated from the fractional concentrations of the precision gas, just as described previously for manual calibrations. If whole blood is used as the control material, then Po_2 and Pco_2, but not pH, can be checked. Blood is ideal for quality control of the gas electrodes because its viscosity and gas exchange properties are the same as patient samples. No other control material provides the oxygen-carrying capacity of whole blood, so for the most precise control of the Po_2 electrode, tonometry is the method of choice. Unless the buffering capacity of the blood to be tonometered is known, however, the pH cannot be accurately calculated. Tonometry of a bicarbonate-based buffer using a known fractional concentraiton of CO_2 allows both gas and pH electrodes to be controlled, but the gas exchange characteristics of the buffer differ from whole blood. Tonometry can be performed inexpensively using pooled waste blood and small amounts of precision gas, with control of pH accomplished by tonometry of a buffer. Normally, three levels of control materials are used to provide checks over the physiologic range of the electrodes, so three precision gas mixtures are required. Accuracy of tonometry is highly dependent on a standardized technique. Sampling syringes must be lubricated and then flushed with the precision gas. Careful attention to the preparation and sampling from the tonometer is required to obtain reliable results, and is somewhat dependent on individual technique. Problems that sometimes

occur with tonometry include contamination of the precision gas caused by leaky connections, improper thermostating of the chamber, or inadequate gas flow to reach equilibrium.

2. *Commercially prepared controls.* Commercially prepared controls fall into three general categories: blood-based, aqueous, or fluorocarbon-based. The blood-based matrix consists of a solution containing buffered human red cells. The aqueous-based is usually a bicarbonate buffer; the fluorocarbon-based is a perfluorinated compound that has enhanced oxygen-dissolving characteristics. These control materials are packaged in sealed-glass ampules to 2- to 3-ml volume, and they require minimum preparation for use. The blood-based material requires refrigerated storage, incubation at 37° C for several minutes, and agitation before use. The aqueous and fluorocarbon-based controls can be stored under refrigeration for long periods, or at room temperature for day-to-day use. Most aqueous and fluorocarbon-based controls have shelf lives of 1 year, and simply require agitation for 10 to 15 seconds before use. Multiple levels of these materials are used to provide control over the range of values clinically seen. Although commercially prepared controls may be considerably more expensive than tonometered samples, they are convenient to use and less susceptible to handling errors. One difficulty associated with aqueous controls (and to a lesser extent with fluorocarbon solutions) is poor precision of the P_{O_2}, especially at low partial pressures. This results in such a wide range of "expected" values that the control may be of limited clinical usefulness. Some of these difficulties may be overcome by careful statistical handling of the P_{O_2} quality control data as described later in this section.

With all of the quality control methodologies described, a sound method of interpretation of the results of "control runs" is necessary to translate the controls into information that will allow the technologist to maintain or repair a poorly operating electrode. The most common method for detecting "out-of-control" blood gas electrodes is to use the control mean $\pm$ 2 standard deviation (SD) statistical concept, with a data base of at least 30 control runs (see Appendix for a sample calculation). One SD on either side of the mean in a normal distribution will include about 67% of the points, while 2 SDs will include 95%, and 3 SDs will include 99.7%. Any quality control value that falls within $\pm$ 2 SDs of the mean can be considered "in control." If the control value falls between 2 and 3 SDs from the mean, there is only a 5% chance that the run is in control. This normal variability that occurs when multiple measurements are performed is termed "random error," and one out of 20 control runs can be expected to be in the two to three SD range and still be acceptable. To distinguish true "out-of-control" situations from random errors, more complex sets of rules have been developed. The most widely used rules are those proposed by Westgard (see the Selected Bibliography). These rules are a subset of many statistical models that are used together to provide the greatest probability for detecting real errors and rejecting false errors.

This approach to quality control is termed the multiple-rule method, and usually requires two or more control levels be evaluated on the same measurement device (electrode). The multiple-rule method is applied:

1. When one control observation exceeds the mean ± 2 SD, a "warning" condition exists.
2. When one control observation exceeds the mean ± 3 SD, an "out-of-control" condition exists.
3. When two consecutive control observations exceed the mean + 2 SD or the mean − 2 SD, an "out-of-control" condition exists.
4. When the range of differences between consecutive control runs exceeds 4 SDs, an "out-of-control" condition exists.
5. When four consecutive control observations exceed the mean + 1 SD or the mean − 1 SD, an "out-of-control" condition exists.
6. When 10 consecutive control observations fall on the same side of the mean (±), an "out-of-control" condition exists.

The multiple-rule method attempts to detect marked changes in electrode performance, sometimes referred to as a "shift" by examining how far from the mean a single control value falls (rules 1 and 2). "Trends" in the performance of the electrode are detected by examining the recent history of control runs (rules 3 to 6). Similar rules may be applied to more than one level of control material by linking. For example, if three different levels of PO_2 controls are all between 2 and 3 SDs higher than their respective means, it is unlikely that the PO_2 electrode is in control. One problem with using a strict statistical approach is that when outliers (values more than 2 SDs from the mean) are repeatedly rejected, the standard deviation tends to become smaller, so that eventually good data may be rejected. This situation can be managed by including data into the data base that is clinically acceptable. With the multiple-rule approach, it is necessary to evaluate not only the mean and standard deviation of the current control run, but to keep a control history as well. This is usually accomplished by means of a control chart (Fig. 11-5). To adequately control an instrument such as a blood gas analyzer, three levels of control materials are normally used. The three levels of control for each of the three electrodes (pH, PCO_2, and PO_2) require that 9 means and 9 SDs be calculated for each instrument, and tracking consecutive control runs can become quite cumbersome. To automate this procedure, computerized quality control data reduction programs are commonly employed. Such programs are available from professional organizations as well as commercial vendors. Some computerized laboratory information systems also support statistical data bases for evaluation of control runs. The chief advantages of such programs is that data storage is simplified, all necessary statistics can be maintained, and sets of rules such as those outlined can be applied easily to each control run to detect errors. This type of recordkeeping for quality control and instrument maintenance is required by many accrediting agencies and by some states.

Quality control of blood gas analyzers should be performed on a sched-

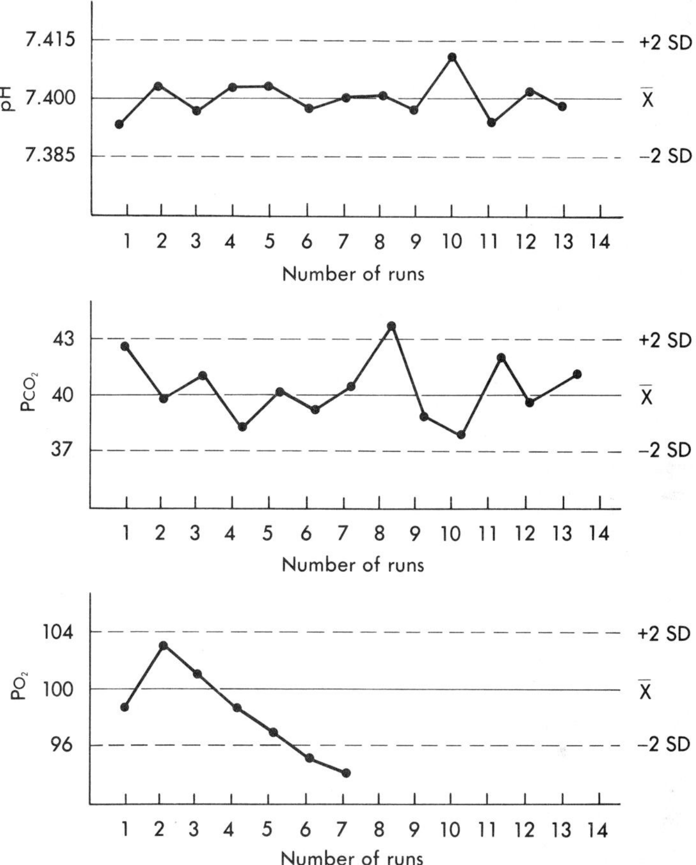

Fig. 11-5 Blood gas quality control charts—three examples of Shewhart/Levey-Jennings charts (pH, P_{CO_2}, and P_{O_2}) on which the mean for a specific control material is plotted as a solid line and the $\pm$ 2 standard deviation (SD) lines are dotted. The left axis on each graph is labeled with the actual mean and 2 SD values. Consecutive control "runs" are plotted along the horizontal axis. On the pH control chart, all of the values vary about the mean in a regular fashion—the electrode appears "in control" for the 13 measurements plotted. The P_{CO_2} chart shows a slightly different pattern: individual control values vary more than the pH, and run 8 shows a value outside of the 2 SD range. In this case, the value is probably a "random" error, because it is the only control value outside the $\pm$ 2 SD limits and because subsequent controls show normal variability about the mean. The P_{O_2} chart shows a "trend" of decreasing control values until runs 6 and 7 both produce values more than 2 SD below the mean; this pattern suggests that the electrode is malfunctioning and needs to be serviced. By applying strict rules to the interpretation of consecutive control runs (with or without charts), most "out-of-control" situations can be detected.

ule commensurate with the number of specimens analyzed. For most laboratories, controls must be performed daily or more often. In busy laboratories, multiple levels of controls may be required on each shift or whenever electrode maintenance is performed. Quality control runs establish the precision of the electrodes so that blood gas interpretation can be related to a range of values. If the variability of a Po_2 electrode is found to be ± 6 mm Hg (2 SDs), then each Po_2 result can be interpreted within a range of 6 mm Hg above or below the reported value.

Several other techniques related to quality control of blood gas analyzers are commonly employed. Interlaboratory proficiency testing consists of the analysis of unknown control specimens from a single source so that an individual laboratory can be compared to other laboratories using both the same and different methodologies. Results of proficiency tests are also reported as means and SDs for each type of instrument participating in the program. Proficiency testing does not establish a level of precision, as does day-to-day quality control, but provides a measure of the absolute accuracy of the individual laboratory. It is possible for a laboratory to have an acceptable level of precision, as determined by daily control runs, but to be inaccurate when compared with other laboratories. Proficiency testing often detects systematic errors that occur because of faulty calibration techniques, contaminated buffers, or procedural errors. Multiple levels of unknowns are usually provided to check the typical ranges of values seen in clinical practice. Proficiency testing programs are available from professional organizations such as the College of American Pathologists and the American Thoracic Society as well as from commercial vendors, and are required by most accrediting agencies.

Comparison of either controls or random samples on multiple instruments provides another means of quality control. Because many blood gas laboratories have two or more instruments, interinstrument comparisons provide a type of proficiency testing that yields immediate information. Similarly, monitoring either controls or samples by independent methods may provide a means of checking the accuracy of a particular instrument. For example, measurement of pH by means of an automated blood gas analyzer and a manual pH electrode could be used to verify the accuracy of the automated calibration system.

Common problems

Some of the common problems encountered in the blood gas laboratory that are detected by quality control and proficiency testing are:

- *Electrode malfunction.* The most common causes of "out-of-control" situations relate to problems arising from the gas and pH electrodes. Protein and blood product buildup on the membranes covering the electrodes are quite common and can usually be remedied by careful cleaning. Leaks in the membranes themselves and depletion of electrolyte solution also commonly lead to electrode drift.

- *Temperature control.* Failure of the water or air bath to maintain the measuring chamber at 37° C, or thermometer inaccuracy, may lead to unacceptable electrode performance. Temperature control systems should be checked routinely against a thermometer certified by the National Bureau of Standards.
- *Improper calibration.* Improper manual calibration, either one- or two-point, is often related to operator error. Analysis of quality control data may determine if the technologist is performing calibration or sampling incorrectly. Problems arising from automatic calibration almost always relate to the instrument trying to perform a calibration with inadequate buffer, or to a poorly functioning electrode.
- *Reagent contamination or loss.* Contamination of calibration buffers and gases leads to inaccurate calibration and sample analysis. Quality control data which are consistently high or low may indicate a problem with reagents. Analysis of the buffers, reagents, or gases by an independent method may be required to detect deficiencies.
- *Mechanical problems.* A common source of error is the mechanism responsible for pumping or aspirating the sample into the measuring chamber. Leaks in pump tubing or poorly functioning pumps allow calibrating solutions, controls, and patient samples all to be contaminated. If air bubbles are introduced during analysis, gas tensions may be in error while pH determinations may be acceptable, but large changes in P_{CO_2} can cause alterations in the pH. Inadequate rinsing of the measuring chamber may also occur with pump problems or improperly functioning valves. This usually results in blood clotting in the transport tubing or measuring chamber.
- *Improper sampling technique.* Questionable results may be caused by failure to collect arterial specimens anaerobically, failure to properly store the sample in ice water, and bubbles in the specimen. Excess heparin typically results in a dilution of the sample with changes in the P_{O_2} and P_{CO_2}. Improperly iced blood gas specimens exhibit changes in pH, P_{CO_2}, and P_{O_2}; red and white blood cells consume O_2 and produce CO_2, with a reduction in the pH. Air bubbles in the specimen shift the gas tensions in the sample toward room air; low P_{O_2} values move toward 150 mm Hg while P_{O_2} values above 150 mm Hg are reduced. Another common problem related to sampling is obtaining a venous specimen inadvertently. Adequately functioning electrodes, as demonstrated by good quality control, can detect poor sampling techniques, as opposed to actual clinical abnormalities.

CRITERIA FOR THE ACCEPTABILITY OF PULMONARY FUNCTION STUDIES

Quality assurance in the pulmonary function laboratory focuses not only on the instrumentation used, equipment calibration, and application of control signals, but on careful attention to the testing technique (sampling) employed. In terms of pulmonary function testing, "sampling" technique is best defined as the procedures used to obtain patient data. This includes the effort and cooperation of the subject, the instruction and encouragement provided by the technologist, as well as the proper performance of the equipment. Application of objective criteria to determine the validity of the data is one means of providing high quality results.

The criteria described in the sections that follow are arranged by test category. Standards for spirometry and the single-breath D_{LCO} have been set forth by the American Thoracic Society, but guidelines for other tests are much less standardized. In each of the test categories, a common method is employed; in applying the criteria, the following steps should be generally followed:

1. Examine the printed or displayed tracing whenever available. A direct recording, such as a kymograph tracing for spirometry, is ideal; computer-generated graphics, either printed or on a video display, may be used as well. Compare the observed tracing with the characteristics of an acceptable curve.
2. Look at the numerical data; are the results reproducible? Are the best two values of multiple efforts within 5% of one another?
3. Are key indicators for a particular test procedure present (such as minimum change in a gas concentration, or timing of a maneuver)? The key indicators to look for vary with the exact methodology employed for each category of test.
4. Are the results of different categories of test consistent (i.e., do spirometry, lung volumes, D_{LCO}, and blood gas analysis all point to a similar interpretation)?

These general guidelines are the basis for applying the criteria to individual sets of patient data.

CRITERIA FOR ACCEPTABILITY OF SPIROMETRY

The following criteria may be used to judge the acceptability of tests derived from the forced expiratory volume (FEV) maneuver:

1. The volume-time tracing should show maximal effort, with a smooth curve; there should be no coughing or hesitation at the beginning of the maneuver. The tracing should show at least 6 seconds of forced effort. An obvious plateau with no volume change for at least 2 seconds should be achieved. Some subjects with severe obstruction may continue exhalation well past 15 seconds, so 6 seconds is simply a minimum. In severe obstruction, very low flows may be observed at the end of expiration, and continuation of the maneuver will not appreciably change the interpretation. The FEV maneuver may be terminated if the subject cannot continue for clinical reasons, such as excessive coughing or dizziness.
2. The start-of-test should be abrupt and unhesitating; on any maneuver that displays a "slow" start, the back-extrapolated volume

should be calculated and the $FEV_{1.0}$ and all other flows should be adjusted (Fig. 11-6). If the volume of back-extrapolation is greater than 5% (or 0.1 L, whichever is greater) of the measured FVC, then the maneuver is not acceptable and should not be included for reporting purposes.

3. A minimum of three acceptable tests should be obtained; both the FVC values and the $FEV_{1.0}$ values of the two largest acceptable tests should be within 5%, or 100 ml, whichever is larger. These may be calculated:

$$\frac{\text{2nd largest FVC}}{\text{largest FVC}} \times 100$$

The same calculaton is applied for the $FEV_{1.0}$. If the two largest acceptable tests are not within 5% (or 100 ml), then the maneuver

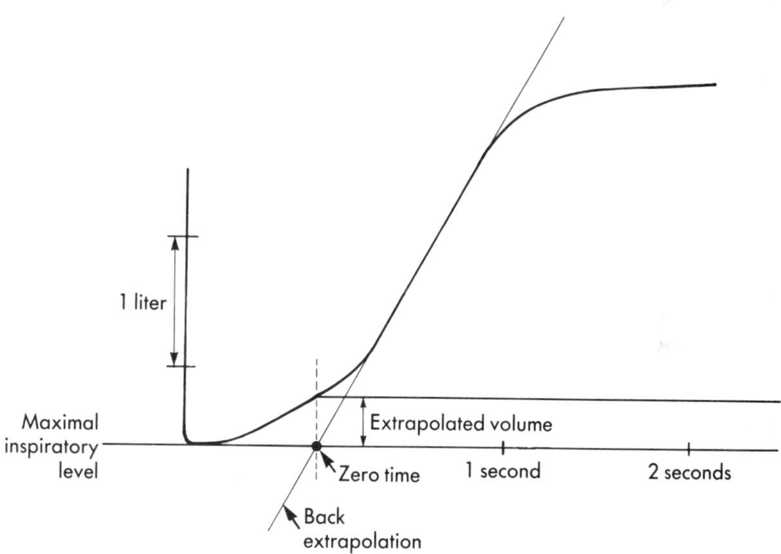

Fig. 11-6 Back-extrapolation of a volume-time spirogram. Back-extrapolation is a means of correcting measurements made from a spirogram that does not show a sharp deflection from the baseline maximal inspiratory level. A straight line drawn through the steepest part of a volume-time tracing is extended to cross the volume baseline. The point of intersection is the back-extrapolated time zero, and timed intervals (such as $FEV_{1.0}$) are measured from this starting point rather than from the initial deflection from the baseline or from the point of maximal flow. The perpendicular distance (slashed line) from the zero time point to the volume-time tracing defines the back-extrapolated volume. To accurately determine the zero time point, the extrapolated volume should be less than 5% of the FVC, or 100 ml, whichever is greater. Tracings with larger extrapolated volumes may be considered invalid.

should be repeated up to a maximum of eight attempts, until the criteria are met. The reproducibility criteria should be applied only after the maneuver has been deemed acceptable with regard to start-of-test and effort. Individual spirometric maneuvers should not be rejected solely because they are not reproducible. Bronchospasm or fatigue may affect reproducibility. The interpretation should include comments regarding the reproducibility, or lack of it, for the test maneuvers. The only criteria for eliminating a test completely is failure to obtain two acceptable maneuvers after at least eight attempts.

4. The MEFV curve, if obtained, should show reproducible flows at similar lung volumes. The PEFR (peak flow) should be consistent, and is a good indicator of subject effort. Superimposing MEFV curves, or displaying them side-by-side, offers a simple means of checking reproducibility. Complete loops should close; i.e., inspiratory and expiratory VC values should be similar.

The largest FVC and the largest $FEV_{1.0}$ (BTPS) should be recorded, after examing the data from all of the acceptable maneuvers, even if the two values do not come from the same curve. Spirometric parameters that are determined by the FVC (such as the $FEF_{25\%-75\%}$) and instantaneous flows ($\dot{V}$) should come from the single "best" test. The "best" test is that maneuver with the largest sum of FVC and $FEV_{1.0}$ (Table 11-2). One problem with using these criteria for spirometry reporting is that if a single volume-time or flow-volume tracing is stored for inclusion in the final report, it may not contain all of the data that appear on the report. It is advisable to maintain recordings (or raw data) for all acceptable maneuvers. Other methods of selecting the "best" test that have been suggested include using

Table 11-2 Comparison of spirometry efforts

Test	Trial 1	Trial 2	Trial 3	"Best" test
FVC	5.20	5.30	5.35*	5.35
$FEV_{1.0}$	4.41*	4.35	4.36*	4.41
$FEV_{1.0}$/FVC	85	82	82	82
$FEF_{25\%-75\%}$	3.87	3.92	3.94	3.94
$\dot{V}_{max\ 50}$	3.99	3.95	3.41	3.41
$\dot{V}_{max\ 25}$	1.97	1.95	1.89	189
PEFR	8.39	9.44	9.89	9.89

*These values are keys to selecting the "best" test results. The $FEV_{1.0}$ is taken from Trial 1, even though the largest sum of FVC and $FEV_{1.0}$ occurs in Trial 3. All FVC-dependent flows (average and instantaneous flows) come from Trial 3. It should be noted that the $FEV_{1\%}$ ($FEV_{1.0}$/FVC) is calculated from the $FEV_{1.0}$ of Trial 1 and the FVC of Trial 3. The MEFV curve, if reported, would be the curve from Trial 3 as well.

the PEFR as an indicator of maximal effort, or combining raw data from several MEFV loops to create an "envelope" loop. Using the peak flow may be in error if the FVC and $FEV_{1.0}$ are not also evaluated, because the PEFR is largely effort dependent and occurs at the beginning of the forced expiration. Combining loops to generate an envelope will provide the maximal flow achieved at any lung volume, but again, not all reported data may be depicted.

Spirometry may be performed in either the sitting or standing position by adults or children. There is some evidence that forced expiratory volumes may be larger in the standing position in adults and in children less than 12 years of age. The position used for testing should be indicated on the final report. The use of nose clips is recommended for spirometric measurements that require rebreathing, even if just for a few breaths. Some spirometers record only expiratory flow and require the subject to place the mouthpiece into the mouth after inspiring to TLC; if such is the case, nose clips are usually unnecessary. Care should be taken, however, to ensure that the subject places the mouthpiece into his or her mouth rapidly before beginning the forced expiration to avoid undetectable loss of volume. It may be impossible to accurately calculate the volume of back-extrapolation from a tracing that displays only expiratory flow. In either type of recording system (rebreathing or expiratory flow only), the mechanical recording device should have its pen (or paper) moving at recording speed when the forced expiration begins. Systems that initiate pen or paper movement at the same time as expiration are typically unable to adequately record the start-of-test, and may seriously underrecord expiratory flow.

CRITERIA FOR ACCEPTABILITY OF THE MAXIMUM VOLUNTARY VENTILATION (MVV)

The maximum voluntary ventilation (MVV) maneuver may be considered acceptable if the following criteria are met:

1. The tracing (volume-time) should show a continuous, rhythmic effort for at least 12 seconds. The end-expiratory level should remain fairly constant; if significant air trapping occurs, the end-expiratory volume may increase. On some spirometers, water-sealed types in particular, a leak at the mouthpiece may cause the spirometer volume to decrease, giving the appearance of gas being trapped in the lungs. Most subjects show a change in the end-expiratory level on the first few breaths of the MVV as they adjust to a mechanically efficient lung volume. This change typically shows up on the tracing as a decrease in spirometer volume, because most subjects perform the MVV at a lung volume slightly above FRC. The first three to five breaths may be discarded if the maneuver was continued long enough for a 12-second interval to be measured. Performing the test for 12 to 15 seconds is usually adequate.

2. At least two acceptable maneuvers should be obtained; the results should not differ by more than 10%. If a difference greater than 10% is observed, the test should be repeated until the two best maneuvers are reproducible. Other less strenuous tests may be interposed to minimize fatigue that may accompany repeated MVV trials. Patients with hyperreactive airways may experience bronchospasm or coughing induced by the hyperventilation occurring with the MVV maneuver. A marked decrease in the measured MVV with repeated efforts may be evidence of hyperreactivity and should be noted in the final report.
3. The measured MVV should exceed the largest $FEV_{1.0}$ multiplied by 35. Because there is a good correlation between the two parameters, the effort put forth by the subject can be judged against an acceptable $FEV_{1.0}$ maneuver. If the MVV is much smaller than the $FEV_{1.0} \times 35$, subject effort should be considered along with other conditions that might cause a decreased MVV (see Chapter 3). Similarly, if the MVV exceeds the $FEV_{1.0} \times 35$ by a large amount, the validity of the $FEV_{1.0}$ itself may be questioned.

The "best" test should be the largest MVV observed from an acceptable maneuver. If the subject is unable to perform the MVV for 12 seconds because of coughing, fatigue, or shortness of breath, the fact should be noted on the final report.

CRITERIA FOR ACCEPTABILITY OF THE SLOW VITAL CAPACITY (SVC)

The slow vital capacity (SVC) maneuver may be considered acceptable if the following criteria are met:

1. The end-expiratory volume during the three breaths immediately preceding the VC maneuver should not vary by more than 100 ml. Increasing or decreasing end-expiratory levels usually indicate that the subject is not breathing consistently near FRC, or that a leak is present. Even if the end-expiratory level is constant, the tidal volume (V_T) usually increases when the subject is asked to breath through a mouthpiece with nose clip in place. This increase in V_T will change the inspiratory capacity (IC) or the expiratory reserve volume (ERV), or both, depending on the pattern of breathing that the subject assumes.
2. The subject should expire smoothly to RV and then inspire without interruption to TLC. A plateau (volume) should occur at both maximal expiration and maximal inspiration. The SVC may be measured either from maximal inspiration (inspiratory VC) or from maximal expiration (expiratory VC).
3. At least two acceptable SVC maneuvers should be obtained. The volumes on these trials should be within 5% of one another, or the maneuver should be repeated until the two best results are reproducible.

4. The SVC should be within 5% of the largest FVC. If the SVC is much less than 95% of the FVC, poor effort on the part of the subject may be the cause. If the SVC is much larger than the FVC, it may be due to dynamic compression of the airways during the FVC maneuver or insufficient effort by the subject during the FVC. An SVC that is significantly larger than the FVC may mean that the $FEV_{1\%}$ was overestimated.

Obtaining an acceptable SVC is important, particularly when its subdivisions (IC and ERV) are used in the calculation of residual volume (RV) and total lung capacity (TLC). An excessively large tidal volume (i.e., $V_T < 1.0$ L) or an irregular breathing pattern during the SVC maneuver may reduce the ERV or IC. When a spuriously reduced ERV is subtracted from the FRC, the calculated RV will appear larger than it should. Similarly, if a spuriously reduced IC is added to the FRC, the TLC will be underestimated.

The same criteria should be applied to the SVC if it is done alone or in conjunction with the lung volume determination (by gas dilution or plethysmography). SVC maneuvers done during the He dilution FRC measurement may show slightly low expiratory reserve volumes (ERV) because the subject exhales through the CO_2 absorber. The IC and ERV may be measured from the FVC maneuver if tidal breathing is also recorded; the end-expiratory level should be well defined as in number 1 in the previous list.

CRITERIA FOR ACCEPTABILITY OF LUNG VOLUMES AND PLETHYSMOGRAPHY

Helium dilution FRC

The He dilution FRC determination may be considered acceptable if the following criteria are met:

1. The "system" baseline should be flat, and the He concentraion should be stable up to the point of subject switch-in, indicating that no system leaks are present.
2. The rebreathing pattern should be regular; the tidal breathing pattern should be regular, with successive breaths showing a gradually falling end-tidal level (as O_2 is consumed). A pattern of increasing tidal volume and rate usually indicates inadequate CO_2 absorption; this is uncomfortable and dangerous for the subject, and may affect the He analyzer readings.
3. The test should be continued until the He concentration changes by less than 0.02% over a 30-second interval. If the He analyzer is incapable of readings as small as 0.02%, then 0.05% in 30 seconds may be used. If the He concentration is recorded only every 30 seconds (as in some computerized systems), then the test should be continued for at least 3 minutes, even if the equilibration criteria above is met before then. This avoids a "false" equilibrium that may occur with irregular breathing patterns or frequent addition of O_2.

4. The O_2 consumption, either measured or estimated, should be appropriate for a quietly breathing subject (200 to 400 ml/min). Some systems estimate O_2 consumption during the rebreathing by noting the volume added divided by the time of the test. In the stabilized volume method, the O_2 consumption can be estimated by noting how often (and how much) O_2 is added. During the O_2 bolus method, the rate of fall of the spirometer volume is proportional to the O_2 consumption rate. High O_2 consumption usually indicates a leak; very low or no O_2 consumption means that the subject is receiving O_2 outside the system, also usually indicating a leak.
5. The He equilibration curve, if plotted, should be smooth and regular. The shape of the equilibration curve will depend on the evenness of ventilation, but the curve should show gradually decreasing He concentrations. The curve should be flat at equilibrium.

The time to reach equilibrium should be reported; if the subject fails to achieve equilibrium within 7 minutes, that also should be reported. Extremely large or small FRC values, especially in normal subjects, should be examined carefully with regard to the above criteria. Comparison of the He dilution lung volumes to those obtained by an independent method is helpful. In normal subjects or those with purely restrictive disease, lung volumes by plethysmography, chest x-ray method, or single-breath dilution (as done with $D_{L_{CO}}SB$) should be similar. In subjects with moderate or severe obstruction, He lung volumes should be less than plethysmograph volumes and greater than the volume determined from a single-breath dilution.

If He dilution is the only available method and a questionable value is obtained, the procedure should be repeated, allowing at least 4 minutes between tests to wash residual He out of the subject's lungs.

Nitrogen washout FRC

The N_2 washout lung volume determination may be considered acceptable if the following criteria are met:

1. The washout should show a regular pattern without noticeable increases or abrupt jumps in end-tidal N_2. Individual breaths may vary, particularly in subjects with irregular breathing patterns or uneven ventilation, but the general trend should show gradually falling N_2 concentrations. Leaks in tubing, at the N_2 sampling head, or at the mouthpiece usually allow room air containing N_2 to enter the system. If a Tissot collection system is used, the volume of the spirometer should be constant when the valves are closed to the patient, indicating no leak in the spirometer.
2. Washout times should be appropriate for the type of subject being tested; washout times in normal subjects should be approximately 3 minutes or less. Washout should be complete; i.e., down to approximately 1% N_2 in subjects without obstruction. Incomplete

washout in unobstructed subjects usually indicates a small leak or a contaminated O_2 source. An improperly calibrated or poorly functioning N_2 analyzer may also cause prolonged washout times. In systems that intgegrate a flow signal with the N_2 analyzer signal, changes in the lag time between the two signals can cause inaccurate measurement of the breath-by-breath volume of N_2 washed out.

The washout time should be reported; failure to washout within 7 minutes (or more) should also be noted. Extremely large or small FRC values should be questioned in regard to the previous list. Lung volume determinations by an independent method should compare as described previously for the Helium dilution FRC. If the N_2 washout is the only method available and questionable results are obtained, the test should be repeated after a delay of at least 15 minutes to allow reestablishment of the normal N_2 and O_2 tensions in the lung and body tissues. Longer delays may be necessary if the subject has severe obstruction.

Body plethysmography (VTG)

The thoracic gas volume (VTG) determined using the body plethysmograph may be considered acceptable if the following criteria are met:

1. The displayed or recorded tracing should indicate that the subject panted correctly; the P_{mouth}/P_{box} panting loop should be closed, or nearly closed. The loop should be contained within the pressure range for which the transducers were calibrated; i.e., if full-scale deflection is ± 10 cm H_2O on the mouth pressure axis, then the mouth pressure deflection should not exceed ± 10 cm H_2O. If the oscilloscope or display is calibrated appropriately, pressure signals that exceed the calibration limits will go "off-screen" and will easily be detected. Open loops may indicate compression of gas in the oropharynx, especially with the cheek muscles, or leaks at the mouth. Panting loops that drift across the display usually indicate that thermal equilibrium has not been attained, or that the panting volume is excessive.
2. A minimum of three acceptable panting maneuvers should be obtained. The angles should agree within 10% of the average of the angles measured. This may not always be practical, if only three acceptable tangents are obtained and all three vary significantly. In such cases, the average may be used without rejecting individual maneuvers, but the variability of the angles should be considered when interpreting the reported lung volumes. Visual inspection of the tracings or displays of the panting maneuvers often allows markedly different efforts to be discarded. Computerized systems that allow the mouth shutter to be closed at lung volumes other than at FRC, by continuously tracking the absolute lung volume, may display widely varying angles. For these systems, the calculated FRC values determined from the various panting maneuvers

should be compared, and outliers should be discarded. Most computerized plethysmographs use least squares regression analysis to determine a "best-fit" line through the angle generated by the panting maneuver. The technologist may need to override the computer-generated tangent, depending on the quality of the data obtained from the panting maneuver.

Similar criteria may be applied to measurements of angles for calculation of airway resistance (Raw), except that the angles for open shutter and closed shutter maneuvers are not averaged. Because the $\dot{V}/P_{box}$ angle and P_{mouth}/P_{box} angles are interdependent, airways resistance is derived for each maneuver separately, and then the results of several maneuvers are averaged. In most instances, the closed shutter angles (volume) measured during the resistance maneuvers will be less than those measured to derive thoracic gas volume (VTG) because most subjects pant above FRC. If the subject cannot perform at least three acceptable maneuvers, it should be noted on the report. The thoracic gas volume should be determined from the average of three or more acceptable maneuvers. As described previously in this chapter for the gas dilution techniques, it is often instructive to compare lung volume determinations by two or more independent methods. In subjects with obstructive disease, plethysmographically determined lung volumes usually exceed those measured by the gas dilution techniques, but compare favorably with radiologic volumes.

CRITERIA FOR ACCEPTABILITY OF $DL_{CO}SB$

The American Thoracic Society (ATS) has published guidelines for the standardization of the $DL_{CO}SB$ test (see box on p.323). The $DL_{CO}SB$ maneuver may be considered acceptable if the following criteria are met:

1. The volume-time tracing (see Fig. 5-2) should show a smooth, rapid inspiration from residual volume (RV) to total lung capacity (TLC). The rate of inspiration should be rapid enough so that 90% of the vital capacity is inspired in 2.5 seconds in healthy subjects and in less than 4.0 seconds in patients with obstruction. The breath-hold baseline should be flat, and the exhalation of dead space gas should be rapid and smooth. The volume of dead space should be between 0.75 and 1.00 L. If the subject's vital capacity is less than 2.0 L, the dead space may be reduced to 0.5 L. The tracing should indicate the switch-in to alveolar sampling. Alveolar sample volume should be 0.5 to 1.0 L and the sample should be collected in 3 seconds or less.
2. The volume inspired (VC or VI) should exceed 90% of the largest previously measured vital capacity value, either FVC or SVC. If the inspired volume is less than 90% of the known VC, it may be assumed that the subject either did not exhale to RV, or did not breath-hold at TLC, or both. For purposes of standardization, the breath-hold should be as close to the true TLC as possible. If the

$DL_{CO}SB$ RECOMMENDATIONS*

A. *Equipment*
  1. Volume accuracy same as for spirometry with O_2, CO, He, other gases.
  2. Gas concentrations:

CO	0.3	± 0.05%
He	10.0	± 1.0%
O_2	21.0	± 1.0%

  3. Documented CO and He analyzer linearity.
  4. CO analyzer calibrated at least every 6 months.
  5. Timing mechanism checked quarterly.
  6. Documented instrument dead space (inspiratory/expiratory).
  7. Check for leaks and volume accuracy (3-L calibration) daily.
  8. Validate system by testing healthy nonsmokers.

B. *Technique*
  1. Subject should refrain from smoking for 24 hours before test.
  2. Subject should be instructed carefully before procedure.
  3. Subject should achieve an inspired volume > 90% of VC.
  4. Subject should perform breath-hold for 9 to 11 seconds.
  5. Dead space washout should be 750 to 1000 ml (unless VC < 2.0 L).
  6. Alveolar sample volume should be 500 to 1000 ml.
  7. At least 4 minutes should elapse between repeat tests.

C. *Calculations*
  1. Average at least two acceptable tests.
  2. Use Ogilvie or Meade-Jones methods of timing breath-hold.
  3. Adjust for dead space volumes (instrument and subject).
  4. Determine inspired gas conditions (ATPS or ATPD).
  5. Correct for CO_2 and H_2O absorption.
  6. Report DL/VA in ml CO (STPD)/min/mm Hg per L (BTPS)
  7. Correct for Hb concentration (Cotes method).
  8. Adjustment for COHb (recommended).
  9. Adjustment for altitude (recommended).

*Summarized from American Thoracic Society: Single breath carbon monoxide diffusing capacity (transfer factor)—recommendations for a standard technique, Am Rev Respir Dis 136:1299, 1987.

inspired volume exceeds the best previously determined VC, then that VC should be questioned and may need to be repeated.

3. The breath-holding time should be between 9 and 11 seconds; any tests outside these limits should be discarded. Various methods of timing are employed with the single-breath DL_{CO} (see Chapter 5). Again, for purposes of standardization, the breath-holding time should be kept close to 10 seconds. Rapid inspiration and expiration tend to reduce differences produced by the timing method. In subjects with obstruction, prolonged expiration adds to the time for diffusion to occur and may overestimate diffusing capacity. Reducing the washout volume may shorten the measured breath-hold time, but it may also lead to inaccuracies; sampling earlier will add more dead space gas to the "alveolar" sample, particularly in those subjects who may have increased dead space. The breath-hold itself should be relaxed against either a closed glottis or the valve. A sustained inspiratory effort (Mueller maneuver) will artifactually increase $DL_{CO}SB$ due to an increase in pulmonary capillary blood volume. Excessive positive pressure duing the breath-hold (Valsalva maneuver) tends to reduce pulmonary capillary blood volume and $DL_{CO}SB$. The only practical means of detecting excessive pressure during the breath-hold is careful observation by the technologist conducting the test.
4. Duplicate determinations should be within 10% or 3 ml CO/min/mm Hg (STPD), whichever is greater. The difference between two tests may be calculated:

$$\frac{\text{Test 1} - \text{Test 2}}{\text{Average}} \times 100$$

The reported value should be the average of two or more acceptable maneuvers. The number of acceptable maneuvers that are averaged should be included in the report.

If the subject is unable to perform acceptable maneuvers, that fact should be included in the report, particularly if a $DL_{CO}SB$ value is reported anyway. If a dead space washout volume other than the "standard" 0.75 to 1.00 L is used, it should be noted. The lung volume calculated from the DL_{CO} maneuver (V_A) may be compared to previously measured lung volumes, but must be expressed in liters (BTPS). In normal and even moderately restricted subjects, the V_A correlates reasonably well with the TLC, if the single-breath maneuver is performed acceptably. In subjects with obstruction, the single-breath lung volume may be smaller than lung volumes determined by multiple-breath gas dilution techniques, by radiologic estimation, or by plethysmography. The $DL_{CO}SB$ may be reported using the standard single-breath technique or by calculating the diffusion capacity using an independently determined lung volume in a similar equation.

Corrections for the subject's hemoglobin, COHb, and the altitude at which the measurement is made (see Chapter 5) are recommended but not required. If the Hb is corrected, both the adjusted and unadjusted values should be reported. COHb and altitude corrections, if made, should be documented on the final report for interpretive purposes.

Several conditions affecting the subject may influence the acceptability of the $DL_{CO}SB$. The subject should be instructed to refrain from smoking for 24 hours before the test. The subject should be relaxed and in a sitting position, and should be carefully instructed in each of the required steps of the procedure. For duplicate determinations, at least 4 minutes should elapse between tests to allow test gas to wash out of the subject's lungs.

INFECTION CONTROL

Pulmonary function tests, including blood gas analysis, are often useful in the management of patients with both blood-borne and respiratory pathogens. Reasonable precautions regarding testing techniques and equipment handling can prevent cross-contamination between patients, and between those performing tests and the patient.

General precautions

Each laboratory should have written guidelines, contained in a policy and procedure manual, concerning safety and infection control. These procedures should include, but not be limited to, handwashing techniques, use of protective equipment such as lab coats and gloves, and guidelines for equipment cleaning.

Pulmonary function tests

Pulmonary function testing does not present a significant risk of infection for either patients or technologists, but some potential hazards do exist. Most respiratory pathogens are spread either by contact with contaminated equipment or by an airborne route. Airborne organisms may be contained in droplet nuclei, on epithelial cells that have been shed, or in dust particles. The following guidelines can help reduce the possibility of infection:

1. Disposable mouthpieces and nose clips should be used for spirometry. Reusable mouthpieces should be disinfected or sterilized after each use.
2. Tubing or valves through which subjects rebreathe should be changed after each test, particularly when used for maneuvers such as the FVC where there is a potential for mucus, saliva, or droplet nuclei to contaminate the device. Breathing circuit components should be stored in sealed plastic bags after disinfection.
3. Spirometers should be cleaned in accordance with the manufacturer's recommendations on a schedule commensurate with the frequency of tests done. Flow-based spirometers in which the flow sen-

sor is located at the subject's mouth should be cleaned daily. Other types of pneumotachometers can be disinfected less frequently. Disposable flow sensors should not be reused. Water-sealed spirometers should be drained at least weekly and allowed to dry completely; only distilled water should be used for filling. Bellows and rolling-seal spirometers may be more difficult to disassemble, but they should be disinfected on a routine basis.

4. Bacteria filters may be used in some circuits to prevent equipment contamination, but they may impose increased resistance that will affect maximal flows. Some types of filters show increased resistance after continued use in expired gas. If filters are used for low-flow procedures such as lung volume determinations, their volume must be included in the calculations.
5. Nebulizers, such as those used for bronchodilator or bronchial challenge, and metered dose inhalers offer the greatest potential for cross-contamination. These devices, if reused, should be sterilized to destroy vegetative microorganisms, fungal spores, tubercle bacilli, and some viruses. Preferably, disposable single-use nebulizers should be used. Metered dose devices may be used for bronchodilator studies by using disposable mouthpieces or "spacers" to prevent colonization of the device.
6. Mucous membrane contact may be minimized by the use of gloves or other barriers to remove used mouthpieces or tubing, particularly in subjects with documented infections. Although the risk of transmission from subjects with hepatitis B or human immunodeficiency virus (HIV, or AIDS) via respiratory secretions is slight, there is a risk of acquiring other infections such as tuberculosis or Pneumocystis carinii that occur in infected individuals.
7. Surveillance should include routine cultures of reusable components (i.e., mouthpieces, tubing, valves) following disinfection if the equipment is likely to contact the patient's mucus membranes.

Blood gases

The Centers for Disease Control (CDC) have established universal precautions that apply to personnel handling blood or other body fluids containing blood. Universal precautions apply to blood, semen, vaginal secretions, cerebrospinal fluid (CSF), synovial fluid, pleural fluid, pericardial fluid, and amniotic fluid. Some of these fluids are commonly encountered in the blood gas laboratory. Body fluids to which the universal precautions do not apply include feces, nasal secretions, sputum, sweat, tears, urine, and vomitus, unless they contain visible blood. Some of these fluids are encountered in the pulmonary function laboratory. Although they present an extremely low or nonexistent risk for HIV or hepatitis B, these fluids may be a potential source for nosocomial infections from other non-blood-borne pathogens. Universal precautions do not apply to saliva, but general infection control practices such as use of gloves and handwashing further minimize the minute risk involved in contact with mucous membranes of the mouth.

Universal precautions should be applied in the pulmonary function (blood gas) laboratory:

1. Treat *all* blood and body fluid specimens as potentially contaminated.
2. Exercise care to prevent injuries from needles, scalpels, or other sharp instruments or devices. Do not resheath used needles by hand; do not remove used needles from disposable syringes by hand; do not bend, break, or otherwise manipulate used needles by hand. Use a rubber block or cork to obstruct used needles after arterial punctures. Place used syringes and needles, scalpel blades, and other sharp items in puncture-resistant containers. Locate the containers as close as possible to the area of use.
3. Use protective barriers to prevent exposure to blood, body fluids containing visible blood, and other fluids to which the universal precautions apply. Examples of protective barriers include gloves, gowns, lab coats, masks, and protective eyewear. Gloves should be worn for drawing blood samples, but they cannot prevent penetrating injuries caused by needles or sharp objects. Gloves are also indicated if the technologist has cuts, scratches or other breaks in the skin. Gloves should be worn in situations in which hand contamination with blood may occur, such as obtaining blood from an uncooperative patient, when performing finger/heel sticks on infants, or when receiving training in blood drawing. Maintenance of blood gas analyzers, such as repair of electrodes and emptying of waste containers, should be performed wearing gloves. Examination gloves should be worn for procedures involving contact with mucous membranes. Masks and protective goggles may be indicated for procedures that present a possibility of blood splashing, such as arterial line placement.
4. Immediately and thoroughly wash hands and other skin surfaces that are contaminated with blood or other fluids to which the universal precautions apply. Blood spills should be cleaned up using a solution of 1 part 5% sodium hypochlorite (bleach) in 9 parts of water. Bleach should also be used to rinse sinks used for blood disposal.

SELF-ASSESSMENT QUESTIONS

1. A spirometer is tested by injecting a 3-L volume from a large syringe several times; the results are as follows:

Trial	Volume
1	2.82
2	2.83
3	2.85

Which of the following descriptions are true:
I. The spirometer may have a leak
II. The spirometer is precise
III. The spirometer is accurate within 3%
IV. The spirometer meets American Thoracic Society recommendations
a. I, II, III, IV
b. II, III, IV
c. I, II only
d. III, IV only

2. A 3-L syringe is used to perform quality control on a spirometer; the results of three maneuvers are:

Trial	Volume
1	2.95
2	2.90
3	2.93
	2.93 average

What is the % error of this spirometer:
a. 0.7%
b. 2.3%
c. 5.0%
d. 7.0%

3. According to the American Thoracic Society's recommendations, spirometer quality controls include which of the following:
I. Daily check for leaks
II. Daily check of FVC and $FEV_{1.0}$ of at least one known subject
III. Daily check of volume accuracy with a 3-L syringe
IV. Quarterly calibration checks across the spirometer's range
a. I, II, III, IV
b. I, III, IV
c. II, III
d. I, IV

4. A spirometer recorder that is used for manual calculation of the $FEV_{1.0}$ should have sensitivities of:

Volume	Time
a. 5 mm/L	1 cm/sec
b. 10 mm/L	2 cm/sec
c. 12 mm/L	5 cm/sec
d. 15 mm/L	3 cm/sec

5. An O_2 analyzer is set up to measure a subject's exhaled gas as part of a metabolic study; what gas(es) should be used to calibrate the analyzer:

a 5% CO_2 in room air
b 10% O_2
c Room air and 15% O_2
d Room air and 100% O_2

6. To demonstrate the linearity of a gas analyzer, _____ gas(es) is (are) required?
   a. 1
   b. 2
   c. 3 or more
   d. Room air plus 1

7. Which of the following may be used to perform quality control on a pressure plethysmograph for measuring V_{TG}:
   I. Comparison with gas dilution lung volume determinations
   II. A 3-L syringe with occlusion valve
   III. An isothermal lung analog
   IV. A known subject who has been tested at least 10 times
   a. I, II, III, IV
   b. I, II, III
   c. I, III, IV
   d. II, IV only

8. To calibrate a blood gas analyzer, a gas with 11.0% oxygen and 5.0% CO_2 is used; if the local barometric pressure is 764, the respective calibration partial pressures are:
   a. 84 and 38 mm Hg
   b. 79 and 38 mm Hg
   c. 84 and 40 mm Hg
   d. 79 and 36 mm Hg

9. Which of the following are true regarding the use of tonometry for quality control of blood gas analzers:
   I. Blood may be used to check pH, P_{O_2}, and P_{CO_2} electrodes
   II. Tonometered buffer may be used to check the pH electrode
   III. A precision gas is required for each level of control material
   IV. Tonometry is dependent on the sampling technique employed
   a. I, II, III, IV
   b. I, III, IV
   c. II, III, IV
   d. II, IV only

10. Quality control runs for a P_{O_2} electrode have produced a mean of 58.0 mm Hg with an SD of 2 mm Hg. According to the multiple-rule method, if the next three control runs produce values of 61, 63, and 60 mmHg, the electrode:
    a. Is "out-of-control"
    b. Is "in control"
    c. Is displaying a "random" error
    d. Both b and c

11. A subject performs spirometry, and these results are recorded from three efforts:

	Trial 1	Trial 2	Trial 3
FVC (L)	3.3	3.4	3.5
$FEV_{1.0}$ (L)	2.3	2.5	2.3
$FEF_{25\%-75\%}$ (L/sec)	1.7	1.2	1.3

Which values should be reported for this subject:

FVC ____________
$FEV_{1.0}$ ____________
$FEV_{1\%}$ ____________
$FEF_{25\%075\%}$ ____________

12. According to the recommendations of the American Thoracic Society, the two best FVC values and $FEV_{1.0}$ values should be within:
a. 1% or 50 ml, whichever is greater
b. 3% or 50 ml, whichever is greater
c. 5% or 100 ml, whichever is greater
d. 10% or 300 ml, whichever is greater

13. Which of the following would be indications for rejecting a $DL_{CO}SB$ maneuver:
I. Breath-hold time = 11.6 seconds
II. Volume inspired = 84% of FVC
III. Inspiratory time = 4.1 seconds
IV. Dead space washout volume = 1.0 L
a. I, II, III, IV
b. I, III, IV
c. I, II, III
d. III and IV only

14. Infection control for pulmonary function testing includes which of the following:
I. Use of disposable mouthpieces for spirometry
II. Cleaning and disinfecting of spirometers after each use
III. Sterilization of nebulizers used for inhalation challenge tests
IV. Use of filters for low-flow rebreathing studies
a. I, II, III, IV
b. I, III, IV
c. II, IV
d. II, III

15. Which of the following are contrary to the universal precautions recommended by the Centers for Disease Control (CDC):
a. Resheathing used needles
b. Handling blood without gloves
C. Emptying blood gas waste without gloves
d. All of the above

SELECTED BIBLIOGRAPHY

General references

American Thoracic Society: Standardization of spirometry, Am Rev Respir Dis 119:831, 1979.

American Thoracic Society: Standardization of spirometry—1987 update, Am Rev Respir Dis 136:1285, 1987.

American Thoracic Society: Single breath carbon monoxide diffusing capacity (transfer factor)—recommendations for a standard technique, Am Rev Respir Dis 136:1299, 1987.

Clausen JL, editor: Pulmonary function testing guidelines and controversies, New York, 1982, Academic Press, Inc.

Morris AH et al: Clinical pulmonary function testing, ed 2, Salt Lake City, 1984, Intermountain Thoracic Society.

Calibration and quality control

Clausen JL et al: Interlaboratory comparisons of blood gas measurements, Am Rev Respir Dis 123(suppl):104, 1981.

Gardner RM et al: Spirometry: what paper speed?, Chest 84:161, 1983.

Gardner RM, Hankinson JL, and West BJ: Evaluating commercially available spirometers, Am Rev Respir Dis 121:73, 1980.

Glindmeyer HW et al: A portable adjustable forced vital capacity simulator for routine spirometer calibration, Am Rev Respir Dis 121:599, 1980.

Hankinson JL and Gardner RM: Standard waveforms for spirometer testing, Am Rev Respir Dis 126:362, 1982.

Hankinson JL: Pulmonary function testing in the screening of workers: guidelines for instrumentation, performance, and interpretation. J Occup Med 28:1081, 1986.

Leary ET, Graham G, and Kenny MA: Commercially available blood-gas quality controls compared with tonometered blood, Clin Chem 26:1309, 1980.

Leith DE and Mead J: Principles of body plethysmography, Bethesda, Md, 1974, National Heart, Lung, and Blood Institute—Division of Lung Diseases.

Shigeoka JW: Calibration and quality control of spirometer systems, Respir Care 28:747, 1983.

Shigeoka JW, Gardner RM, and Barkham HW: A portable volume/flow calibrating syringe, Chest 82:598, 1982.

Westgard JO et al: Performance characteristics of rules for internal quality control: probabilities for false rejection and error detection, Clin Chem 23:1857, 1977.

Criteria for acceptability of pulmonary function studies

Office spirometry in clinical practice: ACCP Committee on clinic and office pulmonary function testing: Chest 74:298, 1978.

Ferris BG, editor: Epidemiology standardization project: recommended standardized procedures for pulmonary function testing, Am Rev Respir Dis 118(suppl 2):55, 1978.

Nathan SP, Lebowitz MD, and Knudson RJ: Spirometric testing: number of tests required and selection of data, Chest 76:384, 1979.

Quanjer PH, editor: Standardization of lung function testing, Bull Eur Physiopathol Respir 19(suppl 5), 1983.

Snow M: Determination of functional residual capacity, Respir Care 34:586, 1989.

Sorensen JB et al: Selection of the best spirometric values for interpretation, Am Rev Respir Dis 122:802, 1980.

Townsend MC, Duchene AG, and Fallat RJ: The effects of underrecorded forced expirations on spirometric lung function indexes, Am Rev Respir Dis 126:734, 1982.

Infection control

Centers for Disease Control: Recommendations for prevention of HIV transmission in health-care settings, MMWR 36:3S, 1987.

Centers for Disease Control: Update: universal precautions for prevention of transmission of human immunodeficiency virus, Hepatitis B virus, and other bloodborne pathogens in health-care settings, MMWR 37:377, 1988.

Chatburn RL: Decontamination of respiratory care equipment: what can be done, what should be done, Respir Care 34:98, 1989.

Garner JS and Favero MS: CDC guidelines for the prevention and control of nosocomial infections: guideline for handwashing and hospital environmental control, Am J Infect Control 14:110, 1986.

Simmons BP and Wong ES: Guidelines for prevention of nosocomial pneumonia. Am J Infect Control 11:230, 1983.

Tablan OC, Williams WW, and Martone WJ: Infection control in pulmonary function laboratories, Infect Control 6:442, 1985.

Zibrak JD et al: Infection control in the respiratory management of patients with HIV-related disorders, Respir Care 34:734, 1989.

12

Case Studies

The following cases are presented to illustrate the use of pulmonary function testing, exercise testing, and blood gas analysis to aid in the diagnosis and treatment of various types of pulmonary disorders. Attention should be directed to the subject history accompanying each set of test values to better understand the numeric results. Readers are encouraged to evaluate the History and Testing sections, then to write an interpretation, using the guidelines described, and compare their assessment to the one given in the Interpretation section. The Discussion section explains the comments given in the Interpretation. The first five cases deal with the types of pulmonary function tests typically performed in most hospital laboratories; case 6 is an inhalation challenge test; cases 7, 8, and 9 include exercise test data, interpretations, and discussions. Case 10 is an example of blood gas quality control interpretation.

General guidelines for interpretation provide a framework for a systematic approach to interpreting pulmonary function and blood gas data.

1. *Acceptability of data.* Careful review of tracings and raw data should precede any interpretive steps. Two key elements that should be evaluated include proper equipment function and adequacy of subject effort. Malfunction of spirometers, gas analyzers, or other equipment components can often be discerned from either the tracings recorded or raw data, such as analyzer readings. Subject cooperation and effort can also be evaluated from tracings and raw data. Internal consistency of the data may also be checked to detect problems. For example, the vital capacity (VC) may be measured as part of spirometry, as part of lung volume determination, during the $DL_{CO}SB$ maneuver, and in conjunction with plethysmography. Each of these measures should be internally consistent; the VC measurements need not be identical, but any differences, such as variations between the FVC and SVC, should be accounted for. A report by the technologist performing the study is invaluable if the interpreter is not present for the test. This report can be as simple as a set of notes describing the subject's cooperation and ability to perform the test maneuvers, as well as any potential problems that might affect the reported values. Criteria for acceptability of each test should be determined in advance by the laboratory; guidelines

for standardization, such as those published by the American Thoracic Society (see Chapter 11), should be the basis for these laboratory criteria. Non-acceptability of pulmonary function data should be documented in the interpretation, particularly if the reproducibility of the data is in question.

2. *Measured versus predicted values.* The appropriateness of the predicted values used in the interpretation should be verified. In most instances, this requires that the interpreter be familiar with the variability of the predicted values for each test and with the population from which the predicted values were derived (see Selecting and Using Predicted Values in the Appendix). "Abnormal" values for each test category may be enumerated, after ascertaining that the predicted values are appropriate for the subject tested. Incorrect recording of age, height, or sex commonly result in the wrong predicted values being used. Values outside of predicted limits should be examined in each test category:
   a. spirometry before and after bronchodilator
   b. lung volumes by gas dilution and/or plethysmography
   c. DL_{CO} (single-breath or steady-state)
   d. blood gases
   e. maximal inspiratory and expiratory pressures
   f. airways resistance, conductance, and compliance

   Many computerized systems flag "abnormal" values; the method by which this is done should be determined by the laboratory based on evaluation of normal subjects and subjects with known disease. Other computerized functions that may be helpful include calculation of confidence intervals or percentiles.
3. *Type and severity of dysfunction.* If truly abnormal values are found, some general statement of the pattern of abnormality may be made. The simplest categorization is to describe the pattern as obstructive, restrictive, or as a combination of both. Obstructive diseases are characterized by reduction of maximal expiratory and/or inspiratory flow rates. Obstruction may be accompanied by increases in lung volumes, notably RV, FRC, and TLC. Reduced diffusing capacity and blood gas abnormalities also commonly accompany obstruction. Restrictive diseases are characterized by reduction in lung volumes, particularly the VC and TLC, and may also be accompanied by abnormalities in diffusing capacity and blood gases. The severity of the dysfunction is commonly classified by modifiers attached to the specific physiologic parameter measured, such as "severe reduction in flows," "moderately reduced TLC," "mildly elevated PCO_2"). The use of such modifiers is limited by the variability associated with the particular parameter and may not adequately describe the severity of the disease, functional limi-

tations to the subject, or the risk of morbidity/mortality. If such modifiers are used, the limits of normal for particular tests should be described, particularly if the measured value falls close to the lower limit of normal. Extent of disease is also sometimes described by comparison with changes from previous tests. The variability of a specific physiologic parameter and the variability of the measuring technique combine to determine how large of a change can be considered significant. Subjects with disease often show increased variability in specific parameters, and this must also be considered. Published studies are useful in determining the variation occurring in normal and diseased subjects, but each laboratory has to determine the variability of the test methodology that they employ.

4. *Clinical summary.* A summary statement that relates the acceptability of the data, the abnormal findings, and the type of dysfunction to the subject's clinical history is often useful. In many instances, this summary may be limited more by the history (or lack of it) than by the test data. In some cases, interpretation may include questions such as "Does the subject have any history of exposure to . . ." to assist in relating the observed values to the subject's symptoms. The summary may also include recommendations for further or follow-up testing, as well as suggestions for therapy (i.e., oxygen, bronchodilators).

CASE 1
History

M.B. is a 27-year-old male high school teacher, whose chief complaint is dyspnea on exertion. The subject states that his breathlessness has worsened over the past several months. He has smoked one pack of cigarettes a day for approximately 10 years (10 pack/years). He denies a cough or sputum production. No members of his family have ever had emphysema, asthma, chronic bronchitis, carcinoma, or tuberculosis. There is no history of exposure to extraordinary environmental pollutants.

Pulmonary function testing

A. Personal data

Sex:	Male
Age:	27 yr
Height:	65 in
Weight:	297 lb
BSA:	2.28M^2

B. Spirometry and airway resistance

	Before drug	**Predicted**	**%**
FVC (L)	2.90	4.70	62
$FEV_{1.0}$ (L)	2.47	3.86	64
$FEV_{1\%}$ (%)	85	82	—
$FEF_{25\%-75\%}$ (L/sec)	4.62	4.35	106
$\dot{V}_{max_{50}}$ (L/sec)	4.94	5.82	85
$\dot{V}_{max_{25}}$ (L/sec)	2.49	3.22	77
MVV (L/min)	178	137	130
Raw (cm H_2O/L/sec)	2.33	0.6-2.4	—
SGaw (L/sec/cm H_2O/L)	0.23	0.12-0.50	—

C. Lung volumes (by plethysmograph)

	Before drug	**Predicted**	**%**
VC (L)	2.90	4.70	62
IC (L)	1.96	2.91	67
ERV (L)	0.94	1.80	59
FRC (L)	1.87	3.29	57
RV (L)	0.93	1.49	57
TLC (L)	3.83	6.20	62
RV/TLC (%)	25	24	—

D. Diffusing Capacity (single-breath)

	Before drug	**Predicted**	**%**
DL_{CO} (ml CO/min/mm Hg)	18.8	31.4	60
V_A (L)	3.68	—	—
D_L/V_A	5.11	—	—

E. Blood gases ($F_{I_{O_2}}$ 0.21)

pH	7.44
Pa_{CO_2} (mmHg)	35
Pa_{O_2} (mmHg)	67
Sa_{O_2} (%)	91%
HCO_3^- (mEq/L)	23.6

Interpretation

All data from spirometry, lung volumes, diffusion, and blood gases are acceptable.

Spirometry shows a decreased FVC and $FEV_{1.0}$; flows are within normal limits, as is the MVV. The Raw is near the upper limit of normal but SGaw is normal.

Lung volumes are decreased, with the RV/TLC ratio preserved.

$DL_{CO}SB$ is reduced. pH and Pa_{CO_2} are within normal limits, but the Pa_{O_2} is decreased, representing a widened aleveolar-arterial difference.

Impression: Moderate restrictive lung disease without evidence of obstruction, with mild hypoxemia. Restrictive pattern may be related to subject's weight.

Discussion

This case offers a good example of what might be considered a "pure" restrictive defect. Characteristic of a restrictive process is a proportional decrease in all lung volumes, including FVC and FEV_1 with little or no decrease in any of the flow measurements ($FEF_{25\%-75\%}$, $\dot{V}_{max_{50}}$). Also typical of simple restriction is the well-preserved ratio between $FEV_{1.0}$ and FVC. The volume expired in the first second was in correct proportion to the total volume exhaled, despite the decreases in the absolute volumes of each. The MVV demonstrates the subject's ability to move a normal maximal volume. This may be accomplished in spite of moderately severe restriction by an increase in the rate rather than in the V_T.

The $DL_{CO}SB$ confirms the effect of the decreased lung volume's impairment of gas transfer. The reduction in DL_{CO} is approximately proportional to the decrease in TLC. Another way of expressing this relationship is to divide the DL_{CO} by the lung volume at which the diffusion measurement was made (sometimes called the DL/VA). The ratio in this case is 5.11 ml CO transferred per liter of lung volume. If the predicted $DL_{CO}SB$ is divided by the predicted TLC, a ratio of 5.06 ml CO transferred per liter of lung volume is obtained. The DL/VA may be helpful in defining the contribution of obstructive or restrictive components to reducing the DL_{CO}. In restrictive patterns, the DL/VA ratio is preserved, whereas in obstructive patterns it is decreased.

The widened A-a gradient (approximately 40 mm Hg) is again consistent with reduced lung volumes and is significant, particularly in view of the subject's complaint of exertional dyspnea and his age.

The explanation for the restrictive pattern may well lie in the subject's weight of 297 lb. For his height, he is at approximately 200% of his ideal weight. Obesity is one of the most common causes of restrictive patterns. Further evaluation of this subject might include testing his response to hypoxia and hypercapnia, because chronically obese individuals often display patterns of decreased ventilatory drive resulting in CO_2 retention. The subject does not appear to be retaining CO_2 at this point, and treatment of the obesity might avoid future complications.

CASE 2
History

P.R. is a 21-year-old man in good health. He plays college football and has a chief complaint of shortness of breath following "wind sprints" and similar vigorous exercises. He denies any other symptoms, including cough or sputum production. He has never smoked. His grandfather had "lung problems," but there is no other history of pulmonary disease involving the family. He does state that his brothers and sisters have "hay fever." There is no history of exposure to extraordinary environmental pollutants.

Pulmonary function testing

A. Personal data

Sex:	Male
Age:	21 yr
Height:	73 in
Weight:	180 lb

B. Spirometry and airway resistance

	Before drug	Predicted	%	After drug	%
FVC (L)	6.85	6.04	111	6.73	111
$FEV_{1.0}$ (L)	4.65	4.78	97	5.45	114
$FEV_{1\%}$ (%)	70	79	—	81	—
$FEF_{25\%-75\%}$ (L/sec)	3.90	5.00	78	4.88	97
$\dot{V}_{max_{50}}$ (L/sec)	5.01	6.52	77	6.10	94
$\dot{V}_{max_{25}}$ (L/sec)	2.79	3.75	74	3.25	87
MVV (L/min)	218	166	131	215	130
Raw (cm H_2O/L/sec)	2.10	0.6-2.4	—	1.60	—
SGaw (L/sec/cm H_2O/L)	0.14	0.10-0.39	—	0.18	—

C. Lung volumes (open-circuit method)

	Before drug	Predicted	%
VC (L)	6.58	6.04	109
IC (L)	4.63	3.65	127
ERV (L)	1.95	2.39	82
FRC (L)	3.60	4.33	83
RV (L)	1.65	1.94	85
TLC (L)	8.23	7.98	103
RV/TLC (%)	20	24	—

D. Diffusing capacity (single breath)

	Before drug	Predicted	%
DL_{CO} (ml CO/min/mm Hg)	28.2	34.5	82
VA (L)	7.90	—	—
DL/VA	3.57	4.32	—

E. Blood gases (FI_{O_2} 0.21)

pH	7.41
Pa_{CO_2} (mm Hg)	39
Pa_{O_2} (mm Hg)	94
Sa_{O_2} (%)	97
HCO_3^- (mEq/L)	24.4

Interpretation

All data for spirometry, lung volumes, diffusing capacity, and blood gases are acceptable.

Spirometry is within normal limits except for a decrease in the $FEV_{1\%}$. There is a significant increase in the $FEV_{1.0}$, $\dot{V}_{max_{50}}$, $\dot{V}_{max_{25}}$, $FEV_{1\%}$, and $FEF_{25\%-75\%}$ following administration of the bronchodilator. The MVV is normal, as are the Raw and SGaw. The Raw and SGaw showed a significant improvement following bronchodilator. All lung volumes are within normal limits, as are the blood gases and $DL_{CO}SB$.

Impression: Mild obstructive defect with significant response to bronchodilator; otherwise normal lung function. Evaluation for exercise-induced bronchospasm is recommended.

Discussion

This subject is a good example of an individual with essentially normal, or slightly above normal, values for almost every lung function parameter. The exception is the $FEV_{1\%}$, which is consistent with a mild obstructive pattern. Simple evaluation of the FVC and $FEV_{1.0}$ in relation to their predicted values might give the impression that this subject is normal. But the $FEV_{1\%}$ indicates that the subject, whose lung volumes are slightly larger than normal, expired a disproportionately small volume in the first second. The slightly decreased values for $FEF_{25\%-75\%}$, $\dot{V}_{max_{50}}$, and $\dot{V}_{max_{25}}$ also point to an obstructive process. In addition, there is a significant (17%) increase in $FEV_{1.0}$ following administration of a beta-adrenergic bronchodilator. This is particulary significant in view of the subject's main symptom of shortness of breath following exercise. The subject appears to exhibit reversible airway obstruction triggered by exercise.

Further evaluation of P.R. included an exercise test to try to demonstrate exercise-induced asthma (EIA). After 6 minutes of treadmill jogging at 88% of his predicted maximal heart rate, the subject's $FEV_{1.0}$ began to fall; it reached a low value of 4.10 ($FEV_{1\%}$ of 62%) 5 minutes after termination of the test. Scattered wheezes were heard on auscultation. The obstruction was readily reversed by inhaled bronchodilator.

Measurement of the closing volume (CV) by the SBN_2 method revealed a CV/VC ratio of 16% (predicted 8.1%), further pointing to the presence of small airways abnormality. Methacholine challenge testing was deferred, because the obstructive defect was adequately demonstrated by the exercise test.

CASE 3

History

F.H. is 1 47-year-old loading dock foreman, whose chief complaint is shortness of breath on moderate exertion. He claims that his dyspnea has become worse recently, but that it has been present for more than 5 years.

F.H. has smoked 1½ packs of cigarettes a day since age 15 (48 pack/years). He admits to a cough on arising and states that he produces a "small amount of grayish sputum" usually in the morning. F.H.'s father had tuberculosis, and one brother had multiple cases of pneumonia as a child and now has bronchiectasis. He denies any extraordinary exposure to environmental dusts or fumes.

Pulmonary function testing

A. Personal data

Sex:	Male
Age:	47 yr
Height:	70 in
Weight:	185 lb

B. Spirometry and airway resistance

	Before drug	Predicted	%	After drug	% change
FVC (L)	4.01	4.97	81	4.49	90
$FEV_{1.0}$ (L)	2.05	3.67	56	2.20	60
$FEV_{1\%}$ (%)	51	74	—	49	—
$FEF_{25\%-75\%}$ (L/sec)	1.20	3.69	33	1.30	35
$\dot{V}_{max_{50}}$ (L/sec)	1.35	5.54	24	1.67	30
$\dot{V}_{max_{25}}$ (L/sec)	0.55	2.58	21	1.02	40
MVV (L/min)	71	136	52	85	63
Raw (cm H_2O/L/sec)	3.10	0.6-2.4	—	2.90	—
SGaw (L/sec/cm H_2O/L)	0.07	0.11-0.42	—	0.08	—

C. Lung volumes (by plethysmograph)

	Before drug	Predicted	%
VC (L)	4.01	4.97	81
IC (L)	2.71	3.18	85
ERV (L)	1.30	1.76	74
FRC (L)	4.60	3.94	117
RV (L)	3.30	2.18	151
TLC (L)	7.31	7.12	103
RV/TLC (%)	45	31	—

D. Diffusing capacity (single-breath)

	Before drug	Predicted	%
DL_{CO} (ml CO/min/mm Hg)	6.7	29.1	23
VA	7.16		
DL/VA	0.94		

E. Blood gases ($F_{I_{O_2}}$ 0.21)

pH	7.37
Pa_{CO_2} (mm Hg)	51
Pa_{O_2} (mm Hg)	54
Sa_{O_2} (%)	86%
HCO_3^- (mEq/L)	32
Hb (gm%)	18.3 vol%

Interpretation

All data were acceptable; the breath-hold time on the $D_{L_{CO}}$ was longer than acceptable (11.2 seconds) due to prolonged expiratory time.

The subject has a decreased $FEV_{1.0}$ with only a slightly decreased FVC. The $FEF_{25\%-75\%}$ is decreased, as are the $\dot{V}_{max_{50}}$ and $\dot{V}_{max_{25}}$. The MVV is reduced, and the Raw is slightly above the expected. SGaw is below the lower limit of normal. There is little or no response to the bronchodilator.

Lung volumes shown an increased RV, with concomitant increases in the FRC and TLC. The RV/TLC is elevated.

The $D_{L_{CO}}$ is reduced, and the D_L/V_A is less than 1. The arterial blood gases reveal a compensated respiratory acidosis with moderate hypoxemia and an elevated Hb.

Impression: Moderate airway obstruction with minimal response to inhaled bronchodilator; moderate air trapping is present, and diffusing capacity is markedly reduced. There is hypoxemia and hypercapnia with polycythemia.

Discussion

F.H. typifies a smoker who has developed a moderate degree of airway obstruction. His spirometry reveals the extent of the obstruction: $FEV_{1.0}$, 56% of predicted; $FEF_{25\%-75\%}$, 33% of predicted; and MVV, 52% of predicted. The FVC is relatively well preserved and even increased following inhalation of the bronchodilator. The $FEF_{25\%-75\%}$, despite being 33% of predicted, must be interpreted cautiously because of the variability in normal subjects for this measure. The 95% confidence limits for this subject would include values between 1.45 L/sec and 5.93 L/sec—a large range (see the Appendix for predicted values and the SEE). Flows do not increase significantly following the bronchodilator. The $FEV_{1\%}$ actually decreases as a result of a larger increase in the FVC than in the $FEV_{1.0}$. This pattern occurs rather commonly in irreversible obstructive disease. The MVV is reduced, as might be expected. To ascertain that a valid MVV maneuver was obtained, the $FEV_{1.0}$ may be multiplied by a factor of 40; if the MVV approximates the resulting value, as it does here, it represents good effort on the part of the subject. The Raw is slightly increased, consistent with moderate airway obstruction and a productive cough. Specific conductance is less than the lower limit of normal, consistent with increased resistance and increased lung volumes.

The lung volumes reveal air trapping, as indicated by the increased RV and RV/TLC ratio. The RV has increased at the expense of the VC; the remaining lung volumes (i.e., TLC, FRC) are not far from the expected values.

The DL_{CO} is markedly reduced, presumably as a result of mismatching of ventilation and perfusion caused by airway obstruction. The loss of diffusing capacity per liter of lung volume (0.94) is typical of moderate or severe obstructive disease. This DL/V_A may be contrasted to the value presented in Case 1, in which the DL_{CO} was reduced but the ratio was close to the expected, indicating a restrictive defect. In the present case, the ratio is low, consistent with decreased DL_{CO} attributed to factors other than loss of lung volume. In addition, the low DL_{CO} (23% of predicted) may indicate that oxygenation may be further impaired during exercise, although it is not possible to predict the extent of desaturation that might occur. Although the DL_{CO} is sometimes used to distinguish "pure" emphysema (decreased DL_{CO}) from "pure" bronchitis (normal DL_{CO}), in many instances the diseases overlap in such a way as to seriously limit the usefulness of this type of distinction.

The blood gas results reveal resting hypoxemia consistent with ventilation-perfusion mismatching. There is a slightly elevated Hb, which may be secondary to the hypoxemia. In addition, there is a mild degree of CO_2 retention with renal compensation.

The lung function of this subject exemplifies the pattern seen in chronic obstructive airway disease of the mixed emphysematous and chronic bronchitic type. Although air trapping (increased RV) is consistent with emphysematous changes, it may be present in bronchitis and asthma, particularly during acute exacerbations.

Further evaluation of F.H. included a chest x-ray film and a ventilation-perfusion ($\dot{V}/\dot{Q}$) scan. The chest film showed increased hilar markings and right ventricular enlargement. The $\dot{V}/\dot{Q}$ scan showed areas of low $\dot{V}/\dot{Q}$ in both lower lobes, perhaps explaining the hypoxemia. He was recommended for exercise evaluation to determine whether further desaturation occurred with an increased work load and to determine his potential for pulmonary rehabilitation.

CASE 4

History

R.B. is a 37-year-old pipe fitter whose chief complaint is shortness of breath at rest and on exertion. His dyspnea has worsened in the past 6 months, so much so that he is no longer able to work. Additional symptoms include a dry cough, and he admits to some sputum production when he has a "chest cold." He has smoked one pack of cigarettes a day since age 18 (19 pack/years). He quit smoking about 3 weeks before the tests. His father died of emphysema, and his mother died of lung cancer. His only brother is in good health. His occupational exposure includes working for the past 13 years in the assembly room of a boiler plant, where boilers are put together. He admits to seldom using the respirators provided despite the "dusty" environment.

Pulmonary function testing

A. Personal data

Sex:	Male
Age:	37 yr
Height:	69 in
Weight:	143 lb

B. Spirometry

	Before drug	Predicted	%	After drug	%
FVC (L)	3.04	5.05	60	3.10	61
$FEV_{1.0}$ (L)	2.03	3.90	52	2.26	58
$FEV_{1\%}$ (%)	67	77	—	73	—
$FEF_{25\%-75\%}$	1.30	4.09	32	1.60	39
$\dot{V}_{max_{50}}$ (L/sec)	2.12	5.78	37	2.42	42
$\dot{V}_{max_{25}}$ (L/sec)	0.78	2.95	26	1.20	41
$M\dot{V}V$ (L/min)	83	141	59	91	65
Raw (cm H_2O/L/sec)	2.51	0.6-2.4	—	2.47	—
SGaw (L/sec/cm H_2O/L)	0.14	0.11-0.44	—	0.15	—

C. Lung volumes (by plethysmograph)

	Before drug	Predicted	%
VC (L)	3.04	5.05	60
IC (L)	1.62	3.18	51
ERV (L)	1.42	1.87	76
FRC (L)	2.75	3.81	72
RV (L)	.33	1.94	69
TLC (L)	4.37	6.99	63
RV/TLC (%)	30	28	—

D. Diffusing capacity (single-breath)

	Before drug	Predicted	%
$D_{L_{CO}}$ (ml CO/min/mmHg)	8.1	30.6	25
V_A (L)	4.22	—	
D_L/V_A	1.91	4.38	

E. Blood gases ($F_{I_{O_2}}$ 0.21)

pH	7.43
Pa_{CO_2} (mm Hg)	36
Pa_{O_2} (mm Hg)	52
Sa_{O_2} (%)	87%
HCO_3^- (mEq/L)	23.0

Interpretation

All data from spirometry, lung volumes, diffusing capacity and blood gases are acceptable.

Spirometry shows a reduced FVC and $FEV_{1.0}$. The $FEF_{25\%-75\%}$, $\dot{V}_{max_{50}}$, and $\dot{V}_{max_{25}}$ are all reduced. The MVV is low, while the Raw and SGaw are at their respective limits of normal. Response to bronchodilators is minimal, with an increase in the $FEV_{1.0}$ of only 11%. The $\dot{V}_{max_{25}}$ improved somewhat more than the other flows.

The lung volumes are all decreased; the RV/TLC ratio is normal.

The $DL_{CO}SB$ is reduced, as is the DL/VA. The blood gases indicate resting hypoxemia with a normal acid-base status.

Impression: Combined moderate obstructive and restrictive pattern without significant bronchodilator response. Hypoxemia is present and oxygen supplementation is indicated. Further desaturation may occur with exertion.

Discussion

R.B. typifies the subject with combined obstructive and restrictive disease. His spirometry (i.e., $FEF_{25\%-75\%}$, $\dot{V}_{max_{50}}$) indicates that a rather serious obstructive component is present. The $FEV_{1\%}$, however, is close to normal in this case because the FVC is also reduced. Airway narrowing as a result of restriction is sometimes responsible for decreased flows, particularly if the restriction is severe, but R.B.'s symptoms of cough and sputum point to a genuine obstructive process. In addition, he has a smoking and family history that place him at risk. Because the FVC can be reduced in either obstructive or restrictive processes, spirometry alone does not adequately define the exact nature of this subject's disease.

The lung volume measurements confirm the presence of a restrictive component. All lung volumes are reduced in similar proportions, with the reduction in VC matching decreases in FRC, RV, and TLC. The reduced diffusing capacity is presumably a result of the combined disease patterns, as is the moderate hypoxemia on room air. The subject's history and symptoms point to the possibility of either restrictive or obstructive disease, or both. The obstructive component may be related to the subject's smoking history, but the etiology of the restrictive component is less clear. On further investigation, it was learned that the subject's occupation involved exposure to asbestos, which can cause fibrosis and/or carcinoma. Chest x-rays revealed linear calcifications of the diaphragmatic pleura and pleural thickening, as well as fibrotic changes, all consistent with asbestos exposure.

Asbestos bodies were identified from the subject's sputum. Open lung biopsy was deferred, because it was felt that the causes of both the obstructive and restrictive components were adequately identified. Measurement of compliance (CL) could have been used to document the severity of the fibrosis.

CASE 5
History

P.W. is a 27-year-old auto mechanic whose chief complaint is "breathing problems." He describes "attacks" of breathlessness that occur suddenly and then subside. He has no other symptoms and no personal history of lung disease. No other immediate family member has had any lung disease. He has smoked a pack of cigarettes a day for the last 10 years (10 pack/years). He has no unusual environmental exposure, but claims that gasoline fumes sometimes bring on the episodes of shortness of breath.

Pulmonary function testing

A. Personal data

Sex:	Male
Age:	27 yr
Height:	68 in
Weight:	150 lb

B. Spirometry

	Before drug	Predicted	%
FVC (L)	3.80	5.15	74
$FEV_{1.0}$ (L)	3.70	4.13	90
$FEV_{1\%}$ (%)	97	80	—
$FEF_{25\%-75\%}$ (L/sec)	4.62	4.49	103
$\dot{V}_{max_{50}}$ (L/sec)	4.81	6.01	80
$\dot{V}_{max_{25}}$ (L/sec)	3.12	3.33	94
MVV (L/min)	162	146	111

C. Lung volumes (closed-circuit technique)

	Before drug	Predicted	%
VC (L)	4.97	5.15	97
IC (L)	3.30	3.17	104
ERV (L)	1.67	1.98	84
FRC (L)	3.72	3.68	101
RV (L)	2.05	1.70	121
TLC (L)	7.02	6.85	102
RV/TLC (%)	29	25	—

D. Diffusing capacity (single-breath)*

	Before drug	Predicted	%
D_{LCO} (ml CO/min/mm Hg)	18.8	32.2	58
V_A (L)	4.62	—	
D_L/V_A	4.10	4.70	—

*(corrected for COHb)

E. Blood gases ($F_{I_{O_2}}$ 0.21)

pH	7.44
Pa_{CO_2} (mm Hg)	36
Pa_{O_2} (mm Hg)	92
Sa_{O_2} (%)	87.1
COHb (%)	8.3

Interpretation

Spirometry, lung volumes, and $D_{L_{CO}}$ are unacceptable due to poor patient effort or technical errors.

Spirometry shows a reduced forced vital capacity, with all other flows and the MVV being normal. Lung volumes are normal, with a slight increase in the residual volume. The $D_{L_{CO}}$ is reduced. Blood gases are within normal limits, except for a markedly elevated carboxyhemoglobin and concomitant reduction in Sa_{O_2}.

Impression: The spirometry is inconsistent. The FVC and slow VC differ markedly, and the $D_{L_{CO}}$ is inconsistent. Inadequate subject effort or technical errors are present.

Discussion

These test data are good examples of poor reproducibility, particularly on some maneuvers that may be influenced by subject effort.

The spirometric data is seemingly consistent with a mild restrictive process. However, the FVC is much smaller than the slow VC; because the subject cannot "overshoot" on the vital capacity maneuver, the FVC can be presumed to be inaccurate. The FVC might be less than the slow VC in severe obstruction when dynamic compression of the airways may influence the volume expired. The FVC may also be smaller than the SVC if repeated forced expiratory maneuvers induce bronchospasm; however, all of this subject's flows and his MVV appear normal. Flows for which measurement depends on the FVC (i.e. $FEF_{25\%-75\%}$, $\dot{V}_{max_{50}}$) might also be erroneous if the FVC is incorrect. The $FEV_{1.0}$ and MVV do not depend on the FVC, and they appear to be normal.

The lung volumes appear to be normal. Because the closed-circuit technique for determination of FRC requires only tidal breathing, it is unlikely to be influenced by poor effort unless the subject introduces a leak. If the slow VC is used to calculate $FEV_{1\%}$ ($FEV_{1.0}$/SVC rather than $FEV_{1.0}$/FVC), the ratio becomes 74%, in comparison to the 97% estimated from the FVC maneuver itself.

The $D_{L_{CO}}$ is much lower than one might expect, particularly in relation to the "normal" blood gases. An acceptable $D_{L_{CO}}SB$ maneuver depends largely on the subject rapidly inspiring a VC breath from RV. Again, a poor VC effort could result in an underestimate of the true diffusing capacity. The effect of the elevated COHb would be to reduce the driving pressure of CO across the lung and to further reduce the measured $D_{L_{CO}}$, but in this case the $D_{L_{CO}}$ has been corrected for the carboxyhemoglobin.

Because of the inconsistencies in the reported data, further evaluation of the available raw test data was performed. Closer examination of the volume-time spirograms revealed that during the spirometry the subject terminated each FVC maneuver after approximately 2 seconds, hence the discrepancy between FVC and SVC. In addition, each of the three recorded spirograms had widely varying FVCs (the two best were not within 5%), confirming poor subject cooperation. Lack of reproducibility of the FVC maneuvers is not sufficient reason for discarding the test results, provided that at least three acceptable tests are obtained. This subject's FVC maneuvers lasted only 2 seconds, and thus did not meet the criteria of continuing for at least 6 seconds or showing an obvious plateau (i.e., no volume change for at least 2 seconds). The DL_{CO} maneuver also showed inconsistent inspiratory volumes, with the largest VC equalling only 66% of the slow vital capacity.

Careful attention to these inaccuracies at the time of the test might have prevented the inconsistencies from appearing on the final report. The subject was requested to return for a second test. (Criteria for determining acceptability of various tests may be found in Chapter 11).

CASE 6

History

M.M. is a 39-year-old secretary who has recently begun experiencing episodes of "choking and coughing." She was referred by an industrial health specialist who suspected some sort of reactive airways involvement. She relates that cigarette smoke and strong odors seem to bring on the episodes. She has never smoked, and has no history of lung disease. She had some childhood allergies that disappeared at puberty. There is no history of any lung involvement in her immediate family. She is not currently on any medications.

Pulmonary function testing

A. Personal data

Sex:	Female
Age:	39 yr
Height:	66 in
Weight:	130 lb

B. Spirometry

	Before drug	Predicted	%
FVC (L)	3.71	3.80	98
$FEV_{1.0}$ (L)	2.80	2.97	94
$FEV_{1\%}$ (%)	75	78	—
$FEF_{25\%-75\%}$ (L/sec)	2.99	3.34	90
$\dot{V}_{max_{50}}$ (L/sec)	3.93	4.62	85
$\dot{V}_{max_{25}}$ (L/sec)	1.01	2.36	43
MVV (L/min)	106.4	109.7	97
Raw (cm H_2O/L/sec)	2.51	0.6-2.4	—
SGaw (L/sec/cm H_2O/L)	0.12	0.14-0.56	—

C. Lung volumes (by plethysmograph)

	Before drug	Predicted	%
VC (L)	3.70	3.80	97
IC (L)	2.03	2.60	78
ERV (L)	1.67	1.20	139
FRC (L)	3.11	3.00	104
RV (L)	1.44	1.80	80
TLC (L)	5.14	5.60	92
RV/TLC (%)	28	32	—

D. Diffusing capacity (single-breath)

	Before drug	Predicted	%
DL_{CO} (ml CO/min/mmHg)	18.9	21.9	86
VA (L)	4.99	—	
DL/VA	3.79	3.91	—

E. Blood gases (FI_{O_2} 0.21)

pH	7.43
Pa_{CO_2} (mm Hg)	37
Pa_{O_2} (mm Hg)	98
Sa_{O_2} (%)	97.3%
HCO_3^- (mEq/L)	23.3

Methacholine challenge

Methacholine (mg/ml)	$FEV_{1.0}$	% Control	Cumulative Breaths	Cumulative Units/5 Breaths
Baseline	2.97	—	—	—
Control	2.92	100	—	—
0.075	2.93	100	5	0.375
0.150	2.90	99	10	1.125
0.310	2.75	94	15	2.68
0.62	2.41	83	20	5.78
1.25	1.99	68	25	12.00

One methacholine unit is arbitrarily defined as 1 mg/ml of methacholine in diluent.

Interpretation

Spirometry, lung volumes, diffusing capacity, and blood gas data are all acceptable, as are the data collected during the inhalation challenge.

Spirometry is within normal limits, except for the $\dot{V}_{max_{25}}$, which is reduced. The Raw and SGaw are at their respective limits of normal, consistent with some air flow obstruction. Lung volumes are within normal limits, although the ERV is larger than expected. The DL_{CO} and blood gases are normal.

The methacholine challenge test is positive, with a PD_{20} of 1.25 mg/ml, representing a total dose of 12 methacholine units. The test was terminated because the subject's $FEV_{1.0}$ fell below 80% of the control value. Wheezing was present on auscultation for the last two methacholine dosages, and the subject experienced symptoms similar to her chief complaint when the test became positive.

Impression: Normal lung function with a positive methacholine challenge, consistent with reactive airways disease.

Discussion

This subject is an ideal candidate for an inhalation challenge test. Her baseline pulmonary function studies are normal, with possible small airways involvement. Her complaint of episodic coughing and choking suggests some form of hyperreactive airways abnormality. Many subjects who develop an asthmatic response to inhaled irritants complain of cough as the primary symptom, while wheezing may or may not be present; if it is, it is usually heard on auscultation.

If obvious airways obstruction were present on the baseline spirometry (i.e., $FEV_{1\%}$ less than predicted), the challenge test would have been contraindicated. A simple before- and after-bronchodilator trial might have sufficed to demonstrate reversible obstruction. Methacholine challenge testing may be used in subjects who have known obstruction to quantify the degree of airway hyperreactivity, but in this case the objective of the test was to simply determine if the subject had hyperreactivity.

The $FEV_{1.0}$ is commonly used as the index of obstruction for inhalation challenge tests because it is simple to perform and highly reproducible. Other parameters may also be evaluated, since the forced expiratory maneuver is repeated at each dosage. The $FEF_{25\%-75\%}$, $\dot{V}_{max_{50}}$, $\dot{V}_{max_{25}}$, Raw, and SGaw are sometimes used to define the extent of airway reactivity. The SGaw is sensitive and reproducible, and it is often used to quantify changes occurring during challenge testing. The variability of the $FEF_{25\%-75\%}$, $\dot{V}_{max_{50}}$, and $\dot{V}_{max_{25}}$ make interpretation of changes during challenge testing somewhat difficult. In some instances, the peak expiratory flow rate (PEFR) may fall as the challenge is performed, particularly if the large airways are involved.

Some caution should be applied in interpreting the results of a methacholine challenge test. The subject should be largely symptom-free at the time of the test, and should not be using beta-adrenergic or methylxanthine bronchodilators that might influence the results. These conditions were met in this subject, and because the $FEV_{1.0}$ fell precipitously at a moderate methacholine dosage, the test can be interpreted as positive with some certainty. To better manage this patient, a portable peak flow meter was dispensed. The subject was instructed in its use, and the peak flow using it correlated well with that from baseline spirometry. She was requested to use the device when the symptoms appeared, and follow its use with a metered dose inhaler. Subsequent reports indicated that her peak flow fell in excess of the level demonstrated on the challenge, but that the symptoms were promptly relieved with use of the inhaler.

CASE 7
History

T.S. is a 65-year-old man with a history of COPD who was referred for exercise evaluation for pulmonary rehabilitation. He admits experiencing shortness of breath and dyspnea on exertion, and claims that these have grown worse during the last year. He has a smoking history of 72 pack/years and has recently quit smoking. A chest x-ray is normal except for some flattening of the diaphragms. Family history and occupational exposure were not significant.

Pulmonary function testing

A. Personal data

Sex:	Male
Age:	65 yr
Height:	69 in
Weight:	125 lb

B. Spirometry

	Before drug	Predicted	%	After drug	% change
FVC (L)	2.42	4.35	56	2.51	4
$FEV_{1.0}$ (L)	1.20	3.01	40	1.30	8
$FEV_{1\%}$ (%)	50	69	—	25	—
$FEF_{25\%-75\%}$ (L/sec)	0.77	2.83	27	0.85	10
$\dot{V}_{max_{50}}$ (L/sec)	1.37	4.94	28	1.51	10
$\dot{V}_{max_{25}}$ (L/sec)	0.59	1.80	33	0.57	−3
MVV (L/min)	45	118	38	48	7
Raw (cm H_2O/L/sec)	2.80	0.6-2.4	—	2.71	−3
SGaw (L/sec/cm H_2O/L)	0.07	0.11-0.44	—	0.07	0

C. Lung volumes (by plethysmograph)

	Before drug	Predicted	%
VC (L)	2.42	4.35	56
IC (L)	1.74	2.96	59
ERV (L)	0.68	1.39	49
FRC (L)	5.11	3.81	134
RV (L)	4.43	2.42	183
TLC (L)	6.85	6.77	101
RV/TLC (%)	65	36	—

D. Diffusing capacity (single-breath)

	Before drug	Predicted	%
DL_{CO} (ml CO/min/mm Hg)	11.8	25.7	46
VA (L)	1.76	—	
DL/VA	1.76	3.79	—

Interpretation (pulmonary function study)

Seven acceptable FVC maneuvers were obtained but the two best FVCs were not within 5%; otherwise, lung volumes and diffusing capacity tests were acceptable.

The spirometry is consistent with severe obstructive lung disease without significant response to bronchodilators. Lung volumes show marked air trapping with residual volume replacement of the vital capacity. The diffusing capacity is severely reduced.

Interpretation (exercise evaluation)

The exercise test (see Table 12-1) was terminated because the subject exceeded 85% of his age-related predicted maximum HR, and he was experiencing shortness of breath. His maximum $\dot{V}E$ exceeded his MVV slightly. VT increased with exercise, as did VD, and the VD/VT fell slightly. His gas exchange shows a $\dot{V}O_2$ of 1.2 L/min, which is approximately 57% of expected. $\dot{V}CO_2$ rose so that an R slightly greater than 1 occurred at the highest work load. The ventilatory equivalent for oxygen ($\dot{V}E/\dot{V}_{O_2}$) is elevated, and the O_2 pulse is slightly reduced.

Blood gases during exercise revealed a mild hypoxemia that worsened slightly with exercise. Saturation remained adequate. No hypercapnia or acidosis occurred.

No arrhythmias or ischemic changes were observed. The highest HR achieved was 88% of his predicted maximum. There was mild systolic hypertension.

Impression: (1) Marked aerobic impairment; (2) ventilatory limitation with hypoxemia; and (3) inappropriate cardiovascular response for the work load achieved.

Discussion

T.S. walked a total of 15 minutes on the treadmill, reaching a rate of 3 MPH at 8% grade. This equalled an energy production of 5.08 METS as a maximum.

His ventilatory pattern is characteristic of a subject with moderate airway obstruction. His respiratory rate is elevated at the beginning of the procedure, falls slightly, and then increases, particularly at the last two levels of work. The minute ventilation increases dramatically from Level 1 (rest) to Level 2, then increases slowly until the last two levels. The $\dot{V}A$

Table 12-1 Exercise test—case 7

Exercise level	1	2	3	4	5	6
Work load						
MPH	0	1.5	2	2	2.5	3
%Grade	0	0	4	8	8	8
Duration (min)	10	3	3	3	3	3
METS	1	3.144	3.365	4.030	4.459	5.082
Ventilation						
f (b/min)	30	24	26	30	36	39
$\dot{V}_E$ (L BTPS)	13.52	24.83	27.57	33.30	48.08	51.98
$\dot{V}_A$ (L BTPS)	5.99	14.37	17.34	21.57	31.64	34.31
V_T (L BTPS)	0.451	1.035	1.055	1.110	1.335	1.340
V_D (L BTPS)	0.251	0.436	0.391	0.392	0.457	0.456
V_D/V_T	0.556	0.421	0.371	0.352	0.342	0.340
Gas exchange						
$\dot{V}O_2$ (L STPD)	0.237	0.745	0.797	0.954	1.056	1.204
$\dot{V}CO_2$ (L STPD)	0.244	0.655	0.733	0.896	1.044	1.298
R	1.030	0.880	0.920	0.940	0.989	1.078
$\dot{V}_E/\dot{V}O_2$ (L/L)	57	33.35	34.60	34.90	45.53	43.18
$\dot{V}O_2$/HR (ml/beat)	2.786	7.838	8.390	9.090	8.516	8.916
Blood gases						
pH	7.47	7.43	7.42	7.39	7.39	7.38
Pa_{CO_2} (mm Hg)	33	35	34	36	33	35
Pa_{O_2} (mm Hg)	74	72	72	70	73	68
Sa_{O_2} (%)	95.5	95	95	94	94	93
$P(A\text{-}a)_{O_2}$ (mm Hg)	36	31	38	38	41	46
Hemodynamics						
HR (beats/min)	85	95	95	105	124	135
Sys BP (mm Hg)	124	162	178	194	200	210
Dias BP (mm Hg)	90	86	90	100	104	108

increases in approximately the same pattern. His V_T increases to about 1 L and stays near that level throughout the test. This is a fairly normal response. Healthy subjects generally accomplish increases in ventilation by increasing their V_T until they are using about 60% of their VC. Further increases are obtained by increasing the rate of breathing. In this case, the subject immediately increased his V_T to 50% to 60% of his VC, then increased $\dot{V}_E$ by raising his rate, particularly at the end of the test. Because his MVV was measured as 45 L/min (and the $FEV_{1.0} \times 35$ was 42 L/min), the subject exceeded the maximal level of total ventilation that might have been expected. The VD rose during the exercise and fluctuated somewhat. The VD/VT ratio decreased slightly, as might be expected (even with moderate obstruction), since the VT increased more rapidly than the VD.

At the resting exercise level (level 1) the subject has an R slightly greater than 1.0; the $\dot{V}CO_2$ is elevated in relation to $\dot{V}O_2$. The subject also has a slight respiratory alkalosis, indicating hyperventilation. This pattern is not uncommon in resting subjects before beginning exercise. Once he begins walking on the treadmill, his gas exchange parameters return to a normal pattern and show a steady increase in both $\dot{V}O_2$ and $\dot{V}CO_2$, with an R exceeding 1.0 at the final level. The subject may have reached his anaerobic threshold at this point, although the arterial pH is well within normal limits. The marked increase in $\dot{V}E$ during the last two levels is presumably a result of the increased $\dot{V}CO_2$ from anaerobic metabolism. The ventilatory equivalent for oxygen is inappropriately high at rest (level 1), as might be expected for someone with moderate airway obstruction. The $\dot{V}E/\dot{V}_{O_2}$ falls to lower levels during the first few stages of exercise, but rises again at the higher work loads. At all levels, the subject is performing an abnormally high level of ventilation for the amount of work being performed, consistent again with airway obstruction. The O_2 pulse ($\dot{V}O_2$/HR) rose with exercise, but not as high as might be expected (10 to 15 ml/beat). This suggests an inappropriate cardiovascular response. Because O_2 pulse is a function of the SV and the $C(a\text{-}v)_{O_2}$, it is uncertain which factor was responsible for the low ratio of $\dot{V}O_2$/HR is this case. Cardiac pathology usually results in decreased SV, while deconditioning results in a low $C(a\text{-}v)_{O_2}$ caused by poor extraction of O_2 at the muscle level. Because the subject's HR and BP rose to near maximal levels without arrhythmias or ST segment changes on the ECG, there may be some element of deconditioning involved.

Despite a ventilatory limitation to exercise, the arterial blood gas levels did not change dramatically. The pH was slightly alkalotic at rest (hyperventilation); it fell with exercise, but remained within a normal range. The Pa_{CO_2} stayed fairly constant, while the Pa_{O_2}, slightly low at rest, fell minimally. The subject used his remaining cardiopulmonary reserves to maintain normal blood gas levels.

In summary, the subject demonstrated a marked reduction in his exercise capacity ($\dot{V}O_2$max = 57% of predicted) caused primarily by a ventilatory limitation, but with possible evidence of deconditioning. His rehabilitation program was subsequently directed toward conditioning exercises within the limits of the subject's pulmonary system.

CASE 8
History

J.Y. is 69-year-old woman with a history of chronic bronchitis who was referred for exercise evaluation. She complained of shortness of breath on exertion. Her smoking history is 56 pack/years, but she quit more than 1 year before this test. Her chest x-ray is consistent with chronic bronchitis, showing increased vascular markings and an enlarged heart. She had no significant family history or occupational exposure. She admitted to a morning cough that produced thick white sputum.

Pulmonary function testing

A. Personal data

Sex:	Female
Age:	69 yr
Height:	64 in
Weight:	128 lb

B. Spirometry

	Before drug	Predicted	%
FVC (L)	1.30	2.85	46
$FEV_{1.0}$ (L)	0.73	2.04	36
$FEV_{1\%}$ (%)	56	72	—
$FEF_{25\%-75\%}$ (L/sec)	0.43	2.32	18
$\dot{V}_{max_{50}}$ (L/sec)	0.55	3.80	14
$\dot{V}_{max_{25}}$ (L/sec)	0.25	1.27	20
MVV (L/min)	31	85	36
Raw (cm H_2O/L/sec)	2.77	0.6-2.4	—
SGaw (L/sec/cm H_2O/L)	0.09	0.15-0.60	—

C. Lung volumes (by plethysmograph)

	Before drug	Predicted	%
VC (L)	1.30	2.85	46
IC (L)	1.08	1.99	54
ERV (L)	0.23	0.86	26
FRC (L)	3.78	2.77	137
RV (L)	3.55	1.91	186
TLC (L)	4.85	4.76	102
RV/TLC (%)	73	40	—

D. Diffusing capacity (single-breath)

	Before drug	Predicted	%
DL_{CO} (ml CO/min/mm Hg)	8.3	17.4	48
VA (L)	4.70	—	
DL/VA	1.77	3.77	—

A multistage exercise test was performed with a treadmill and an arterial catheter in place. Level 1 was a 10-minute baseline at rest (see Table 12-2).

Interpretation (pulmonary function study)

All spirometry data were acceptable, as were the data for the diffusing capacity. Several plethysmographic lung volume maneuvers had to be discarded before three acceptable measurements were obtained.

Spirometry is consistent with obstructive airway disease. Lung volumes indicate air trapping with a normal TLC. The diffusing capacity is reduced. Blood gas analysis and bronchodilator studies were deferred because this study immediately preceded the exercise test.

Interpretation (exercise evaluation)

The reason for termination of the test was a systolic BP of 250 mm Hg. The subject's respiratory rate increased from 12 to 33 breaths/min, with an increase in ventilation from 8 to 22 L/min. The V_T was relatively fixed, at about 700 ml. $\dot{V}_A$ increased in proportion to $\dot{V}_E$.

Table 12-2 Exercise test—case 8

Exercise level	1	2	3
Work load			
MPH	0	1.5	3
%Grade	0	0	0
Duration (min)	10	3	3
METS	1	3.3	3.4
Ventilation			
f (breaths/min)	12	27	33
$\dot{V}_E$ (L BTPS)	8.020	21.220	22.630
$\dot{V}_A$ (L BTPS)	4.17	11.671	12.447
V_T (L BTPS)	0.668	0.768	0.686
V_D (L BTPS)	0.321	0.350	0.309
V_D/V_T	0.48	0.45	0.45
Gas exchange			
$\dot{V}O_2$ (L STPD)	0.160	0.530	0.548
$\dot{V}CO_2$ (L STPD)	0.149	0.489	0.498
R	0.930	0.923	0.908
$\dot{V}_E/\dot{V}O_2$ (L/L)	50.14	40.04	41.28
$\dot{V}O_2$/HR (ml/beat)	2.459	5.047	5.221
Blood gases			
pH	7.48	7.42	7.41
Pa_{CO_2} (mm Hg)	34	39	37
Pa_{O_2} (mm Hg)	74	60	63
Sa_{O_2} (%)	94.9	89.9	91.0
$P(A\text{-}a)_{O_2}$ (mm Hg)	39	48	45
Hemodynamics			
HR (beats/min)	65	105	105
Systolic BP (mm Hg)	160	212	250
Diastolic BP (mm Hg)	80	100	102

Her $\dot{V}O_2$ rose to only 0.548 L/min, which was 34% of the predicted maximum (1.634). Her ventilatory equivalent for O_2 ($\dot{V}E/\dot{V}_{O_2}$) remained elevated throughout the test. Her O_2 pulse was low, but elevated normally with exercise, though not to maximal levels.

Blood gas studies indicate a mild hypoxemia during exercise with an increased A-a gradient ($P(A\text{-}a)_{O_2}$). Pa_{CO_2} rose slightly, and the pH changed accordingly, but without evidence of anaerobic metabolism.

Her HR rose to 105 beats/min, which is only 72% of her age-related predicted maximum. The systolic BP rose dramatically from 160/80 to 250/102, at which point the test was terminated. There were no arrhythmias, ST segment changes, or other evidence of ischemia noted.

Impression: (1) Exercise limited by marked hypertension; (2) ventilatory reserve is present despite moderately severe airway obstruction; and (3) mild impairment of oxygenation during exercise, but not significantly limiting.

Discussion

J.Y. presents an example of an individual with well-documented airway obstruction in whom exercise limitation is caused primarily by an inappropriate cardiovascular response.

Comparison of her maximal ventilation (22.63 L/min) with her MVV (31 L/min) indicates the presence of some ventilatory reserve, although the markedly reduced MVV suggests that there must be at least some ventilatory limitation to work. Her VT, both at rest and during the mild exercise, remained relatively fixed near 700 ml. Because this volume was 50% to 60% of her VC, she increased her ventilation by increasing her rate, as might be expected. Her VD/VT ratio decreased only slightly, probably as a direct result of the fixed VT. When both the VT and VD increase proportionately, the VD/VT ratio does not decrease. This pattern may be consistent with pulmonary vascular disorders, which are probably not in evidence here, because neither the VT nor the VD increased significantly.

J.Y. has marked aerobic impairment, as indicated by the low level of work achieved ($\dot{V}O_2$ = 0.548 L/min) at 3.0 MPH and 0% grade on the treadmill. Her R appears to fall, perhaps because of the mild hyperventilation at the resting level. Her ventilation is inappropriately elevated for the work loads evaluated, as shown by the $\dot{V}E/\dot{V}O_2$. This pattern is consistent with the increased VD/VT ratio (high ventilation required to maintain adequate $\dot{V}A$). The O_2 pulse ($\dot{V}O_2$/HR) is low at rest, and increased only slightly during the mild exercise. The maximal O_2 pulse that might have been attained can be estimated by dividing her predicted $\dot{V}_{O_{2max}}$ by her predicted maximum HR (× 1000); in this case, 1.634/148 (× 1000) = 11. J.Y. failed to increase her O_2 pulse because she was limited by other factors at an HR significantly lower than her predicted maximum. In this instance, an inappropriate rise in systolic BP (to 250 mm Hg) led to termination of the test. Peripheral vasodilatation normally redirects the cardiac output to exercising muscles. The hypertensive response observed here indicates a failure of this mechanism. Both local lesions (as in claudication) and diffuse disease (as in essential hypertension) can result in anaerobic metabolism at the muscle level with subsequent metabolic acidosis, stimulation of respiration, and dyspnea. J.Y. did not develop a frank acidosis (pH of 7.41) or dyspnea during the test. Her presenting complaint of increasing shortness of breath may well have been related to both the hypertensive response and her pulmonary limitations.

Because of the results of the exercise evaluation and her slight hypertension at rest, the subject was referred for further evaluation of her hypertension.

CASE 9
History

C.J. is a 53-year-old office worker who was referred for evaluation of shortness of breath. She has a 44 pack/year history of smoking and continued to smoke up to the time of her test. She admits a morning cough that produces thick white sputum, approximately 50 to 100 ml per day. Her chest x-ray shows increased vascular markings and mild hyperinflation. She was taking no medications at the time of this test. No familial history of lung disease or cancer was found, and she had no unusual environmental exposure.

Pulmonary function testing

A. Personal data

Sex:	Female
Age:	53 yr
Height:	65 in
Weight:	131 lb

B. Spirometry

	Before drug	Predicted	%	After drug	%
FVC	3.24	3.35	97	3.34	100
$FEV_{1.0}$ (L)	1.49	2.53	59	1.56	62
$FEV_{1\%}$ (%)	46	75	—	47	—
$FEF_{25\%-75\%}$ (L/sec)	0.79	2.86	27	1.19	42
$\dot{V}_{max_{50}}$ (L/sec)	1.99	4.24	47	2.25	53
$\dot{V}_{max_{25}}$ (L/sec)	0.68	1.86	37	0.99	53
MVV (L/min)	52	97.9	53	55	56
Raw (cm H_2O/L/sec)	2.22	0.6-2.4	—	2.10	—
SGaw (L/sec/cm H_2O/L)	0.12	0.14-0.58	—	0.13	—

C. Lung volumes (by plethysmograph)

	Before drug	Predicted	%
VC (L)	3.27	3.35	98
IC (L)	1.80	2.31	78
ERV (L)	0.99	1.04	95
FRC (L)	3.54	2.88	123
RV (L)	2.55	1.84	136
TLC (L)	5.82	5.20	112
RV/TLC (%)	44	35	—

D. Diffusing capacity (single-breath)

	Before drug	Predicted	%
$D_{L_{CO}}$ (ml CO/min/mm Hg)	8.8	20.0	44
V_A (L)	5.67	—	
D_L/V_A	1.55	3.85	—

E. Blood gases ($F_{I_{O_2}}$ 0.21)

pH	7.38
Pa_{CO_2} (mm Hg)	43
Pa_{O_2} (mm Hg)	59
Sa_{O_2} (%)	85.1
COHb (%)	5.7

Interpretation (pulmonary function study)

All spirometry, lung volume, diffusing capacity, and blood gas measurements were acceptable.

Spirometry shows an obstructive process, with a well preserved FVC. There is only a 5% improvement in the $FEV_{1.0}$ following bronchodilator.

Lung volumes by plethysmography show an increased FRC and RV consistent with air trapping. The TLC is close to normal, so there is little hyperinflation.

The $D_{L_{CO}}$SB is reduced. Arterial blood gases on air show hypoxemia that is complicated by an elevated COHb.

Impression: Moderately severe obstructive disease with no significant response to bronchodilators. Air trapping is present, and the $D_{L_{CO}}$ is severely reduced. Exercise evaluation for oxygen desaturation is recommended.

Three days later, a treadmill exercise test was performed with an arterial catheter in place; the test was repeated with oxygen supplementation. Gas with an $F_{I_{O_2}}$ of 0.28 was prepared in a meteorological balloon for the portion of the exercise test on O_2 (see Table 12-3).

Interpretation (exercise evaluation)

The exercise test was performed in two parts; the first part of the test was terminated because the subject's Pa_{O_2} fell to 46 mm Hg (Sa_{O_2} = 77.3). The second phase, on oxygen, was terminated because of shortness of breath on

Table 12-3 Exercise test—case 9

Exercise level	1	2	3	4	5
	Air			Oxygen	
Workload					
MPH	0	1.5	0	1.5	2
%Grade	0	0	0	0	4
Duration	10	3	10	3	3
METS	1.48	4.00	1.34	3.11	4.73
Ventilation					
f	16	28	13	20	31
$\dot{V}_E$ (BTPS)	10.20	23.40	6.23	16.59	27.81
$\dot{V}_A$ (BTPS)	6.02	14.74	3.74	10.45	17.80
V_T (BTPS)	0.638	0.836	0.479	0.830	0.897
V_D (BTPS)	0.262	0.309	0.190	0.307	0.323
V_D/V_T	0.41	0.37	0.40	0.37	0.36
Gas exchange					
$\dot{V}O_2$	0.310	0.835	0.279	0.649	0.986
$\dot{V}CO_2$	0.303	0.743	0.251	0.617	0.976
R	0.98	0.89	0.90	0.95	0.99
$\dot{V}_E/\dot{V}O_2$	32.90	28.00	22.33	25.50	28.20
$\dot{V}O_2$/HR	3.44	7.59	3.29	6.18	8.57
Pulse oximeter					
Sp_{O_2}	92	87	97	93	93
Blood gases					
pH	7.45	7.39	7.39	7.38	7.36
Pa_{O_2}	34	39	44	45	46
Pa_{O_2}	61	47	84	71	66
Sa_{O_2}	87.4	77.3	91.4	88.9	87.0
COHb	5.1	4.7	4.8	4.7	4.6
$P(A\text{-}a)_{O_2}$	51	56	64	78	84
Hemodynamics					
HR	90	110	92	105	115
Systolic BP	130	145	134	145	150
Diastolic BP	85	88	90	90	90

the part of the subject. The subject tolerated very low work loads even with supplementary oxygen.

Ventilation was slightly elevated at rest but increased in a normal fashion. On O_2, ventilation was slightly lower both at rest and at similar work loads. The V_D/V_T ratio was mildly elevated but decreased with exercise, on both air and oxygen. The subject's minute ventilation was significantly lower than the observed MVV (51% of the post-bronchodilator value), indicating some ventilatory reserve.

The subject achieved a maximal V_{O_2} of only 0.986 on oxygen, which is 53% of her age-related predicted (1.858), consistent with moderately severe exercise impairment. The ventilatory equivalent for O_2 is within normal limits, and the O_2 pulse increased normally, although not to maximal limits.

Blood gas analysis during exercise showed borderline hypoxemia at rest due to a Pa_{O_2} of 61 mm Hg in combination with an elevated COHb. The Pa_{O_2} fell markedly with only slight exertion to 47 mm Hg. On oxygen (F_{IO_2} = 0.28), the Pa_{O_2} improved to 84 mm Hg at rest, but decreased with increasing work loads. The Pa_{CO_2} increased slightly during oxygen breathing, possibly as a result of respiratory depression. The COHb was elevated, probably due to the subject's continued smoking. Pulse oximetry (Sp_{O_2}) during exercise shows readings higher than the actual saturation, presumably as a result of the subject's COHb.

The heart rate and blood pressure responses were appropriate for the work loads achieved breathing both air and oxygen. The low maximal HR suggests an exercise limitation other than cardiovascular pathology or deconditioning. The ECG was unremarkable.

Impression: Moderately severe exercise impairment due primarily to desaturation during exercise. Some ventilatory limitation is probably present as well. The desaturation is aggravated by an elevated COHb. The subject should begin a formal effort toward smoking cessation and use oxygen at 1 to 2 L/min for exertion. A follow-up evaluation is recommended 1 to 3 months following smoking cessation.

Discussion

This patient typifies the subject with obstructive lung disease in whom derangement of blood gases plays a larger role in exercise limitation than does impaired ventilation. C.J.'s ventilation and gas exchange are fairly normal at rest and at 1.5 MPH, 0% Grade. The P_{O_2} is low, however, and falls precipitously with just a small increase in work load. In fact, the decrease is severe enough to warrant concern about the level of desaturation that might occur with simple daily activities or during sleep. The elevated carboxyhemoglobin further impairs O_2 delivery. Although an ear oximeter was used during the exercise test, it read spuriously high due to the elevated COHb. Even if the pulse oximeter readings are corrected for the carboxyhemoglobin, there is still a discrepancy between Sp_{O_2} and Sa_{O_2}

during exercise; this "error" on the part of the pulse oximeter may be due to changes in blood flow at the sensor site or motion artifact during exercise. The pattern of desaturation follows that which might be expected based on the poor diffusing capacity recorded on the pulmonary function studies.

To better elucidate the processes responsible for desaturation and to evaluate the efficacy of oxygen therapy, a controlled trial of walking while breathing supplementary O_2 was performed. The subject breathed from a balloon containing a gas analyzed to have an FI_{O_2} of 0.28. The most notable change was the increase in resting Pa_{O_2} from 61 to 84 mm Hg. The pattern of desaturation persisted, however, in that the O_2 tension fell dramatically, just as when the subject breathed room air. Because of the elevated baseline, the PaO_2 remained above the level at which serious symptoms of hypoxemia might occur (approximately 55 mm Hg). Breathing supplementary oxygen may also be responsible for the decrease in total ventilation, at rest and during exercise, exhibited by the patient. The mild increase in Pa_{CO_2} might be further evidence of an increased sensitivity of the subject to hypoxemia, which becomes blunted when O_2 is breathed. Abnormal $\dot{V}/\dot{Q}$ is the most likely explanation of the pattern of desaturation observed in the subject, particularly in view of the bronchitic component of her obstructive disease.

The subject, while breathing oxygen, did not desaturate to the point where hypoxemia might be considered as a cause of the exercise limitation. Neither did she increase her ventilation to her maximal level. This might suggest that deconditioning was responsible for the low maximal work load achieved, but her heart rate and blood pressure did not rise to levels typically seen with significant deconditioning. Other possible causes for the low work load achieved while breathing oxygen might be inadequate subject effort, the development of bronchospasm, or a greatly increased work of breathing.

The subject was referred for pulmonary rehabilitation, which included smoking cessation, bronchial hygiene, and exercise with supplementary oxygen.

CASE 10

This case concerns the use of blood gas quality control to detect analytical errors.

Background

F.F. is a 30-year-old fireman referred for pulmonary function testing and measurement of arterial blood gases as part of a five-year physical exam required by his fire district. He has no extraordinary symptoms or history suggestive of pulmonary disease. He has never smoked. He performed all portions of the spirometry, lung volumes, and DL_{CO} maneuvers acceptably, and all results were within normal limits for his age and height.

Blood gases	(F_{IO_2} 0.21)
pH	7.41
P_{CO_2} (mm Hg)	39
P_{O_2} (mm Hg)	54
Sa_{O_2} (%)	96.0
COHb (%)	1.2
HCO_3^- (mEq/L)	24.1

Because of the low arterial P_{O_2} in an otherwise normal subject, and because the Sa_{O_2} (measured discretely by co-oximetry) showed a normal saturation, the functioning of the P_{O_2} electrode of the automated blood gas analyzer was questioned.

A review of the two most recent automatic calibrations revealed the following:

	Calibration	Expected	Drift
09:00			
pH	7.387	7.384	0.003
P_{CO_2} (mm Hg)	39.1	38.6	0.5
P_{O_2} (mm Hg)	132.0	140.1	−8.1
10:00			
pH	7.383	7.384	−0.001
P_{CO_2} (mm Hg)	38.4	38.6	−0.2
P_{O_2} (mm Hg)	151.2	140.1	11.1

For each of the automatic calibrations, the instrument analyzes a calibration gas or buffer and compares the measured value to an expected value. The drift is simply the amount of adjustment that must be applied to a particular electrode to bring it within calibration limits. The excessive drift exhibited by the P_{O_2} electrode prompted a review of the most recent quality control runs performed on the analyzer.

Blood gas quality control (five most recent runs)

Control	Mean	SD	Runs*				
			1	2	3	4	5
Level A	45	±2	46	47	49	42	50
Level B	100	±2	101	99	97	96	105
Level C	150	±3	147	151	151	149	143

*Control runs performed every 8 hours

Discussion

The findings in this case regarding the function of the O_2 electrode are not unusual. In this instance, an abnormally low P_{O_2} in an otherwise healthy individual with normal lung function suggested that an analytical error had occurred. If the subject had presented with evidence of lung disease or abnormalities in his pulmonary function parameters, the inaccuracy of the measurement of Po_2 might have gone unnoticed, or it might have led to inappropriate therapy.

The excessive drift of the oxygen electrode should have prompted the immediate attention of the technologist performing the blood gas analyses. A common problem with automated analyzers is their apparent simplicity. Because calibrations are performed automatically on a predetermined schedule, there is a tendency to overlook the corrections which the analyzer makes. Normally, the analyzer adjusts the zero and gain of each electrode to correct for small changes that occur in electrode performance due to buildup of protein at the tip, electrolyte exhaustion, or slight temperature alterations. In the event of a large change in electrode performance, such as electrode failure, the instrument may attempt to correct the electrode's output just as it would for a smaller change that occurs normally. Some microprocessor-controlled analyzers report a large "drift" in electrode performance as an error, while others simply report the "drift." In this case, the reported drifts signaled that the Po_2 electrode was fluctuating, with one calibration reading high, while the next read lower than the expected value.

The change in electrode performance should have been detected by the routine quality control run even before the excessive drift observed during the automatic calibrations. The blood gas quality control used in the laboratory consisted of multiple levels of control materials for which means and standard deviations had been determined. Examination of control runs 1 through 4 reveals acceptable electrode performance; all values are within ± 2 SD of the established mean. Run 5 (the most recent run), however, shows values that are all two or more standard deviations away from the mean. If run 5 is compared to the mean in any of the individual levels of control (Levels A, B, or C), each value appears to be between 2 and 3 standard deviations from the mean. Such values might be expected to occur 5% of the time simply due to the random error associated with sampling. If run 5 is considered in conjunction with the previous four runs, and multiple rules (see Chapter 11) are applied, then the electrode is clearly "out-of-control." When multiple levels of controls are evaluated, the finding of more than one control value outside of 2 SD suggests an out-of-control situation. For both level A and level B, there is a change of 4 standard deviations from run 4 to run 5; changes of this magnitude are not consistent with random error, and are detected only when a control history is kept. Similarly, there are inconsistencies within run 5 across the three level of controls. Levels A and B both show control values that are more than 2 SD above their respective means, while level C shows a value that is more than 2 SD below its mean. This pattern suggests fluctuating electrode performance, as was subsequently displayed during the automatic calibrations.

The Po_2 electrode was removed from the instrument, remembraned, filled with fresh electrolyte, and the tip polished with an abrasive to expose the platinum cathode. The instrument was recalibrated, and multiple levels of controls were run. All Po_2 values fell within 2 SD of the established means. The subject's blood, which had been kept in an ice water bath, was reanalyzed, and a Po_2 of 89 mm Hg was obtained.

SELECTED BIBLIOGRAPHY

Pulmonary function interpretation

American Thoracic Society: Conference on normal values and interpretations, Am Rev Respir Dis 1989 (in press).

Bates DV, Macklem PT, and Christie RV: Respiratory function in disease, ed 2, Philadelphia, 1971, WB Saunders Co.

Becklake MR and Permutt S: Evaluation of tests of lung function for "screening" of early detection of chronic obstructive lung disease, In Macklem PT and Permutt S, editors: The lung in transition between health and disease, New York, 1979, Marcel Dekker, Inc.

Clausen JL: Clinical interpretation of pulmonary function tests. Respir Care, 34:638, 1989.

Morris AH et al: Clinical pulmonary function testing, ed 2, Salt Lake City, 1984 Intermountain Thoracic Society.

West JB: Pulmonary pathophysiology—the essentials, ed 2, Baltimore, 1983, Williams & Wilkins.

Exercise test interpretation

American College of Sports Medicine: Guidelines for graded exercise testing and exercise prescription, ed 2, Philadelphia, 1980, Lea & Febiger.

Astrand PO and Rodahl K: Textbook of work physiology, ed 2, New York, 1977, McGraw-Hill, Inc.

Bell CW: Pulmonary rehabilitation and exercise testing. In Wilson PK, Bell CW, and Norton AC, editors: Rehabilitation of the heart and lungs, Fullerton, Calif., 1980, Beckman Instruments.

Jones NL: Clinical exercise testing, ed 3, Philadelphia, 1988, WB Saunders Co.

Jones NL: Exercise testing in pulmonary evaluation: rationale, methods, and the normal respiratory response to exercise, N Engl J Med 293:541, 647, 1975.

Kattus AA: Exercise testing and training of apparently healthy individuals, New York, 1972, American Heart Association.

Spiro SG: Exercise testing in clinical medicine, Br J Dis Chest 71:145, 1977.

Wasserman K, and Whipp BJ: Exercise physiology in health and disease, Am Rev Respir Dis 112:219, 1975.

Blood gas interpretation

Shapiro BA: Clinical applications of blood gases, Chicago, 1989, Year book Medical Publishers, Inc.

Appendix

SYMBOLS AND ABBREVIATIONS USED IN PULMONARY FUNCTION TESTING

(Where two symbols are given, both are commonly used)

General symbols

P	Pressure, blood or gas
V	Gas volume
$\dot{V}$	Gas volume per unit time, or flow
F	Fractional concentration of gas
I	Inspired
E	Expired
A	Alveolar
T	Tidal
D	Dead space
Q	Blood volume
$\dot{Q}$	Blood flow
C	Content in blood
S	Saturation
a	Arterial
c	Capillary
v	Venous
$\bar{v}$	Mixed venous
BTPS	Body temperature and pressure, saturated with water vapor
ATPS	Ambient temperature, pressure, saturated with water vapor
STPD	0° C, 760 mm Hg, dry

Lung volumes

VC	Vital capacity
SVC	Slow vital capacity
IC	Inspiratory capacity
IRV	Inspiratory reserve volume
ERV	Expiratory reserve volume (FRC − RV)
FRC	Functional residual capacity (ERV + RV)
RV	Residual volume
TLC	Total lung capacity (VC + RV)

RV/TLC (%)	Residual volume to total lung capacity ratio expressed as a percentage
V_{TG}	Thoracic gas volume
V_T	Tidal volume
V_A	Alveolar volume
V_D	Dead space volume
V_L	Actual lung volume

Ventilation and ventilatory control

$\dot{V}_E$	Expired volume per minute (BTPS)
$\dot{V}_A$	Alveolar ventilation per minute (BTPS)
$\dot{V}_D$	Dead space ventilation per minute (BTPS)
f_b, f	Respiratory rate per minute
V_D/V_T	Ratio of dead space to tidal volume
MSVC	Maximum sustainable ventilatory capacity
P_{100}, $P_{0.1}$	Pressure in the first 100 milliseconds of an occluded breath

Spirometry

FVC	Forced vital capacity with maximally forced expiratory effort
FIVC	Forced inspiratory vital capacity with maximally forced inspiratory effort
FEV_T	Forced expiratory volume for a specific interval T
$FEV_T/FVC\%$, $FEV_{T\%}$	Forced expiratory volume to forced vital capacity ratio expressed as a percentage
FEF_X	Forced expiratory flow related to some specific portion of the FVC, denoted as subscript X, referring to the amount of FVC already exhaled at the time of measurement
$FEF_{200\text{-}1200}$	Forced expiratory flow between 200 ml and 1200 ml of the FVC (formerly the MEFR)
$FEF_{25\%\text{-}75\%}$	Forced expiratory flow during the middle half of the FVC (formerly the MMF)
PEFR	Peak expiratory flow rate
MEFV	Maximum expiratory flow-volume curve
PEFV	Partial expiratory flow-volume curve
$\dot{V}_{max_X}$	Forced expiratory flow related to the actual volume of the lungs denoted by subscript X, which refers to the amount of lung volume remaining when measurement is made
MVV_X	Maximal voluntary ventilation as the volume of air expired in a specified interval, denoted by subscript X (formerly MBC)
$Viso\dot{V}$	Volume of isoflow

Pulmonary mechanics

C	Compliance, volume change per unit of pressure change
Cdyn	Dynamic compliance, measured during breathing
Cst	Static compliance, measured during periods of no air flow

CRS	Compliance of the respiratory system
C/VL	Specific compliance
FDC	Frequency dependence of compliance (Cdyn/Cst × 100)
Raw	Airway resistance, pressure per unit of flow
Gaw	Airway conductance, flow per unit of pressure (1/Raw)
Raw/VL, SRaw	Specific resistance
Gaw/VL, SGaw	Specific conductance
MEP	Maximum expiratory pressure
MIP	Maximum inspiratory pressure

Gas distribution

$\Delta N_{2_{750\text{-}1250}}$	Change in percent N_2 over the 750 to 1250 ml portion of the SBN_2 test
SBN_2, SBO_2	Single-breath nitrogen elimination
Slope of Phase III	Slope of best-fit line through alveolar portion of the SBN_2 from 30% of VC to onset of Phase IV
CV	Closing volume
CV/VC (%)	Closing volume to vital capacity ratio expressed as a percentage
CC	Closing capacity
CC/TLC (%)	Closing capacity to total lung capacity ratio expressed as a percentage
IDI	Index of distribution of inspired gas (from 7-minute N_2 test)

Diffusion

DL_{CO}	Diffusing capacity for carbon monoxide
1/Dm	Diffusion resistance of the alveolocapillary membrane
$1/\theta Vc$	Diffusion resistance of the red cell and Hb reaction rate
DL/VA, DL/VL	Specific diffusion per unit of alveolar lung volume

Exercise and metabolic studies

$\dot{V}O_2$	Oxygen consumption per minute (STPD)
METS	Multiples of the resting oxygen uptake
$\dot{V}CO_2$	Carbon dioxide production per minute (STPD)
$\dot{V}E/\dot{V}O_2$	Ventilatory equivalent for oxygen
$\dot{V}E/\dot{V}CO_2$	Ventilatory equilvalent for CO_2
$\dot{V}O_2$/HR	Oxygen pulse
KPM	Kilopond-meters, a unit of power output
R, RER	Respiratory exchange ratio
RQ	Respiratory quotient
REE	Resting energy expenditure
Kcal	Kilocalorie

Blood gases and monitoring

P_{AO_2}	Alveolar oxygen tension
Pa_{O_2}	Arterial oxygen tension
$P\bar{v}_{O_2}$	Mixed venous oxygen tension

tcP_{O_2}	Transcutaneous oxygen tension
Sa_{O_2}	Arterial oxygen saturation
$S\bar{v}_{O_2}$	Mixed venous oxygen saturation
Sp_{O_2}	Pulse oximeter saturation
Ca_{O_2}	Arterial oxygen content
$C\bar{v}_{O_2}$	Mixed venous oxygen content
$P(A\text{-}a)_{O_2}$	Alveolar-arterial O_2 tension difference
$C(a\text{-}\bar{v})O_2$	Arterial-venous O_2 content difference
$P_{A_{CO_2}}$	Alveolar carbon dioxide tension
Pa_{CO_2}	Arterial carbon dioxide tension
$P_{ET_{CO_2}}$	End-tidal carbon dioxide tension
tcP_{CO_2}	Transcutaneous carbon dioxide tension
pH	Negative logarithm of the H^+ concentration used as a positive number
HCO_3^-	Plasma bicarbonate concentration
BE	Base excess, base deficit
COHb	Carboxyhemoglobin
MetHb	Methemoglobin
P_{50}	Partial pressure of O_2 at which hemoglobin is 50% saturated

TYPICAL VALUES FOR PULMONARY FUNCTION TESTS

(Values are for a healthy young man, 1.7 m^2 body surface area)

Test	Value
Lung volumes (BTPS)	
IC	3600 ml
ERV	1200 ml
VC	4800 ml
RV	1200 ml
FRC	2400 ml
V_{TG}	2400 ml
TLC	6000 ml
(RV/TLC) × 100	20%
Ventilation (BTPS)	
V_T	500 ml
f	12 breaths/min
$\dot{V}_E$	6 L/min
V_D	150 ml
$\dot{V}_A$	4200 ml/min
V_D/V_T	0.30
Pulmonary mechanics	
FVC	4800 ml
$FEV_{0.5\%}$	60%
$FEV_{1.0\%}$	83%
$FEV_{2.0\%}$	94%

$FEV_{3.0\%}$	97%
$FEF_{200-1200}$	6 L/sec
$FEF_{25\%-75\%}$	4.7 L/sec
MVV	170 L/min
CL	0.2 L/cm H_2O
CLT	0.1 L/cm H_2
Raw	1.5 cm H_2/L/sec
SGaw	0.25 L/sec/cm H_2O
MIP	130 cm H_2O
MEP	250 cm H_2O
Gas distribution	
SBN_2	Less than 1.5% N_2
7-minute N_2	Less than 2.5% N_2
IDI (ideal lung = 1.0)	1.8
Diffusion	
$DL_{CO}SB$	25 ml CO/min/mm Hg
DL/VA	4.2 ml CO/min/mm Hg/L
Blood gases and related tests	
$\dot{V}A/\dot{Q}C$	0.8
$\dot{Q}S/\dot{Q}T$	Less than 7%
pH	7.40
Pa_{CO_2}	40 mm Hg
HCO_3^-	24.0 mEq/L
Pa_{O_2}	95 mm Hg
Sa_{O_2}	97%
COHb	Less than 1.5%
MetHb	Less than 1.5%

SELECTING AND USING PREDICTED VALUES

Predicted values for each of the many components of pulmonary function testing are derived from a statistical analysis of a population of "normal" subjects. These subjects are usually classified as normal on the basis of the absence of history or symptoms of lung disease in themselves and their families. In addition, minimal exposure to risk factors (i.e., smoking, environmental pollution) is usually considered in selecting "normals." In some studies, smokers were included as "normals," and this most likely affected the resulting predicted values.

All pulmonary function parameters vary in the normal population, some much more than others. The arterial pH and Pa_{CO_2} have a very narrow range in normal subjects, unlike the $FEF_{25\%-75\%}$, which may vary by almost 2 L/sec. This variability must be taken into account in the interpretation of individual pulmonary function parameters, when a measured value is compared to a predicted normal value. Most parameters "regress" (i.e., vary) in a predictable fashion in relation to one or more physical factors. The physical characteristics that most influence pulmonary function are:

Age
Sex
Height (standing/sitting)
Race or ethnic origin
Weight or body surface area

The altitude at which subjects reside also influences their lung function development. By analyzing each parameter in regard to the subject's physical characteristics, regression equations can be generated to predict the "normal" value. Most regression analyses presume that lung function changes are *linearly* related to the physical characteristics (i.e., age, height), but this may not always be the case, particularly in subjects at the extremes, such as those who are very old or young, or very tall or short.

Race or ethnic origin influences stature and body proportions. Lung function parameters, particularly lung volumes and DL_{CO}, differ appreciably among races. Some computerized pulmonary function systems allow proportional changes to be applied to predicted values derived from normal caucasians to "correct" the predicted value. Although the lung function differences among races is well documented, there is no clear cut "correction factor" that would seem to apply. Many laboratories lower the predicted values for lung volumes (i.e., FVC, TLC) by factors of 10% to 15% for blacks. Race-specific regression equations may be used if they produce predicted values representative of normal subjects in the population that the laboratory tests.

Several common methods of using predicted values are:

1. Tables of normal values
2. Nomograms
3. Graphs
4. Regression equations

When a calculator or computer is unavailable or not practical, tables, nomograms, or graphs may be used. However, the widespread use of calculators and computers allows the employment of even complex regression equations, as well as analysis of a measured value in relation to the predicted in terms of variability.

Establishing a lower limit of normal is commonly done in one of several ways. Many clinicians use a fixed percentage of the predicted value (measured/predicted $\times$ 100) to determine the degree of abnormality, often with $\pm$ 20% as the limit of normal. This method is simple and produces acceptable lower levels of normals in adults for FVC, $FEV_{1.0}$, TLC, and $DL_{CO}SB$. The fixed percentage of predicted produces erroneous lower limits, however, for the $FEF_{25\%-75\%}$, for instantaneous flows ($\dot{V}_{max}$), and in children. A more precise approach is to define a lower limit based on the predicted value and the variability. Assuming that the lung function parameter varies in normal fashion (a Gaussian or bell-shaped distribution curve), the mean $\pm$1.96 SD defines the 95% confidence limits. Statistically, 95% of the normal population falls within 1.96 SD of the mean; therefore, if a subject's measured value is outside of the range (mean $\pm$ 1.96 SD), there is less than a 5% chance that the parameter is normal. Certain pulmonary function parameters require consideration of only the lower limit of normal (below the mean). In such a case (sometimes referred to as a one-tailed distribution), 1.65 SD may be used to define the exact value below which there is less than a 5% chance of normality. Those parameters that can be abnormal by being either too high or too low (i.e., RV, TLC, Pa_{CO_2}) must use the 1.96 SD method.

A more sophisticated means of representing the abnormality is to express the difference between the predicted value and the subject's measured value in terms of confidence intervals (CI). In this method, the difference between predicted and measured values is divided by the value representing one CI (either 1.96 or 1.65 SDs, as noted previously) and expressing the result as a ratio:

$$\frac{\text{Predicted} - \text{Measured}}{\text{CI}}$$

Using this method, a normal value is always less than or equal to 1.00, while abnormal values are greater than 1.00. The degree of abnormality can also be quantified by relating the confidence interval ratio to the degree of obstruction or restriction. For example, the $FEV_{1\%}$ may be evaluated:

	$FEV_{1\%}$ (CI)
Normal	<1 CI
Mild obstruction	>1 < 2 CI
Moderate obstruction	>2 <4 CI
Severe obstruction	>4 CI

Degrees of abnormality are not always expressed in terms of whole units of confidence intervals. Parameters that display a wide variability, such as the $FEF_{25\%-75\%}$ may have confidence intervals that in some instances are larger than the expected value, resulting in a lower limit of normal that is zero or even negative; although statistically valid, the use of the CI may not be applicable in every situation.

A third method of determining lower limits of normal uses 95th percentiles. The 95th percentile for any pulmonary function parameter may be calculated as the percent of the predicted value above which 95% of the healthy population falls. Although the 95th percentile method requires a large sample population, it does not require that the pulmonary function parameter be normally distributed throughout the population. Lower limits of normal by the 95th percentile method are usually expressed in relation to specific age groupings. Both the CI and 95th percentile methods yield similar results for lower limits of normal, if the parameter is normally distributed in the population.

In selecting predicted values, individual laboratories should attempt to choose studies that closely approximate the type of population that will be tested. The following factors may be considerations in selecting values to be used as normals:

1. What type of equipment was used for the population study; does it comply with the most recent recommendations (1987) of the American Thoracic Society (see Chapter 11)?
2. Were the methodologies (instrumentation and procedures) used in the reference study similar to those to be employed, particularly for flows, lung volumes, and DL_{CO}?
3. How large was the sample population? What age ranges were included? Did the study generate different regressions for different ethnic origins? Did the study include smokers or other "at-risk" individuals as normals?
4. Are standard deviations, standard errors of estimate, or 95th percentiles available, so that lower limits of normal can be defined?
5. Was the study performed at a different altitude, or under different environmental conditions?
6. Do predicted values generated using the study's regressions differ markedly from other published reports?

Every laboratory should perform measurements on 20 or more individuals who are free of cardiopulmonary disease, and who represent a cross-section of the population that the laboratory normally tests. Measured values from these subjects may then be compared with predicted values from various reference equations. The equations with the smallest average differences and the smallest range of differences should be selected. This type of evaluation based on a small number of subjects may not show marked differences between equations for parameters such as the FVC and $FEV_{1.0}$, but may show noticeable discrepancies for DL_{CO} and maximal flow measurements. Equations for similar tests (i.e., spirometry, lung volumes) should all be taken from one reference, as much as possible. If many subjects fall outside the limits of normal, the laboratory may question its testing methodology, the selection of the normal subjects, or the prediction equations selected.

Although there are no universally accepted predicted values, several excellent studies are available to provide a diverse combination of regressions so that many of the considerations discussed above can be addressed. The reference equations included here represent some of the more widely used regressions and compare favorably with other published studies. Other acceptable studies are included with the references, and laboratories are encouraged to evaluate these and other equations in selecting predicted values.

PREDICTION REGRESSIONS FOR PULMONARY FUNCTION TESTS

(All values BTPS unless otherwise stated)*

Test	Formula	SD	Source
VC, SVC (L)			
Males	0.148H − 0.025A − 4.24	0.58	1
Females	0.115H − 0.024A − 2.85	0.52	1
FRC (L)			
Males	0.130H − 5.16	—	2
Females	0.119H − 4.85	—	2
RV (L)			
Males	0.069H + 0.017A − 3.45	—	3
Females	0.081H + 0.009A − 3.90	—	3
Derived Lung Volumes			
	TLC (L) = VC + RV		
	IC (L) = TLC − FRC		
	ERV (L) = VC − IC		
FVC (L)			
Males	(same as VC)		1
Females	(same as VC)		1
$FEV_{0.5}$ (L)			
Males	0.24 + 0.02H − 0.024A	0.51	4
$FEV_{1.0}$ (L)			
Males	0.092H − 0.032A − 1.260	0.55	1
Females	0.089H − 0.024A − 1.93	0.47	1
$FEF_{200\text{-}1200}$ (L/sec)			
Males	0.109H − 0.047A + 2.010	1.66	1
Females	0.145H − 0.036A − 2.532	1.19	1
$FEF_{25\%\text{-}75\%}$ (L/sec)			
Males	0.047H − 0.045A + 2.513	1.12	1
Females	0.060H − 0.030A + 0.551	0.80	1
PEFR (L/sec)			
Males	0.144H − 0.024A + 0.225	—	5
Females	0.090H − 0.018A + 1.130	—	5

*H is height in inches; A is age in years; PB is barometric pressure.

$\dot{V}_{max\ 75}$ (L/sec)			
Males	0.090H − 0.020A + 2.726	—	5
Females	0.069H − 0.019A + 2.147	—	5
$\dot{V}_{max\ 50}$ (L/sec)			
Males	0.065H − 0.030A + 2.403	—	5
Females	0.062H − 0.035A + 1.426	—	5
$\dot{V}_{max\ 25}$ (L/sec)			
Males	0.036H − 0.041A + 1.984	—	5
Females	0.023H − 0.035A + 2.216	—	5
MVV (L/min)			
Males	3.03H − 0.816A − 37.9	—	5
Females	2.14H − 0.685A − 4.87	—	5
CV/VC (%)			
Males	0.357A + 0.562	4.15	6
Females	0.293A + 2.812	4.90	6
CC/TLC (%)			
Males	0.496A + 14.878	4.09	6
Females	0.536A + 14.420	4.43	6
Viso$\dot{V}$/FVC (%)			
All ages	0.450A + 4.69	5.27	7
>50 years	0.303A + 13.43	4.31	7
$DL_{CO}SB$ (ml CO/min/mm Hg STPD)			
Males	0.250H − 0.177A + 19.93	—	8
Females	0.284H − 0.177A + 7.72	—	8
Maximal expiratory pressure (cm H_2O)			
Males	268 − 1.03A	—	9
Females	170 − 0.53A	—	9
Maximal inspiratory pressure (cm H_2O)			
Males	143 − 0.55A	—	9
Females	104 − 0.51A	—	9
$\dot{V}_{O_{2max}}$ (L/min STPD)			
Males	4.2 − 0.032A	0.4	10
Females	2.6 − 0.014A	0.4	10
HR_{max} (beats/min)			
Males and Females	210 − 0.65A	10-15	10
Pa_{O_2} (mm Hg)			
Males and Females	−0.279A + 0.113PB + 14.632	—	11

SOURCES FOR PREDICTION REGRESSIONS

1. Morris JF, Koski A, and Johnson LC: Spirometric standards for healthy non-smoking adults, Am Rev Respir Dis 103:57, 1971.
2. Bates DV, Macklem PT, and Christie RV: Respiratory function in disease, ed 2, Philadelphia, 1971, WB Saunders Co.
3. Goldman HI and Becklake MR: Respiratory function tests: normal values at median altitudes and the prediction of normal results, Am Rev Tuberculosis 79:457, 1959.
4. Kory RC, Callahan R, and Syner JC: The Veterans Administration-Army cooperative study of pulmonary function: I. Clinical spirometry in normal men, Am J Med 30:243, 1961.
5. Cherniack RM and Raber MD: Normal standards for ventilatory function using an automated wedge spirometer, Am Rev Respir Dis 106:38, 1972.
6. Buist SA and Ross BB: Predicted values for closing volumes using a modified single-breath nitrogen test, Am Rev Respir Dis 111:405, 1975.
7. Gelb AF et al: Sensitivity of volume of isoflow in the detection of mild airway obstruction, Am Rev Respir Dis 112:401, 1975.
8. Gaensler EA and Wright GW: Evaluation of respiratory impairment, Arch Environ Health 12:146, 1966.
9. Black LF and Hyatt RE: Maximal respiratory pressures: normal values and relationship to age and sex, Am Rev Respir Dis 99:696, 1969.
10. Jones NL et al: Clinical exercise testing, ed 2, Philadelphia, 1983, WB Saunders Co.
11. Morris AH et al: Clinical pulmonary function testing, ed 2, Salt Lake City, 1984, Intermountain Thoracic Society.

ADDITIONAL RECOMMENDED SOURCES FOR PULMONARY FUNCTION PREDICTED VALUES

Spirometry

Crapo RO, Morris AH, and Gardner RM: Reference spirometric values using techniques and equipment that meet ATS recommendations, Am Rev Respir Dis 123:659, 1981.

Knudson RJ, Slatin RC, and Lebowitz MD: The maximal expiratory flow-volume curve: normal standards, variability, and effects of age, Am Rev Respir Dis 113:587, 1976.

Quanjer PH, editor: Report of Working Party—European Community for Coal and Steel: Standardized lung function testing, Bull Eur Physiopathol Respir 19(suppl 5):7, 1983.

Schoenberg JB, Beck GJ, and Bouhuys A: Growth and decay of pulmonary function in healthy blacks and whites, Respir Physiol 33:367, 1978.

Lung volumes

Crapo RO et al: Lung volumes in healthy non-smoking adults, Bull Eur Physiopathol Respir 18:419, 1982.

Grimby G and Soderholm B: Spirometric studies in normal subjects: III. Static lung volumes and maximum voluntary ventilation in adults with a note on physical fitness, Acta Med Scand 173:199, 1963.

Diffusing capacity

Bates DV, Macklem PT, and Christie RV: Repiratory function in disease, Philadelphia, 1971, WB Saunders Co.

Crapo RO and Morris AH: Standardized single-breath normal values for carbon monoxide diffusing capacity, Am Rev Respir Dis 123:185, 1981.

Pediatric pulmonary function

Hsu KHK et al: Ventilatory functions of normal children and young adults—Mexican-American, white, and black. I. Spirometry, J Pediatr 95:14, 1979.

Polgar G and Promadhat V: Pulmonary function testing in children: techniques and standards, Philadelphia, 1971, WB Saunders Co.

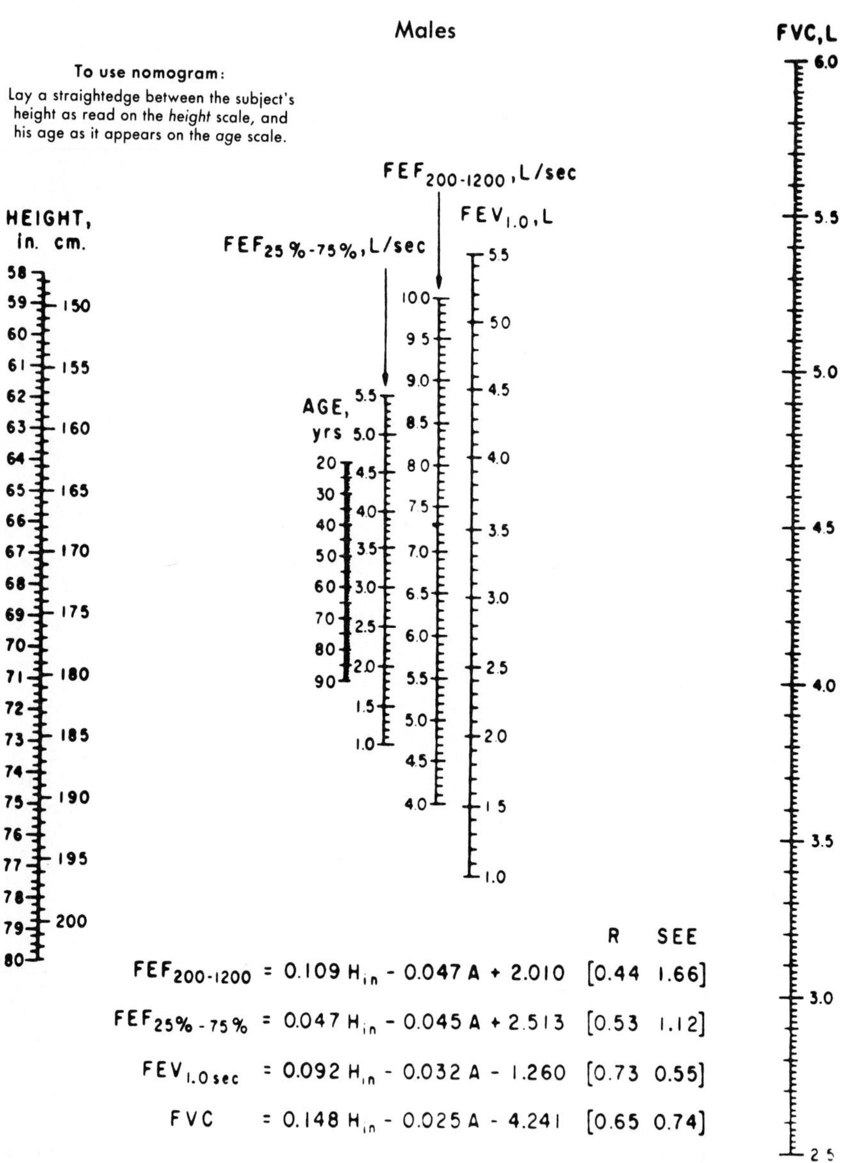

Fig. A-1 Prediction nomograms (BTPS), spirometric values in normal males. (From Morris JF, Koski WA, and Johnson LD: Am Rev Respir Dis 103(1):57, 1971.)

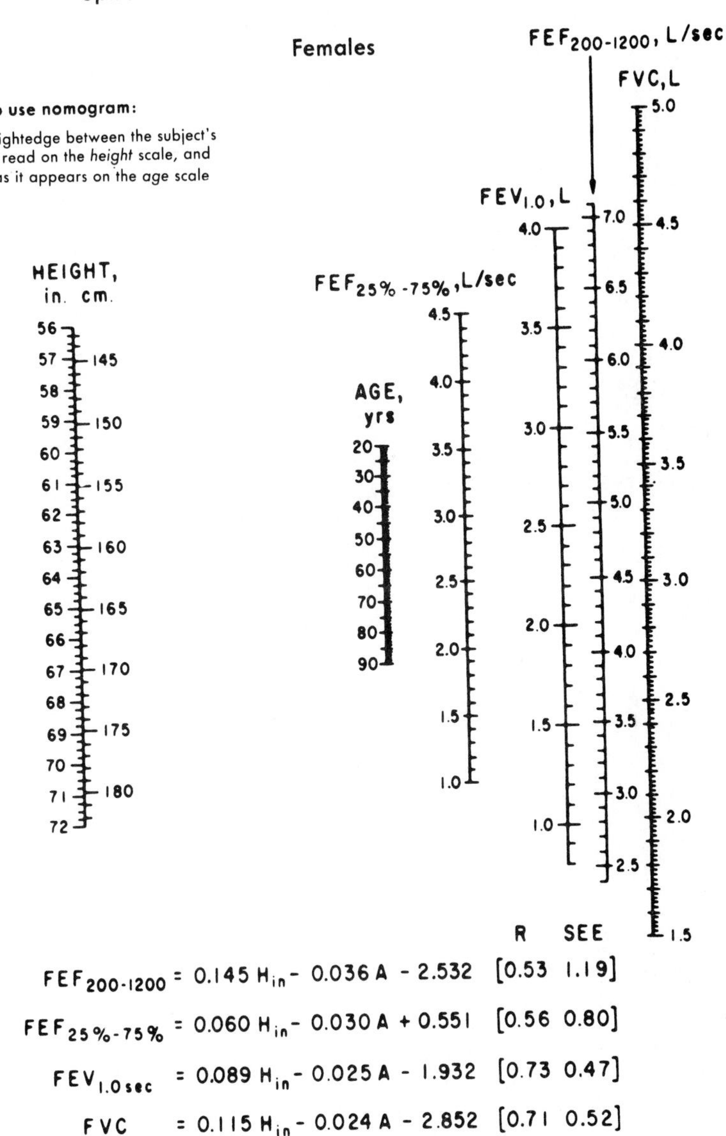

Fig. A-2 Prediction nomograms (BTPS), spirometric values in normal females. (From Morris JF, Koski WA, and Johnson LD: Am Rev Respir Dis 103(1):57, 1971.)

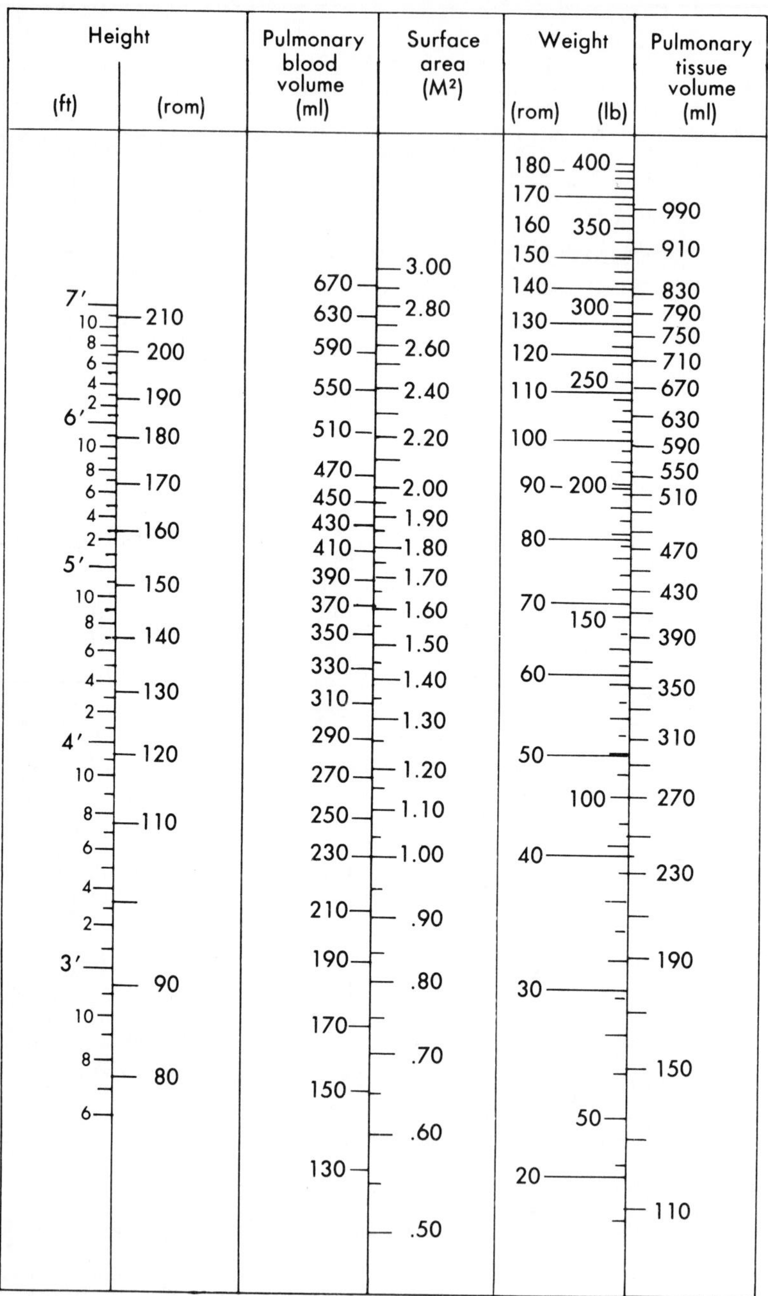

Fig. A-3 Pulmonary tissue/blood volume nomogram (for use with the radiologic method of estimating TLC {see Chapter 1}). (From Ferris BG: Am Rev Respir Dis 118(suppl):109, 1978.)

NORMAL VALUES FOR PULMONARY FUNCTION STUDIES IN CHILDREN

(All values BTPS unless otherwise noted)*

Test	Formula	SD	Source
(Children 42-59 inches, 5-17 years)			
FVC (L)			
Males	0.094H − 3.04	0.176	1
Females	0.077H − 2.37	0.171	1
$FEV_{1.0}$ (L)			
Males	0.085H − 2.86	0.159	1
Females	0.074H − 2.48	0.166	1
$FEF_{25\%-75\%}$ (L)			
Males	0.094H − 2.61	0.388	1
Females	0.087H − 2.39	0.347	1
PEFR (L/Sec)			
Males	0.161H − 5.88	0.451	1
Females	0.130H − 4.51	0.487	1
MVV (L/Min)			
Males and Females	3.81H − 134	—	1
(Children 60-78 inches, 5-17 years)			
FVC (L)			
Males	0.174A + 0.164H − 9.43	0.354	1
Females	0.102A + 0.117H − 5.87	0.287	1
$FEV_{1.0}$ (L/Sec)			
Males	0.126A + 0.143H − 7.86	0.303	1
Females	0.085A + 0.100H − 4.94	0.290	1
$FEF_{25\%-75\%}$ (L/Sec)			
Males	0.126A + 0.135H − 6.50	0.612	1
Females	0.083A + 0.093H − 3.50	0.621	1
PEFR (L/Sec)			
Males	0.205A + 0.181H − 9.54	0.780	1
Females	0.139A + 0.100H − 4.12	0.798	1
MVV (L/Min)			
Males and Females	3.81H − 134	—	1

*H is height in inches; A is age in years.

SVC (L)			
Males	(same as FVC)		1
Females	(same as FVC)		1
FRC (L)			
Males and Females	$0.067 \times e^{0.05334H}$	—	2
RV (L)			
Males and Females	$0.033 \times e^{0.05334H}$	—	2

Derived lung volumes (L)

$$TLC = VC + RV$$
$$IC = TLC - FRC$$
$$ERV = VC - IC$$

$D_{L_{CO}}$SB (ml CO/min/mm Hg STPD)			
Males and Females	0.693 − 20.13	—	3

SOURCES FOR NORMAL VALUES

1. Dickman ML, Schmidt CD, and Gardner RM: Spirometric standards for normal children and adolescents (ages 5 years through 18 years), Am Rev Respir Dis 104:680, 1971.
2. Weng TR and Levison H: Standards of pulmonary function in children, Am Rev Respir Dis 99:879, 1969.
3. Gaensler EA and Wright GW: Evaluation of respiratory impairment, Arch Environ Health 12:146, 1966.

(see also Additional Recommended Sources for Pulmonary Function Predicted Values)

SUMMARY CURVES FOR PREDICTING NORMAL VALUES IN CHILDREN

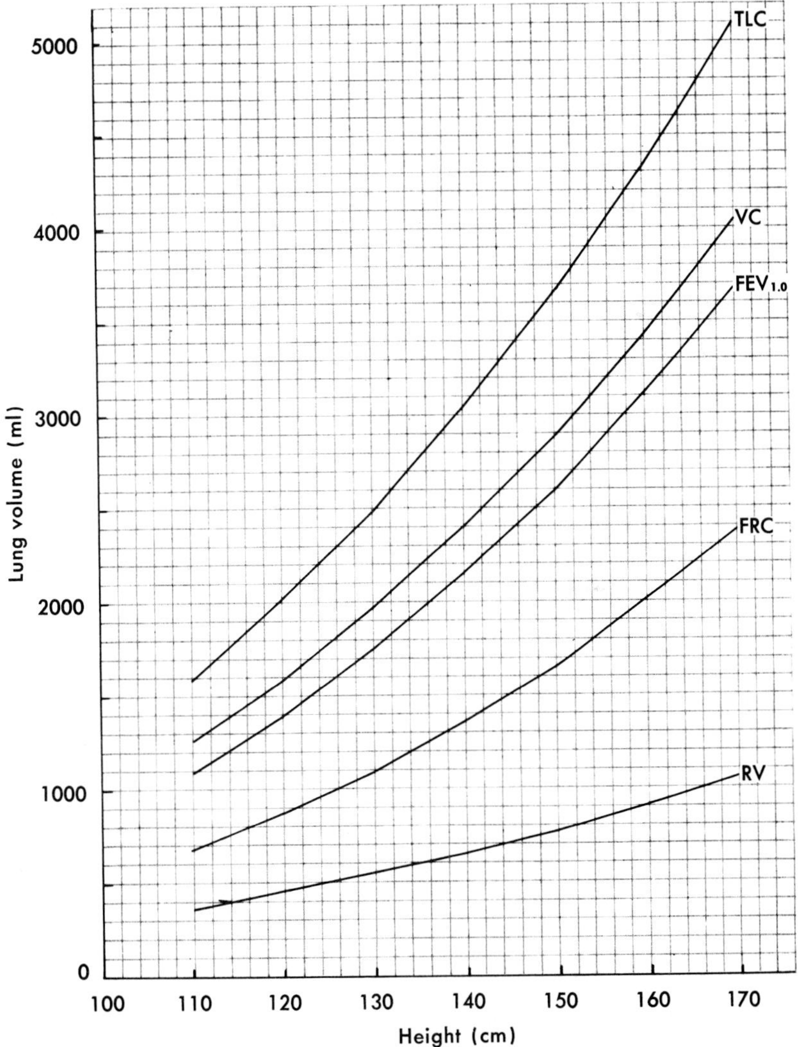

Fig. A-4 Summary curves for lung volumes, in milliliters, for boys, as a function of height in centimeters. Summary curves are derived from regression equations from several different studies. (From Polgar G and Promadhat V: Pulmonary function testing in children, Philadelphia, 1971, WB Saunders Co.)

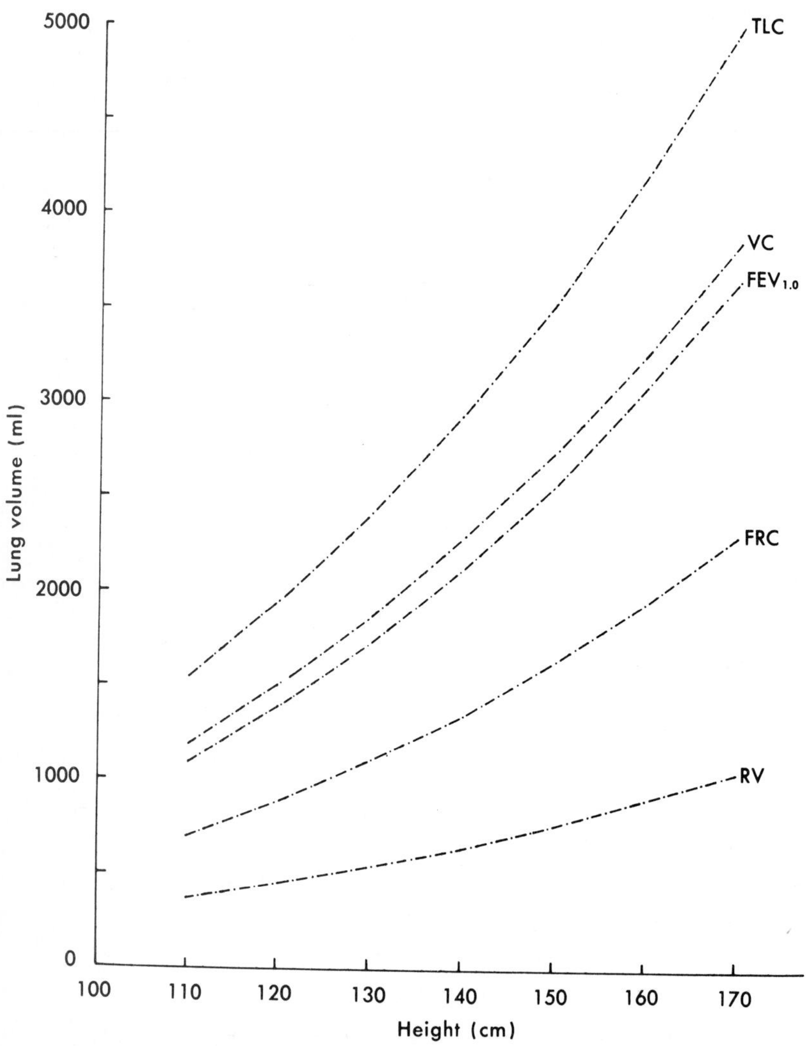

Fig. A-5 Summary curves for lung volumes, in milliliters, for girls, as a function of height in centimeters. Summary curves are derived from regression equations from several different studies. (From Polgar G and Promadhat V: Pulmonary function testing in children, Philadelphia, 1971, WB Saunders Co.)

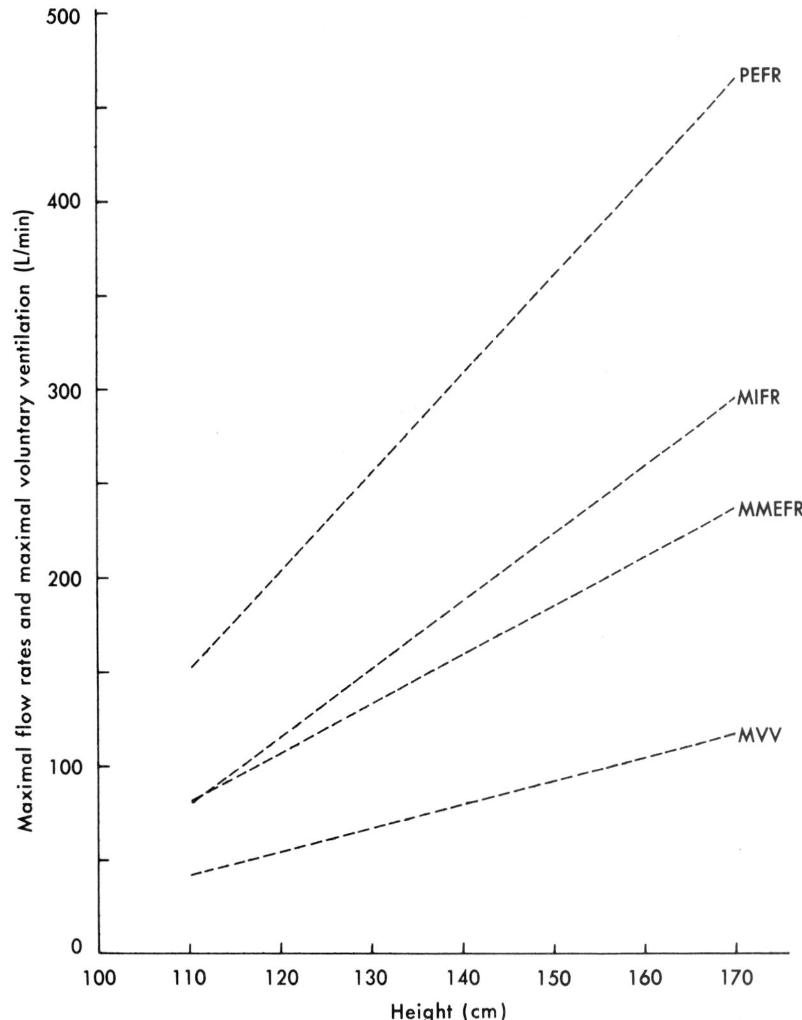

Fig. A-6 Summary curves for maximal mid-expiratory flow rate ($FEF_{25\%-75\%}$), peak expiratory flow rate (PEFR), maximal voluntary ventilation (MVV), and maximal inspiratory flow rate (MIFR) in liters per minute as a function of height for boys and girls. Summary curves are derived from regression equations from several different studies. (From Polgar G and Promadhat V: Pulmonary function testing in children, Philadelphia, 1971, WB Saunders Co.)

FACTORS FOR CONVERTING GAS VOLUMES FROM ATPS TO BTPS

$$\text{Volume (BTPS)} = \text{Volume (ATPS)} \times \frac{P_B - P_{H_2O}}{P_B - 47} \times \frac{310}{273 + T}$$

where:

P_B = Barometric pressure, in mm Hg
P_{H_2O} = Vapor pressure of water at spirometer temperature
T = Temperature centigrade
47 = Vapor pressure of water at 37°C
310 = Absolute body temperature

Most of the factors of this equation can be combined to give an approximate value for a conversion factor; local P_B causes slight differences.

Conversion factor	Gas temperature (°C)	P_{H_2O} (mm Hg)
1.112	18	15.6
1.107	19	16.5
1.102	20	17.5
1.096	21	18.7
1.091	22	19.8
1.085	23	21.1
1.080	24	22.4
1.075	25	23.8
1.068	26	23.8
1.063	27	26.7
1.057	28	28.3
1.051	29	30.0
1.045	30	31.8
1.039	31	31.8
1.032	32	35.7
1.026	33	35.7
1.020	34	35.7
1.014	35	42.2
1.007	36	44.6
1.000	37	47.0

CONVERTING GAS VOLUMES FROM ATPS TO STPD

$$\text{Volume (STPD)} = \text{Volume (ATPS)} \times \frac{P_B - P_{H_2O}}{760} \times \frac{273}{273 + T}$$

where:

P_B = Barometric pressure
P_{H_2O} = Water vapor pressure at spirometer temperature
T = Temperature of the spirometer
760 = Standard barometric pressure at sea level
273 = Absolute temperature equal to 0° C

SI (SYSTÈME INTERNATIONAL) UNITS

Conversion factors for units of measurement commonly used in pulmonary function testing. (Except for temperature, to convert a value expressed in conventional units to its equivalent in SI units, multiply the conventional units by the conversion factor; to convert from SI to conventional units, divide by the factor.)

Measurement	Conventional unit	SI unit	Conversion factor
Temperature	°C	°K	°C+273.15
Length	inch (in)	meter (M)	0.0254
	foot (ft)	M	0.3048
Area	in^2	cm^2	6.452
	ft^2	M^2	0.0929
Volume	ft^3	L	28.32
Pressure	cm H_2O	kilopascal (kPa)	0.09806
	mm Hg (torr)	kPa	0.1333
	pounds/in^2 (psi)	kPa	6.895
Work	kilogram meter (kg M)	joule (J)	9.807
Power	kg M/min	(J)	0.1634
Energy	kilocalorie (Kcal)	(J)	4185.0
Compliance	L/cm H_2O	L/kPa	10.20
Resistance	cm H_2O/L/sec	kPa/L/sec	0.09806

SOME USEFUL EQUATIONS

Alveolar air equation

It is often necessary to ascertain the composition of alveolar gas. Estimations of the partial pressure of CO_2, N_2, and H_2O can be done rather easily, but the $P_{A_{O_2}}$ is somewhat more difficult to obtain. The most practical application of the alveolar air equation is determination of $P_{A_{O_2}}$ as required for calculation of the percent shunt. The formula for the alveolar equation is as follows:

$$P_{A_{O_2}} = (F_{I_{O_2}} \times (P_B - 47)) - Pa_{CO_2} \frac{(F_{I_{O_2}} + 1 - F_{I_{O_2}})}{R}$$

where:

$F_{I_{O_2}}$ = Fractional concentration of O_2 inspired
P_B = Barometric pressure
47 = Partial pressure of water vapor at 37°C
Pa_{CO_2} = Arterial CO_2 tension, presumed equal to alveolar CO_2 tension
R = Respiratory exchange ratio ($\dot{V}_{CO_2}/\dot{V}_{O_2}$)

If the fraction of inspired O_2 is 1.0, the entire factor in the right-hand parentheses becomes one. R usually varies between 0.70 and 1.00 and can usually be assumed to be about 0.80.

Poiseuille's law

Poiseuille's law describes the flow of gas through a tube. The law has many applications in pulmonary physiology, notably insofar as it applies to laminar flow of gas through the conducting airways. It is also used in pneumotachography to relate flow and pressure changes within a tube. The law is stated thus:

$$\Delta P = \frac{\dot{V}8nl}{\pi r^4}$$

where:

ΔP = Change in pressure from one end of the tube to the other
$\dot{V}$ = Flow through the tube
n = Coefficient of viscosity of the gas
l = Length of the tube
r = Radius of the tube

The equation can be rearranged thus:

$$\frac{\Delta P}{\dot{V}} = \frac{8nl}{\pi r^4}$$

Here, the ratio of the pressure difference at the ends of the tube (ΔP) and the flow through the tube ($\dot{V}$), which defines resistance, is equated to the remaining variables, notably the length and radius of the tube. The resistance varies directly with the length of the conducting tube and inversely with the 4th power of the radius. A twofold increase in the length of the tube doubles the resistance, whereas a reduction of the radius by half increases the pressure differential 16 times. In the airways, abnormal narrowing by mucous secretions or other lesions can cause significant increases in airway resistance. Poiseuille's law holds true for any round tube in which laminar flow is possible, and pneumotachography is based directly on this law (see the discussion of pressure differential flow sensors, in Chapter 9). Because the length and radius of a pressure differential flow sensor remain constant and the viscosity of respiratory gases varies only slightly, all of the variables in Poiseuille's equation can be reduced to a constant except ΔP and $\dot{V}$. By rearranging:

$$\dot{V} = \frac{\Delta P}{K_R}$$

where

K_R = A resistance constant based primarily on the length and radius of the tube

Using this equation, all that is necessary to measure the $\dot{V}$ is a means of determining the pressure differential; this is easily accomplished by means of pressure transducers.

Thoracic gas volume equation

Measurement of the VTG with the body plethysmograph is based on Boyle's law:

$$P_1V_1 = P_2V_2$$

or by expanding:

$$P_1V_1 = (P_1 + \Delta P)(V_1 + \Delta V)$$

where

P_1 = Initial pressure in the lungs (713 mm Hg or 970 cm H_2O)
V_1 = VTG or thoracic gas volume
ΔV = Change in lung volume
ΔP = Change in lung pressure

Then by rearranging:

$$P_1\,\Delta V + V_1\,\Delta P + \Delta V\,\Delta P = 0$$

Solving for V_1:

$$V_1 = -\frac{\Delta V}{\Delta P}(P_1 + \Delta P)$$

Because ΔP is small compared with P_1, $P_1 + \Delta P \cong P_1$, therefore:

$$V_1 = -\frac{P_1(\Delta V)}{\Delta P}$$

In terms of the plethysmographic method (and disregarding the sign):

$$V_{TG} = 970\,\frac{(\Delta V)}{(\Delta P)}$$

A sloping line is recorded on an oscilloscope and represents the change in mouth pressure per unit change in box volume, $(\Delta P)/(\Delta V)$ or λV_{TG}, as the subject breathes against an occluded airway. The equation then becomes:

$$V_{TG} = \frac{970}{\lambda V_{TG}}$$

This is the working form of the equation to which box pressure and mouth pressure calibration factors are added (see the Sample Calculations section, later in the Appendix). Simple measurements of the slope of the trace allows rapid calculation of VTG.

Fick's law of diffusion (modified)

In reference to gas exchange across a membrane, Fick's law states that:

$$\dot{V}_{gas} = \frac{A}{T} \times D \times (P_1 - P_2)$$

where

$$\begin{aligned} A &= \text{Area of the membrane} \\ T &= \text{Thickness of the membrane} \\ P_1 - P_2 &= \text{Pressure gradient across the membrane} \\ D &= \text{Diffusion constant} \end{aligned}$$

D is related to the molecular weight and solubility of the gas to which it refers by:

$$D \propto \frac{\text{Solubility}}{\sqrt{\text{Molecular Weight}}}$$

Because A and T remain relatively constant in the lung system:

$$D_L \propto \frac{\dot{V}_{gas}}{P_A - P_C}$$

where

$$\begin{aligned} D_L &= \text{Diffusion constant for the lung} \\ P_A &= \text{Alveolar gas pressure} \\ P_C &= \text{Capillary gas pressure} \end{aligned}$$

When D_L is measured with carbon monoxide (CO), the capillary partial pressure is assumed to be zero, thus:

$$D_L = \frac{\dot{V}_{CO}}{P_{A_{CO}}}$$

All CO methods of measuring D_L use this basic equation. The single-breath and steady-state methods differ in that the former measures $\dot{V}_{CO}$ during breath-holding, while the latter measures it during "normal" breathing. The steady-state methods vary by the way in which they measure $P_{A_{CO}}$.

Fick principle (cardiac output determination)

The Fick principle relates $\dot{V}O_2$ to the arterial-mixed venous O_2 content difference ($C[a\text{-}\bar{v}]_{O_2}$) to determine cardiac output ($\dot{Q}$):

$$\dot{Q}_T = \frac{\dot{V}O_2}{Ca_{O_2} - C\bar{v}_{O_2}}$$

This equation forms the basis for determining various fractions of the cardiac output, namely, the shunt fraction ($\dot{Q}_S$) and the fraction participating in ideal gas exchange ($\dot{Q}_C$). The relationship between $\dot{Q}_S$ and the total cardiac output $\dot{Q}_T$ can be expressed as a ratio using the concept of O_2 content differences:

$$\frac{\dot{Q}_S}{\dot{Q}_T} = \frac{Cc_{O_2} - Ca_{O_2}}{Cc_{O_2} - C\bar{v}_{O_2}}$$

where

$Cc_{O_2} - Ca_{O_2}$ = Content difference between pulmonary end capillary blood, Cc_{O_2}, and arterial blood, Ca_{O_2}, which increases when blood passes through the pulmonary system without coming into contact with alveolar gas (a shunt)

$Cc_{O_2} - C\bar{v}_{O_2}$ = Content difference between blood returning to the lungs by way of the pulmonary artery and the pulmonary end-capillary blood; the total change reflecting the arterialization of mixed venous blood

In a system in which all blood equilibrates with alveolar gas, Cc_{O_2} and Ca_{O_2} become identical, no matter what the value of the denominator, so that the ratio becomes zero and the shunt must be zero. As more blood fails to equilibrate, the numerator becomes larger in relation to the denominator and is reflected by an increased $\dot{Q}s/\dot{Q}_T$.

Because true pulmonary end-capillary O_2 content, Cc_{O_2}, is practically impossible to sample and represents a mathematical entity rather than an actual phenomenon, a modified form of the equation is used clinically (as described in Chapter 6):

$$\frac{\dot{Q}s}{\dot{Q}_T} = \frac{(P_{A_{O_2}} - Pa_{O_2})(0.0031)}{(C[a\text{-}\bar{v}]_{O_2}) + (P_{A_{O_2}} - Pa_{O_2})(0.0031)}$$

where

$P_{A_{O_2}} - Pa_{O_2}$ = Tension difference of O_2 between the alveoli and arterial blood

0.0031 = Solubility factor to convert O_2 tension to volumes percent

The equation is implemented by having the subject breathe 100% O_2 long enough to completely saturate the Hb (Pa_{O_2} greater than 150 mm Hg). Therefore, the only difference between pulmonary end-capillary blood (assumed to be in equilibrium with the $P_{A_{O_2}}$) and arterial blood exists in the difference in O_2 content in the dissolved form. Again, this is related to the normal a-$\bar{v}$ content difference ($C[a\text{-}\bar{v}]_{O_2}$) plus the actual dissolved content difference, denoted by the same term in both numerator and denominator. A ratio is thus derived between the content difference of shunted blood and the total difference, in this case determined by using dissolved O_2 differences. $P_{A_{O_2}}$ is determined by the alveolar air equation outlined previously in the Appendix.

Calculated bicarbonate (HCO_3^-)

The bicarbonate concentration in plasma can be calculated from the Henderson-Hasselbalch equation if the pH and P_{CO_2} are known:

$$pH = pK + \log\frac{(HCO_3^-)}{(H_2CO_3)}$$

The working form of the equation becomes:

$$(HCO_3^-) = 0.0306 \times P_{CO_2} \times 10^{((pH-6.161)/0.9524)}$$

where:

HCO_3^- = Bicarbonate concentration, in mEq/L
0.0306 = Solubility coefficient for CO_2
6.161 = The pK for carbonic acid
0.9524 = An empirically determined constant

The total CO_2 concentration can then be determined by summing the HCO_3^- and the dissolved CO_2:

$$T_{CO_2} = 0.0306 \times P_{CO_2} + (HCO_3^-)$$

Calculated oxygen saturation

Although it is preferable to actually measure oxygen saturation (see Chapter 6), the saturation of Hb with O_2 can be calculated if the pH and P_{O_2} are known. Assuming that the Hb is normal (i.e., having a P_{50} of 26.6), the saturation may be calculated:

$$\text{Saturation} = \frac{Z^{2.60}}{(26.6)^{2.60} + Z^{2.60}} \times 100$$

where:

$Z = P_{O_2} \times 10^{(-0.48(7.40-pH))}$
P_{O_2} = The partial pressure of O_2 in the sample
pH = The hydrogen ion concentration (−log) in the sample
−0.48 = The Bohr factor (normal blood)

Because of the assumptions concerning normality of the hemoglobin as well as its P_{50}, calculated saturations may be in error if the true factors are unknown.

SAMPLE CALCULATIONS

Open-circuit FRC determination (N_2 washout) (see Chapter 1)

FRC:	Unknown
$\%N_{2_{final}}$:	6% (0.06 as a fraction)
$\%N_{2_{alveolar\ 1}}$:	76% (0.76 as a fraction)
$\%N_{2_{alveolar\ 2}}$:	1% (0.01 as a fraction)
Vol. expired: (VE)	27.5 L
Test time (T):	7 minutes
Blood/tissue N_2 washout factor:	0.04 L/min (N_2 correction factor)
Spirometer temperature:	24°C
System deadspace (VD)	1.0 L

$$1.\ \text{FRC} = \frac{[\%N_{2_{final}} \times (V_E + V_D)] - (T \times N_2\ \text{correction})}{\%N_{2_{alveolar\ 1}} - \%N_{2_{alveolar\ 2}}}$$

2. $= \frac{[0.06 \times (27.5 + 1.0\text{ L})] - (7.0\text{ min} \times 0.04\text{ L/min})}{0.76 - 0.01}$

3. $= \frac{(0.06 \times 28.5) - (0.28\text{ L})}{0.75}$

4. $= \frac{1.71\text{ L} - 0.28\text{ L}}{0.75}$

5. $= \frac{1.43}{0.75}$

6. FRC = 2.00 L (ATPS)

This value is ATPS and must be corrected to BPTS. The spirometer temperature was 24° C; thus using the appropriate correction factor from p. 384:

7. FRC (BTPS) = 1.91 × 1.08
8. FRC (BTPS) = 2.06

Closed-circuit FRC determination (Helium dilution) (see Chapter 1)

FRC:	Unknown
He_{added}:	0.5 L
$\%He_{initial}$:	9.5% (0.095 as a fraction)
$\%He_{final}$:	5.5% (0.055 as a fraction)
He absorption correction:	0.1 L
Spirometer temperature:	24° C

1. $FRC = \left[\frac{(\%He_{initial} - \%He_{final})}{\%He_{final}} \times \text{Initial volume}\right] - \text{He correction}$

2. $= \text{Initial Volume} = \frac{He_{added}}{\%He_{initial}}$
(spirometry and circuitry)
$= \frac{0.5L}{0.095}$
$= 5.26\text{ L}$

3. $FRC = \left[\frac{(0.095 - 0.055)}{0.055} \times 5.26\text{ L}\right] - 0.1\text{ L}$

4. $= (0.73 \times 5.26\text{ L}) - 0.1\text{ L}$

5. $= 3.84\text{ L} - 0.1\text{ L}$

6. FRC = 3.74 L (ATPS)

Correcting to BTPS with appropriate correction factor from p. 384:

7. FRC (BTPS) = 3.74 × 1.08
8. FRC (BTPS) = 4.04 L

Single-breath DL_{CO} (see Chapter 5)

Volume inspired (VI):	4.0 L
FI_{CO}:	0.3% (0.003 as a fraction)
$FA_{CO_{T2}}$:	0.125% (0.00125 as a fraction)
FI_{He}:	10.0% (0.10 as a fraction)
FE_{He}:	7.5% (0.075 as a fraction
PB:	760 mm Hg
Breath-hold time ($T_2 - T_1$):	10.0 sec
Spirometer temperature:	25° C

1. $$DL_{CO}SB = \frac{VA \times 60}{(PB - 47)(T_2 - T_1)} \times \text{Ln}\frac{(FA_{CO_{T1}})}{(FA_{CO_{T2}})}$$

2. $$VA = \frac{VI}{FE_{He}/FI_{He}}$$

$$= \frac{4.0\text{ L}}{0.075/0.10} = 5.33\text{ L (5333 ml)}$$

3. $$FA_{CO_{T1}} = FI_{CO} \times FE_{He}/FI_{He}$$

$$= 0.003 \times 0.075/0.10 = 0.0025$$

4. $$DL_{CO}SB = \frac{5333\text{ ml} \times 60}{(713) \times (10.0)} \times \text{Ln}\frac{(0.0025)}{(0.00125)}$$

5. $$= \frac{319980}{7130} \times \text{Ln (1.8)}$$

6. $$= 44.9\text{ ml/min/mm Hg} \times (0.5878)$$

7. $$= 26.38\text{ ml CO/min/mm Hg (ATPS)}$$

This value is ATPS and is normally converted to STPS (0° C, 760 mm Hg, dry). The correction factor can be calculated:

8. $$\frac{273}{273 + T°\text{ C}} \times \frac{PB - P_{H_2O}\ T°\text{ C}}{760} = \text{Correction factor}$$

where

T° C = Spirometer temperature

P_{H_2O} T° C = Partial pressure of water vapor at the spirometer temperature (in this case: 24 mm Hg at 25° C)

9. $$\frac{273}{273 + 25} \times \frac{760 - 24}{760} = \text{Correction factor}$$

10. $0.916 \times 0.968 = 0.887$

11. (26.38 ml CO/min/mm Hg) × (0.887) = 23.4 ml CO/min/mm Hg (STPD)

Thoracic gas volume (VTG) (Chapter 1)

(Data for VTG and Raw are from the same subject)

VTG:	Unknown

VTG Tangents:	0.71 (angle 35.4)
	0.73 (angle 36.1)
	0.73 (angle 36.1)
PB:	755 mm Hg
Subject Weight:	71 Kg
P_{mouth} Calibration:	10 cm H_2O/cm
P_{box} Calibration:	30 ml/cm
Dead space correction:	100 ml
Plethysmograph volume:	530 L

1. Average VTG tangent (TAN)

$$\begin{array}{r} 0.71 \\ 0.73 \\ +\ \underline{0.73} \\ 2.17 / 3 = 0.72 \text{ (avg.)} \end{array}$$

2. Pressure correction

$$\begin{aligned} PB_{corr} &= (PB - 47) \times 1.36 \\ &= (755 \text{ mm Hg} - 47 \text{ mm Hg}) \times 1.36 \\ &= 963 \text{ cm } H_2O \end{aligned}$$

3. Subject volume correction (K)

$$K = \frac{[\text{Pleth volume} - (\text{Subject weight}/1.07)]}{\text{Pleth volume}}$$

$$0.874 = \frac{[530 \text{ L} - (71 \text{ Kg}/1.07)]}{530 \text{ L}}$$

4.
$$\begin{aligned} VTG &= \left(\frac{PB_{corr}}{TAN} \times \frac{P_{box_{cal}}}{P_{mouth_{cal}}} \times K\right) - \text{Dead space} \\ &= \left(\frac{963}{0.72} \times \frac{30}{10} \times 0.874\right) - 100 \\ &= (1338 \times 3 \times 0.874) - 100 \\ &= 3408 \text{ ml or } 3.41 \text{ L} \end{aligned}$$

Airway resistance (Raw) (Chapter 3)

Raw:	Unknown
P_{mouth}/P_{box} TAN:	0.61 (angle = 31)
$\dot{V}/P_{box}$ TAN:	3.0 (angle = 72)
P_{mouth} Calibration:	10 cm H_2O/cm
P_{box} Calibration:	30 ml/cm
$\dot{V}$ Calibration:	1.0 L/sec/cm
R_{sys}:	0.25 cm H_2O/L/sec

1. $$\text{Raw} = \left(\frac{P_{mouth}/P_{box} \text{ TAN}}{\dot{V}/P_{box} \text{ TAN}} \times \frac{P_{mouth_{cal}}}{\dot{V}_{cal}}\right) - R_{sys}$$

2. $= \left(\frac{0.61}{3.0} \times \frac{10}{1.0}\right) - 0.25$

3. $= (0.203 \times 10) - 0.25$

4. $= 1.78$ cm H_2O/L/sec

Normally, several repetitions of the maneuver are performed; unlike the V_{TG}, however, the tangents are not averaged. Because the flow and volume tangents influence each other, the Raw is calculated and then averaged. To calculate the Gaw/V_L (specific airway conductance) the volume at which each Raw maneuver was performed is calculated as for the V_{TG}, using the P_{mouth}/P_{box} tangent from the specific maneuver. For the above example:

1. Gaw/V_L = (1/Raw)/V_{TG}

2. $V_{TG} = \left(\frac{963}{0.61} \times \frac{30}{10} \times 0.874\right) - 100$

3. $= (1579 \times 3 \times 0.874) - 100$

4. = 4040 ml or 4.04 L

Calculating the Gaw/V_L (SGaw):

5. = (1/1.78)/4.04

6. = 0.14 cm H_2O/L/sec/L

The average of several maneuvers is normally reported, again after the SGaw for individual efforts has been calculated.

EXERCISE STUDY (see Chapter 7)*

Volume exhaled (V):	20.0 L (ATPS)
Collection time (sec):	60 sec
Temperature (T):	24°C
$F_{E_{O_2}}$:	17.0% (0.17 as a fraction)
$F_{E_{CO_2}}$:	3.0% (0.03 as a fraction)
f:	25/min
HR:	100/min
Pa_{O_2}	95 mm Hg
Pa_{CO_2}:	35 mm Hg
P_B:	750 mm Hg
Mechanical V_D:	18 ml (0.018 L)
Subject's weight:	55 Kg

The first step is to calculate conversion factors to correct ventilation and gas exchange measurements to BTPS and STPD (this STPD factor is for conversion from BTPS), respectively:

*Values as might be obtained at a submaximal level using either a treadmill or bicycle ergometer.

$$1.\ \text{BTPS factor} = \frac{P_B - P_{H_2O}}{P_B - 47} \times \frac{273 + 37}{273 + T}$$
$$= \frac{721}{703} \times \frac{310}{297}$$
$$= 1.07$$

$$2.\ \text{STPD factor} = \frac{P_B - 47}{760} \times \frac{273}{273 + 37}$$
$$= \frac{703}{760} \times 0.881$$
$$= 0.815$$

Next, parameters of ventilation may be calculated:

$$3.\ \dot{V}_E\ (\text{BTPS}) = \frac{V_{exhaled} \times 60}{\text{Collection time in seconds}} \times \text{BTPS factor}$$
$$= \frac{20.0\ \text{L} \times 60}{60} \times 1.07$$
$$= 21.4\ \text{L (BTPS)}$$

$$4.\ V_T\ (\text{BTPS}) = \frac{\dot{V}_E\ (\text{BTPS})}{f}$$
$$= \frac{21.4}{25}$$
$$= 0.856\ \text{L (BTPS)}$$

$$5.\ V_D\ (\text{BTPS}) = V_T\ (\text{BTPS}) \times \left[1 - \frac{F_{E_{CO_2}} \times (P_B - 47)}{Pa_{CO_2}}\right] - V_{D_{mech}}$$
$$= 0.856 \times \left[1 - \frac{0.03 \times 703}{35}\right] - 0.018$$
$$= .856 \times [1 - 0.603] - 0.018$$
$$= (0.856 \times 0.397) - 0.018$$
$$= 0.340 - 0.018$$
$$= 0.322\ \text{L (BTPS)}$$

$$6.\ \dot{V}_A\ (\text{BTPS}) = \dot{V}_E\ (\text{BTPS}) - [f \times V_D\ (\text{BTPS})]$$
$$= 21.4 - [25 \times 0.322]$$
$$= 21.4 - 8.05$$
$$= 13.4\ \text{L (BTPS)}$$

$$7.\ V_D/V_T = \frac{0.322}{0.856}$$
$$= 0.38\ (\text{or } 38\%)$$

Next, gas exchange parameters are computed:

$$8.\ \dot{V}_E\ (\text{STPD}) = \dot{V}_E\ (\text{BTPS}) \times \text{STPD factor}$$
$$= 21.4 \times 0.815$$
$$= 17.4\ \text{L (STPD)}$$

$$9.\ \dot{V}O_2\ (STPD) = \left[\left(\frac{1 - FE_{O_2} - FE_{CO_2}}{1 - FI_{O_2}} \times FI_{O_2}\right) - FE_{O_2}\right] \times \dot{V}E\ (STPD)$$

$$= \left[\left(\frac{1 - 0.17 - 0.03}{1 - 0.2093} \times 0.2093\right) - 0.17\right] \times 17.4$$

$$= \left[\left(\frac{0.80}{0.79} \times 0.2093\right) - 0.17\right] \times 17.4$$

$$= [(1.01 \times 0.2093) - 0.17] \times 17.4$$

$$= [0.212 - 0.17] \times 17.4$$

$$= 0.042 \times 17.4$$

$$= 0.731\ L\ (STPD)$$

$$10.\ \dot{V}CO_2\ (STPD) = (FE_{CO_2} - 0.0003) \times \dot{V}E\ (STPD)$$

$$= (0.03 - 0.0003) \times 17.4$$

$$= 0.297 \times 17.4$$

$$= 0.517\ L\ (STPD)$$

$$11.\quad R = \frac{\dot{V}CO_2\ (STPD)}{\dot{V}O_2\ (STPD)}$$

$$= \frac{0.517}{0.731}$$

$$= 0.71$$

$$12.\quad \dot{V}E/\dot{V}O_2 = \frac{\dot{V}E\ (BTPS)}{\dot{V}O_2\ (STPD)}$$

$$= \frac{21.4}{0.731}$$

$$= 29.3\ L/L\ \dot{V}O_2$$

$$13.\quad \dot{V}O_2/HR = \frac{\dot{V}O_2\ (STPD)}{HR} \times 1000$$

$$= \frac{0.731}{100} \times 1000$$

$$= 7.31\ ml\ O_2/beat$$

The calculation of energy expenditure at any particular work load is described by the term METS, for multiples of the resting $\dot{V}O_2$; the MET level for any work load can be calculated by one of two methods. In each method:

$$14.\quad METS = \frac{\dot{V}O_2\ (STPD)\ exercise}{\dot{V}O_2\ (STPD)\ rest}$$

but the means of estimating $\dot{V}O_2$ (STPD) at rest differs. $\dot{V}O_2$ (STPD) rest can be measured, or it may be estimated as 0.0035 L/min/kg (3.5 ml/kg). Using the second method in this example:

$$METS = \frac{0.731}{0.0035 \times 55}$$

$$= 3.80$$

If the subject measured $\dot{V}O_2$ at rest had been 0.225 L/min (STPD), then:

$$\text{METS} = \frac{0.731}{0.225} = 3.25$$

CALCULATION OF THE MEAN AND STANDARD DEVIATION

The mean ($\overline{X}$) and standard deviation (SD) are computed to determine the variability of a series of values. The SD is affected by every value in the series, especially extreme values. If the values are normally distributed (i.e., each value has an equal chance of appearing), the SD may be used to relate any subsequent value to the population of values already obtained. In the laboratory setting, this concept is often applied to determine the variability of a particular measuring device, such as a blood gas electrode or spirometer. By performing multiple measurements of the same quantity (the control), the mean value may be determined and the precision of the device expressed by the SD of the measurements. Assuming that all of the values sampled are normally distributed, 68.3% of the values will be within ± 1 SD of the mean, 95.5% will be within ± 2 SD, and 99.7% within ± 3 SD. Once the mean and standard deviation have been determined for a particular series of measurements, subsequent values may be checked to see if they are "in control." Values between 2 SD and 3 SD from the mean should occur only 5% of the time, and values more than 3 SD from the mean should occur less than 1% of the time. The mean ($\overline{X}$) is calculated:

$$\overline{X} = \frac{\Sigma(X)}{N}$$

where

Σ = A symbol meaning "the sum of"
X = Individual data values
N = Number of items sampled

The standard deviation (SD) is calculated:

$$SD = \sqrt{\frac{\Sigma(x^2)}{N}}$$

where

x^2 = Deviations from the mean ($X - \overline{X}$) squared
N = Number of items sampled

If the SD is computed from a sample (usually 30 items or less), N − 1 is substituted for N.

Example calculation of the mean and SD for a series of P_{CO_2} values:

Sample #	P_{CO_2} (mm Hg) (X)	Deviation from mean (x)	Deviation squared (x^2)
1	39	−0.9	0.81
2	40	0.1	0.01
3	43	3.1	9.61
4	42	2.1	4.41
5	39	−0.9	0.81
6	38	−1.9	3.61
7	40	0.1	0.01
8	41	1.1	1.21
9	38	−1.9	3.61
10	39	−0.9	0.81
Total	399		24.90
Mean	39.9		2.49

$$SD = \sqrt{\frac{24.9}{(10 - 1)}}$$
$$= \sqrt{2.77}$$
$$= 1.66$$

The range of P_{CO_2} values in this example within two standard deviations of the mean is:

39.9 ± (2 × 1.66) or from 36.6 to 43.2 mm Hg

ANSWERS TO SELF-ASSESSMENT QUESTIONS

Chapter 1

1. 2.71 L (BTPS)
2. b
3. 4.53 L (BTPS)
4. b
5. e
6. a
7. b
8. a
9. b
10. b
11. a
12. b

Chapter 2

1. b
2. a
3. a. 0.6 L (BTPS)
   b. 9 breaths/min
   c. 5.23 L/min (BTPS)
4. b
5. c
6. c
7. d
8. d
9. a. 0.633 L (BTPS)
   b. 0.206 L (BTPS)
   c. 0.325 (32.5%)
10. 5.4 L/min (BTPS)
11. b
12. d

Chapter 3

1. c
2. a
3. b
4. d
5. 100%
6. b
7. d
8. d
9. b
10. b
11. a
12. a

Chapter 4

1. e
2. d
3. d
4. a
5. c
6. a
7. e
8. b
9. a
10. b

Chapter 5

1. c
2. e
3. b
4. c
5. a
6. a
7. d
8. a
9. b
10. c

Chapter 6

1. c
2. e
3. 17.2
4. c
5. b
6. c
7. d
8. e
9. b
10. c

Chapter 7

1. d
2. b
3. d
4. d
5. b
6. c
7. a
8. a
9. c
10. a
11. c
12. e

Chapter 8

1. e
2. a
3. c
4. d
5. b
6. d
7. b
8. c
9. d
10. b
11. c
12. c
13. a
14. b

Chapter 9

1. c
2. b
3. d
4. d
5. d
6. b
7. d
8. d
9. d
10. d
11. b
12. b
13. b
14. c
15. e
16. b

Chapter 10

1. e
2. b
3. d
4. d
5. c
6. a
7. c
8. a
9. c
10. d

Chapter 11

1. c
2. b

3. b
4. b
5. c
6. c
7. c
8. d
9. c
10. c
11. 3.5 L
    2.5 L
    71%
    1.2 L/sec
12. c
13. c
14. b
15. d

Index

H

I

J

K

L

M

Q

T

U

V

W

Z